DUE DATE	RETURN DATE	DUE DATE	RETURN DATE

CONTEMPORARY TOPICS IN MOLECULAR IMMUNOLOGY

VOLUME 9

CONTEMPORARY TOPICS IN MOLECULAR IMMUNOLOGY

A Continuation Order Plan is available for this series. A continuation order will bring delivery of each new volume immediately upon publication. Volumes are billed only upon actual shipment. For further information please contact the publisher.

CONTEMPORARY TOPICS IN MOLECULAR IMMUNOLOGY

VOLUME 9

EDITED BY

F. P. INMAN

East Tennessee State University
Johnson City, Tennessee

and

T. J. KINDT

National Institute of Allergy and Infectious Diseases
National Institutes of Health
Bethesda, Maryland

PLENUM PRESS • NEW YORK AND LONDON

The Library of Congress cataloged the first volume of this title as follows:

Contemporary topics in molecular immunology. v. 2–
New York, Plenum Press, 1973–

    v. illus. 24 cm.

Continues Contemporary topics in immunochemistry.

1. Immunochemistry—Collected works. 2. Immunology—Collected works.

QR180.C635	574.2′9′05	73–648513
ISSN 0090–8800		MARC-S

Volume 1 of this series was published under the title
Contemporary Topics in Immunochemistry

Library of Congress Catalog Card Number 73-648513

ISBN 0-306-41304-3

© 1983 Plenum Press, New York
A Division of Plenum Publishing Corporation
233 Spring Street, New York, N.Y. 10013

Printed in the United States of America

Contributors

John E. Coe *Laboratory of Persistent Viral Diseases*
Rocky Mountain Laboratories
National Institute of Allergy and Infectious Diseases
National Institutes of Health
Public Health Service
U.S. Department of Health and Human Services
Hamilton, Montana

John E. Coligan *Laboratory of Immunogenetics*
National Institute of Allergy and Infectious Diseases
National Institutes of Health
Bethesda, Maryland

Edward S. Kimball *Frederick Cancer Research Facility*
Biological Development Branch
Biological Response Modifiers Program
Division of Cancer Treatment
National Cancer Institute
National Institutes of Health
Frederick, Maryland

Lawrence B. Lachman *Immunex Corporation*
Seattle, Washington

Abby L. Maizel *Department of Pathology*
Division of Pathobiology
M. D. Anderson Hospital and Tumor Institute
Houston, Texas

Henry Metzger *Section on Chemical Immunology*
Arthritis and Rheumatism Branch
National Institute of Arthritis, Diabetes, Digestive and Kidney Diseases
National Institutes of Health
Bethesda, Maryland

Peter J. Morris   *Nuffield Department of Surgery*
                   University of Oxford
                   John Radcliffe Hospital
                   Oxford, United Kingdom

J. R. L. Pink   *Basel Institute for Immunology*
                 Basel, Switzerland

Stuart Rudikoff   *Laboratory of Genetics*
                   National Cancer Institute
                   National Institutes of Health
                   Bethesda, Maryland

Alan Ting   *Nuffield Department of Surgery*
             University of Oxford
             John Radcliffe Hospital
             Oxford, United Kingdom

Preface

Studies concerning the structure and function of cell-surface antigens continue to command the attention of immunologists and biochemists. Some of these membrane-bound molecules are important because of the immunological consequences they evoke in recipients. Others are being studied because they are components of receptors on cells or because they change with various stages of differentiation. Four of the articles in this volume deal with cell membrane components that are involved in immune phenomena.

What are now called the class I histocompatibility antigens were previously referred to as the major transplantation antigens because they were identified as the primary structures responsible for allograft rejection in the mouse. Recent experiments suggest a more general role in the immune system for the class I antigens. Detailed structural studies of these, or indeed of any histocompatibility antigens, are relatively new; the first extensive amino acid sequence information appeared around 1977. The recent information on these cell-surface molecules reviewed by Kimball and Coligan includes much of their own data on the primary protein structure and gives an excellent picture of the ways in which this highly polymorphic family of proteins may show variability. In contrast to this variability, there are portions of the class I antigens that show remarkable conservation of primary structure. The genetic mechanisms that give rise to these conserved and variable portions in a contiguous sequence remain to be explained. There are promising data that point out structure–function relationships, especially with respect to the differential recognition of these molecules by antibodies and T cells. In addition, this review provides an excellent example of the complementary nature of information obtained from protein and DNA sequence studies and how such studies may be used to obtain complete information on various proteins.

In contrast to the detailed chemical analysis of the major histocompatibility complex (MHC) antigens in the article by Kimball and Coligan, the contribution by Morris and Ting points to an extremely important aspect of the application of chemical studies to the MHC antigens. As the dissection of the HLA locus in man becomes finer and the identities of various new antigens are sorted out, much more precise correlations between matching of transplantation donors to recipients and acceptance of allografts can be made. The authors have the experience and ability to bridge the entire field of transplantation and their article encompasses both clinical and immunochemical data in this area. Their data show clearly that matches for the DR antigens are more important than those at the ABC loci in determination of graft survival. Additional relevant factors, including autoimmunity and other B-cell antigens, are discussed and correlated with graft survival. The authors also present pathology data concerning the distribution of HLA-DR antigens in various tissues. These data indicate a fruitful area for future investigations on the chemical aspects of the various antigens encoded within the human MHC.

Do changes in the structure of lymphocyte surface glycoproteins, especially changes in their carbohydrate portions, occur during normal lymphoid differentiation? Information about this question is limited, and pertinent data are available for only a few proteins. Three of the proteins are major glycoprotein constituents of rodent thymocyte membranes: the Thy-1 antigen, a glycosylated leukocyte sialoglycoprotein called W3/13, and a high-molecular-weight glycoprotein known as the leukocyte-common antigen. In his contribution, Pink thoroughly characterizes these glycoproteins and discusses the evidence that the structures change when a thymocyte differentiates into a mature, peripheral T cell. A comparison is drawn between lymphocyte glycoprotein changes and those that occur during red blood cell differentiation. The reader will find Pink's discourse informative and provocative.

Mast cells, basophils, and related tumor lines bind IgE with very high affinity. When the cell-bound IgE subsequently reacts with a multivalent antigen, the cell rapidly degranulates. The degranulation is mediated by a glycoprotein receptor for IgE in the membrane of the responsive cell. The subject of the chapter by Metzger is the IgE receptor, but before the antigen-binding and triggering events can occur, IgE must bind to that receptor. Metzger first describes the recent data from his laboratory regarding the reaction of IgE with its receptor, and some of the data suggest that the receptor interacts with the immunoglobulin well up along the Fc region. New biochemical data are then used to characterize further the α and β chains that comprise the receptor. Some problems related to the structure of the α chains have led to ambiguous results when one examines their composition and substructure. The β chain has not been thoroughly characterized, but Metzger reports its molecular weight and some surprising compositional data. The ratio of α to β chains in the receptor and the relationships between the receptor and the intact cell membrane are also discussed. What is it, however, that relates the occupied receptor to degranulation? Association of receptors prior to degranulation is known to occur, so the most pressing structural–functional problem is defining how association of receptors initiates biochemical events leading to exocytosis. The reader is presented with the limited observations relevant to this question and is given some conceptual approaches to consider.

Three of the contributions discuss soluble proteins that function in immunity. The first of these deals with monokines and lymphokines that regulate lymphocyte proliferation. Another describes recent structural data for antibodies of known specificity. The third concerns the pentraxins, a group of proteins related to human C-reactive protein.

The regulation of T- and B-cell differentiation is being investigated intensively. Antigens and certain lectins initiate a complex series of events that ultimately cause T and B cells to proliferate. Lachman and Maizel describe the lymphocyte regulators interleukin 1 and interleukin 2 (IL-1 and IL-2), which affect various subclasses of T lymphocytes. IL-2 is thought to represent the proximate mitogenic stimulus for certain subsets of T cells, while the monokine IL-1 acts as an amplification factor in the production of IL-2. Recently it was revealed that culture media from lectin-stimulated peripheral blood lymphocytes or antigen-specific helper T cells are capable of promoting S-phase entry in a subpopulation of B lymphocytes. The agent responsible for this is called B-cell growth factor (BCGF). The biochemical evidence that BCGF is an entity distinctly different from other interleukins is described. Although the investigations of the mode of action of human BCGF are in the early stages of development, a biological description of its effect is emerging. Following an activation event, a subpopulation of human B lymphocytes acquires sensitivity to the subsequent effects of growth factors, and a proportion of the population enters the S phase of the cell cycle. The authors relate experiments dealing with the cellular production of BCGF and the role of the factor in the B-cell differentiation response. By utilizing the information in this article, the reader may develop a clear concept of the role of soluble factors in T- and B-cell proliferation as it currently is understood.

Studies of immunoglobulin genes at the DNA level recently have eclipsed investigations of antibody protein structure. One area wherein the study of protein structure continues to dominate is discussed by Rudikoff, who uses up-to-date compilations of amino acid sequences of antibodies with known specificity and idiotypic properties to bring into focus our knowledge of antibody structure and function. The author's scholarly analysis of several of the best-studied systems does give certain answers concerning the relationship of primary structural correlates with binding and idiotypic properties of antibodies. However, the questions that remain from this analysis underscore the need for continued detailed studies of the structure–function relationships of the antibodies. Rudikoff's article directs attention to those systems that will be most fruitfully analyzed in the future and gives an excellent summary of what is actually known about the structure–function relationship in these antibody groups.

Although the existence of C-reactive protein (CRP) has been known for over 50 years, it is only in recent years that its many homologs have been studied. Because members of this protein family are characterized by a pentameric subunit structure, the name *pentraxins* has been suggested. CRP is an acute phase protein that binds to phosphorylcholine in the presence of Ca^{2+} and that also binds to serum complement components. Another prominent member of the pentraxin family, present in the human, is amyloid P component (AP), which is very similar in structure to CRP but different in most binding properties. Coe has chosen to study the hamster homolog of the pentraxin family, which is designated female protein (FP). FP is extremely interesting in that it has closest structural similarity to AP and closest functional similarity to CRP. This study has given new insights into the structure–function relationships within the pentraxin family; new data challenge certain of the previous conclusions concerning peptide structures necessary for binding to the various reactive substances. In addition to this new structural information, the mode of hormonal control of FP provides an excellent model for the study of the control of specific protein synthesis. The female hamster has extraordinarily high levels of this protein, whereas the male has barely detectable levels in normal serum. It is certain that we will be hearing more of this highly conserved family of proteins in the future.

We hope that readers will find this volume as informative as previous entries in the series.

F. P. Inman
T. J. Kindt

Contents

HLA-DR and Renal Transplantation
Peter J. Morris and Alan Ting

Human Immunoregulatory Molecules: Interleukin 1, Interleukin 2, and B-Cell Growth Factor
Lawrence B. Lachman and Abby L. Maizel

Immunoglobulin Structure–Function Correlates: Antigen Binding and Idiotypes
Stuart Rudikoff

Homologs of CRP: A Diverse Family of Proteins with Similar Structure
John E. Coe

Structure of Class I Major Histocompatibility Antigens

Edward S. Kimball

Frederick Cancer Research Facility
Biological Development Branch
Biological Response Modifiers Program
Division of Cancer Treatment
National Cancer Institute
National Institutes of Health
Frederick, Maryland 21701

and

John E. Coligan

Laboratory of Immunogenetics
National Institute of Allergy and Infectious Diseases
National Institutes of Health
Bethesda, Maryland 20205

I. INTRODUCTION

H-2 antigens were discovered by Gorer (1936) as a blood group system associated with histocompatibility between mouse strains. Later research indicated that H-2 antigens were encoded by a series of genes, hence the designation *H-2 complex* (J. Klein, 1975). Similar complexes have been identified in all vertebrates examined (Götze, 1977) and are generally known as major histocompatibility complexes (MHC). It is now known that genes within the MHC influence as many as 60 separate traits (J. Klein, 1975, 1979) with many controlling important immunological functions.

Figure 1 presents a schematic view of our current understanding of the genetic organization of the mouse and human MHCs. The murine *H-2* region is located on chromosome 17 and is approximately 1.5 centimorgans long (Klein,

1

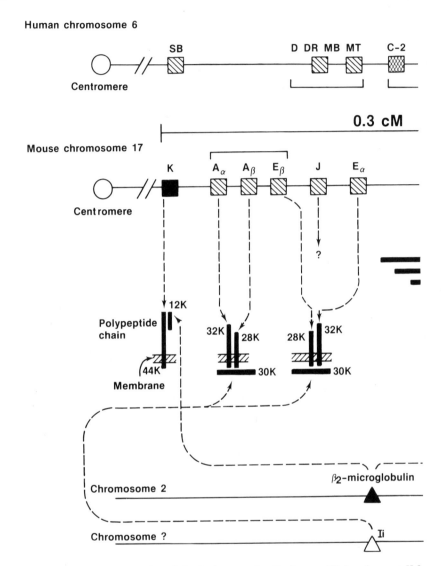

Figure 1. Schematic representation of the loci composing the human *HLA* and mouse *H-2* regions and the corresponding murine products. Brackets and arrows indicate that the order of loci is unknown. Loci designated by the same type of squares belong to the same class: solid squares, class I loci; open squares, class I loci whose products have a different tissue

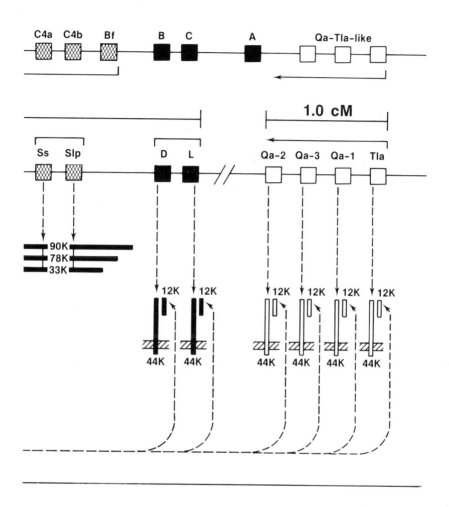

distribution and possibly different functional properties than the classical transplantation antigens K, D, and L; hatched squares, class II loci; cross-hatched squares, class III loci. Class I molecules are associated with β_2M and class II molecules with invariant chain (Ii). Adapted from J. Klein (1981).

1979), while that of humans (*HLA*) is located on chromosome 6 and is 2 centimorgans long (Van Someren *et al.*, 1974). The products of the *H-2K*, *H-2D*, and *H-2L* regions and the *HLA-A*, *HL-B*, and *HL-C* regions are analogous in structure and function, as are those of the murine *I*-region and human *HLA-D/DR* regions. The former are referred to as class I antigens, while the latter are called class II antigens (Götze, 1977; J. Klein, 1979). Class III molecules are complement components.

The class I antigens are defined as noncovalently associated complexes of a 45,000-dalton MHC-encoded glycoprotein and β_2-microglobulin (β_2M), a 12,000-dalton, non-MHC-encoded protein. This definition extends to the Qa and Tl antigens as well, even though these antigens demonstrate different tissue distribution from the classical transplantation antigens H-2K, H-2D, and H-2L and historically have been considered to be products of genes adjacent to, but not a part of, the MHC (see review by Flaherty, 1981). Recent studies on the structures of the Qa and Tl antigens reveal significant homology with H-2 molecules (Soloski *et al.*, 1982; Steinmetz *et al.*, 1981b; Yokoyama *et al.*, 1981), thereby indicating a close evolutionary relationship between these families of antigens. The class II antigens consist of two noncovalently associated, membrane-bound glycoproteins with molecular weights of approximately 32,000–35,000 (α chain) and 25,000–28,000 (β chain). Under certain conditions, a third chain (Ii) of 31,000 daltons, which is structurally invariant regardless of haplotype, can be co-isolated with mouse *I*-region molecules (Jones *et al.*, 1978; Moosic *et al.*, 1980). In regard to function, the class I gene products differ from those of class II in that the former guide cytolytic and the latter regulatory (helper and suppressor) T lymphocytes (J. Klein *et al.*, 1981). This brief description of the MHC provides background information for the subject of the remainder of this chapter—the class I molecules.

Serological analyses of human and murine class I gene products have revealed an unparalleled degree of genetic polymorphism. This polymorphism is reflected in two ways. First, multiple loci encode class I molecules. For example, certain, if not all, strains of mice apparently express at least six *K/D* region alloantigens—in *d* haplotype mice, serological analyses have revealed K^{d1}, K^{d2}, D^d, L^d, R^d, and M^d (see Section X.A). Furthermore, studies on MHC genes suggest the possibility for expression of other, as yet undetected, class I molecules (Steinmetz *et al.*, 1982). Second, in addition to the polymorphism provided by multiple class I loci, each locus can apparently encode one of many alleles; for example, it is estimated that there may be upwards of 100 alleles for each of the *H-2K* and *-D* loci (Duncan *et al.*, 1979). Thus, a completely heterozygous mouse may express 12 or more different *K/D*-region alloantigens.

While the function(s) of class I antigens have not been clearly defined, it would seem likely that the extensive polymorphism of class I molecules is important for species survival. Work by many investigators (see review by Zinkernagel and Doherty, 1979) that indicates foreign molecules, such as viral antigens expressed on the host cell surface, are recognized by cytotoxic T lymphocytes (CTL) in the context of the host's own class I antigens provides evidence about the possible function of these molecules and the role of polymorphism. Accordingly, the recognition of viral antigens in the context of host class I antigens might serve to focus effector immune cells on the source of the virus, the infected cell, rather than on free viral particles, as a more effective means of combating infection. Polymorphism and heterozygosity may serve to maximize the repertoire of associative recognition, i.e., certain allelic products might be more suitable to present a particular antigen rather than other allelic products of that same or another locus.

Studies on the detailed structure of class I antigens were thus undertaken to provide a molecular understanding of their role in immunological processes. Initial structural studies on class I antigens consisted of comparative peptide mapping analyses (Brown *et al.*, 1974). These studies were followed by extensive protein sequence analyses of a number of H-2 (Coligan *et al.*, 1981) and HLA molecules (Lopez de Castro *et al.*, 1982). More recently, the advent of recombinant DNA techniques has led to the molecular cloning of class I genes (Ploegh *et al.*, 1980; Sood *et al.*, 1981; Steinmetz *et al.*, 1981a,b; Kvist *et al.*, 1981; Suggs *et al.*, 1981), which has further advanced our appreciation of the structure and genetic organization of these MHC antigens. Some of the results and ramifications of these structural studies are discussed in this article.

II. ISOLATION OF H-2 AND HLA ANTIGENS

Studies on the structure of major transplantation antigens have had to overcome two difficult problems. First, H-2 and HLA molecules are integral membrane proteins tightly associated with the cell membrane lipid bilayer and hence are not water-soluble. Second, these molecules represent a small fraction of the total cellular components and therefore must be purified from a complex biological mixture. Multiple approaches have been devised by investigators to deal with these problems.

A. Source of Material

An initial decision in pursuing the structural determination of H-2 or HLA antigens is the choice of starting material. In making this decision multiple factors, which include the availability of material and the convenience and expense of obtaining it, must be weighed. In the case of HLA, tissue is readily available at relatively low cost from either cadavers or peripheral blood cells from donors. However, in addition to containing relatively small amounts of antigen, material from these sources usually contains many different types of HLA molecules, which makes it difficult to purify any one type in order to obtain unambiguous structural information.

A more reproducible and less heterogeneous source of relatively large quantities of HLA antigens has been the B-cell lines established by Epstein–Barr virus transformation of human peripheral blood lymphocytes. These cell lines often express 10- to 20-fold greater quantities of HLA than normal cells (McCune et al., 1975). However, kilogram quantities of cells are required to perform structural characterization by classical procedures.

As a source of H-2 antigens, the inbred strains of mice provide a reproducible source of tissue. However, in order to obtain even relatively small amounts (several milligrams) of material, very large numbers of animals must be sacrificed (Henriksen et al., 1979). There are no available murine B-cell lines that are analogous to the human lymphoblastoid cell lines that express relatively large amounts of antigen. Despite this, Freed et al. (1979), Mole et al. (1982), and Rogers et al. (1979) have been able to purify H-2 antigens from murine cell lines in amounts (milligrams) sufficient for preliminary structural studies. However, most structural data concerning H-2 molecules have been obtained using radiochemical methods (discussed in Section II.C).

B. Solubilization

Because HLA and H-2 antigens are integral membrane proteins, tightly associated with the lipid bilayer, methods had to be developed to solubilize these molecules. Of the methods explored, treatment with proteolytic anzymes and nonionic detergents has proven most useful. Some years ago it was demonstrated that most, if not all, of the alloantigenic determinants associated with class I molecules could be solubilized by the treatment of H-2-bearing cells with proteolytic enzymes (Nathenson and Davies, 1966). The success of this procedure depends on the fact that histocompatibility antigens are relatively resistant to mild protease treatment except in a small segment of the molecule near the outer membrane surface (see Section IV.B). Shimada and Nathenson (1969) found that limited digestion with papain yielded up to a 20% recovery of the alloantigenic activity associated with crudely purified membranes of mouse spleen cells. The papain-solubilized molecules are water-soluble, globular proteins that can be readily purified. HLA molecules appear to be more resistant to proteolytic digestion that H-2 antigens (Shimada and Nathenson, 1969), and consequently papain-solubilized HLA antigens (Lopez de Castro et al., 1979; Trägårdh et al., 1980) have been extensively employed for structural studies.

Despite the advantageous solubility properties of the papain-cleaved class I glycoproteins, the yield of such molecules is less than optimal and, in addition, these products represent only a fragment of the intact molecule. In order to gain an appreciation of the biochemical properties of the intact structure and increase the yield of soluble product, solubilization procedures were developed utilizing nondenaturing detergents, mainly Triton X-100 and Nonidet P40 (Hilgert *et al.*, 1969; Schwartz and Nathenson, 1971). In addition to being excellent solubilizing agents for integral membrane proteins, these detergents also tend to preserve HLA and H-2 alloantigenic activity (Schwartz and Nathenson, 1971). In the presence of appropriate concentrations of detergent, the class I glycoproteins are maintained in solution in the form of aggregates, termed mixed micelles, containing both protein and detergent components.

There are, however, some disadvantages of solubilizing histocompatibility antigens with these detergents. These include: (1) their large micelle size, which prevents the use of standard protein separation procedures such as gel filtration; (2) their low critical micelle concentration, which hinders their elimination by dialysis or exchange with other detergents; and (3) their ultraviolet absorbance at 280 nm (except for Brij and a few other detergents), which inhibits the direct detection of proteins by spectrophotometric means. Consequently, most purifications of detergent-solubilized histocompatibility antigens employ immunological reagents (see Section II.C).

C. Purification

The strategies for purification of histocompatibility antigens depend on several factors, some of which have been discussed earlier. As previously mentioned, the advantages of detergent over proteolytic solubilization are increased yield and the production of intact molecules; the disadvantages are the problems caused by the presence of detergent in most separation methods that depend on size and charge. The latter problem can be overcome by resorting to separation with affinity reagents such as lectins (Snary *et al.*, 1974; Dawson *et al.*, 1974) and antibodies (Schwartz and Nathenson, 1971; Ewenstein *et al.*, 1976), whose binding to histocompatibility antigens is usually unaffected by the concentrations of detergent utilized for solubilization.

1. HLA

Since most human alloantisera have low affinity and are multispecific, they are not useful for immunoaffinity purification. Therefore, most purifications for structural studies of HLA antigens have utilized papain-solubilized material (Fig. 2A) (Orr *et al.*, 1979b; Lopez de Castro *et al.*, 1979). The lymphoblastoid cell lines that have been utilized as the source of antigen are selected for homozygosity and for the production of abnormally large amounts of the antigen. Culture techniques designed to produce kilogram amounts of these cells are then employed. As shown in Fig. 2A, the papain-solubilized molecules are then purified by standard biochemical techniques. Trägårdh *et al.* (1980) utilized a

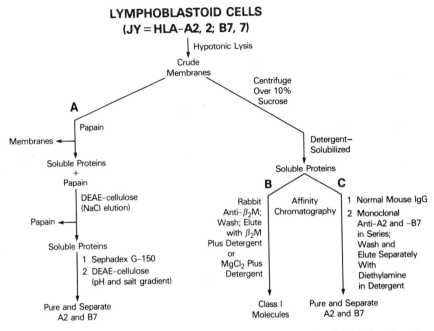

Figure 2. Purification procedures for papain- and detergent-solubilized HLA from lympho-blastoid cell lines.

similar purification scheme to determine the primary structure of pooled HLA molecules isolated from spleens of cadavers.

More recently, immunological reagents have been developed for the purification of intact, detergent-solubilized HLA molecules, as shown in Fig. 2B,C. This development was first made possible by employing purified, high-titered antibodies to $\beta_2 M$ (Fig. 2B). Since $\beta_2 M$ is a constitutive component of HLA antigens, anti-$\beta_2 M$ immunoadsorbents can be used to purify such molecules. However, since all class I moleclues present in a given cell lysate contain $\beta_2 M$, individual HLA antigens must be obtained by further purification. Although HLA-A2 and -B7, which are present in the JY lymphoblastoid cell line, could be separated by DEAE-cellulose chromatography (Lopez de Castro, 1979), most attempts to purify individual H-2 and HLA molecules by conventional separation procedures have met with limited success (Bridgen *et al.*, 1976; Henriksen *et al.*, 1979).

Most recently, the development of monoclonal antibodies has made possible the large-scale purification of specific HLA molecules (Parham, 1979), as shown in Fig. 2C. In addition to the high yield of HLA antigens for structural studies, antigens eluted from the monoclonal antibody columns, if neutralized promptly, retain a significant degree of alloreactivity.

2. H-2

Studies of H-2 class I molecules are hampered by the fact that only small amounts of antigen can be isolated from either tissue or cultured cells, but this problem can be overcome by the fact that high-titered, monospecific alloantisera or monoclonal antibodies are readily available. This combination of circumstances has led to an approach for structural studies of these molecules that utilizes antigens biosynthetically labeled with radioactive amino acids, which are specifically purified by precipitation with either alloantisera (Ewenstein *et al.*, 1976) or, more recently, monoclonal antibodies (Maloy *et al.*, 1980) (Fig. 3). The radiolabeled antigens have usually been obtained from tumor lines because they are metabolically more active than normal cells and can be maintained in

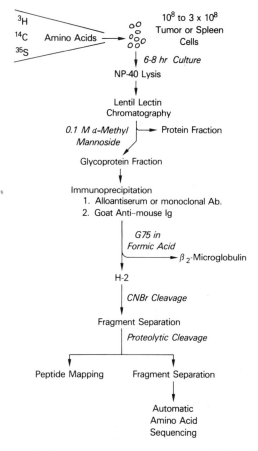

Figure 3. Purification procedure for detergent-solubilized H-2.

culture, thus providing a ready source of material. In addition, tumor lines expressing above-average amounts of the antigen in question can often be obtained (Nairn *et al.*, 1980a). Normal cells, such as spleen cells, can also be utilized as a source of radiolabeled material, although the efficiency of radioactive amino acid incorporation is lower. Initial studies on the structure of H-2 class I molecules (see the review by Vitetta and Capra, 1978) as well as studies on H-2 mutant molecules (see the review by Nairn *et al.*, 1980b) have employed radiolabeled antigens isolated from spleen cells. Details of the methodology employed for sequence analyses of biosynthetically radiolabeled material have recently been reviewed (Coligan and Kindt, 1981; Coligan *et al.*, 1983).

While radiosequence methodology has been valuable for the determination of the primary structure of H-2 class I antigens, the amounts of material isolated are insufficient for biological studies or for studies of three-dimensional structure (a 20% yield of material from 10^8 cells, assuming 5×10^5 molecules/cell, would be approximately 500 ng). However, recent studies employing immunoadsorbent columns prepared with monoclonal antibodies (Stallcup *et al.*, 1981; Mole *et al.*, 1982) indicate the feasibility of purifying milligram amounts of H-2 antigens for such studies.

III. β_2-MICROGLOBULIN

β_2M was first discovered in the urine of patients with renal tubular dysfunction (Berggärd and Bearn, 1968); not until several years later was it found to be an integral component of class I molecules (Nakamuro *et al.*, 1973). Although the function of β_2M is still undefined, a number of studies suggest possible roles for it. Certain investigations suggest that β_2M serves to stabilize the configuration of the class I heavy chains. These include (1) circular dichroism studies (Lancet *et al.*, 1979), which show that isolated heavy chains lose some of their β-pleated structure and assume more of a random coil configuration in the absence of β_2M; (2) immunochemical studies, which demonstrate that HLA alloantisera are less able to recognize the antigen if β_2M has become dissociated from the heavy chain and that antigenic activity can be restored if the heavy chain–β_2M complex is carefully renatured (Krangel *et al.*, 1979, 1980); and (3) studies with Daudi cells, which fail to synthesize β_2M (Arce-Gomez *et al.*, 1978), which reveal that cytoplasmic HLA molecules not associated with β_2M are not recognized by alloantisera but can be recognized by xenoantisera raised against denatured HLA heavy chains (Krangel *et al.*, 1980). In addition to stabilizing the configuration of class I heavy chains, β_2M appears to be necessary for the expression of these chains on the cell surface. Daudi cells are only able to express cytoplasmic HLA (Ploegh *et al.*, 1979), and a mutant murine cell line, $R1(\beta_2^-)$, which like Daudi cells does not synthesize β_2M, fails to express H-2 or Tl (Hyman and Stallings,

1977). Southern blot analysis on DNA from the murine cell line indicates that the β_2M structural gene either is entirely deleted or contains sufficient deletions to render it defective (Parnes and Seidman, 1982).

The complete amino acid sequences for β_2M from a variety of species have been determined (Table I). Homology of β_2M among species ranges between 61% and 74%, except for murine and rat β_2M, which, as might be expected, show greater homology (86%). In other studies, β_2M has been shown to demonstrate significant homology to immunoglobulin light and heavy chain constant region domains, the third extracellular domain of MHC class I molecules, and the second extracellular domain of the β chain of MHC class II molecules. This homology will be discussed in more detail in Section VIII.

As far as is known β_2M is nonpolymorphic in all species except the mouse (Michaelson et al., 1980; Gates et al., 1981). The polymorphism reported for guinea pig β_2M (Cigén et al., 1978) appears to be the result of posttranslational modifications (Wolfe and Cebra, 1980). The discovery of the existence of two β_2M alleles in the mouse, $\beta_2 m^a$ and $\beta_2 m^b$, allowed the gene encoding β_2M to be mapped to chromosome 2 (Michaelson, 1981; Robinson et al., 1981). The β_2M gene is linked to the genes for H-3 (Michaelson, 1981) and Ly-4 (Goding, 1981).

Southern blots with β_2M probes have shown that murine β_2M is encoded by a single gene per haploid genome, indicating that the same β_2M gene encodes the light chain of the various class I molecules (Parnes and Seidman, 1982). Examination of the β_2M gene structure by these investigators showed that the protein is encoded in three exons, which are the signal peptide plus residues 1 and 2, residues 3–95, and residues 96–99, respectively.

IV. CLASS I HEAVY CHAINS

A. Strategy for Sequence Determination

H-2K^b and HLA-B7 were the first class I molecules whose primary structures were studied. The strategy used for determining the complete sequence of the H-2K^b molecule relied on initial isolation of fragments obtained by cyanogen bromide (CNBr) cleavage at Met residues (Coligan et al., 1981). Subsequent amino acid sequence analyses and the use of tryptic overlap peptides permitted the alignment of these fragments. The amino acid sequences of small CNBr fragments (<30 residues) were determined on the intact fragments. Larger CNBr fragments were reduced to smaller fragments by enzymatic cleavage (thrombin, trypsin, V-8 protease) in order to obtain appropriately sized peptides for sequence determination. The alignment of the CNBr peptides of H-2K^b is depicted in Fig. 4. Structural analyses of similarly derived CNBr peptides from other H-2 molecules revealed strong conservation of certain features (Fig. 4). Not only

Table I. Sequences of β_2-Microglobulins Aligned for Homology[a]

```
                    10          20           30          40         50
Bovine      I Q R P P K I Q V Y S R H P P E N G K P N Y L N C Y V Y G F H P P Q I E I D L L K N G E K I K S [J]E Q
Guinea pig  V L H A—R V ———————— A —————Q—F I ————— S ——————————VE ————— K—DNV—M
Rabbit      V——A—NV ————————— A ————— F —————— S ————— D—E ————— V—ENV—
Human       ——T ——————————— A ————— S—F ————— S ————— SD—V ————— D—R—EKV—H
Mouse       ——KT—Q ———————————————— I ————— TQ ———— H ———— QM ————— K—PKV—M
Rat         ——KT—Q ———————————————— F ————— SQ —————————— E ————— K—PNI—M
                                                                             50
```

```
                    60           70            80          90          98
Bovine      S D L S F S K D W S F Y L L S H A E F T P D S K D E Y S C R V K H V T L E Q P R I V K W D R D L
Guinea pig  ——————— T ————— V—A ————— NDS —————— S—I ——— SE—K ————— PNK
Rabbit      —————— N ————— V—T ————— NN—N ——————— KE—MT ————— Y
Human[b]    ——————————— YYT ———— TE ————— A ————— N ————— S—K —————————— M
Mouse[c]    ——M —————————— I—A—T ————— TET—T—A ———— ASMAE—KT—Y ————— M
Rat         ——————————— I—A—T ————— TET—V—A ————————— KE—KT—T ————— M
                                                                90           99
```

[a] The numbering on top refers to the bovine sequence and the numbering below refers to the others. Deletion in the alignment is indicated by []. A solid line indicates identity with the bovine sequence. The sequences were determined by the following investigators: cow, Groves and Greenberg (1982); guinea pig, Wolfe and Cebra (1980); rabbit, Gates et al. (1979); mouse, Gates et al. (1981); human, Cunningham et al. (1973); rat, S. Sundelin, personal communication.

[b] In the initial human β_2M sequence of Cunningham et al. (1973), the molecule was reported to be 100 residues in length owing to an incorrect insertion of a Ser residue at position 67 (Groves and Greenberg, 1982; Suggs et al., 1981).

[c] Murine β_2M is polymorphic at position 85, with C67Bl/6 mice having Ala and all other strains having Asp at this position (Gates et al., 1981; Parnes et al., 1981).

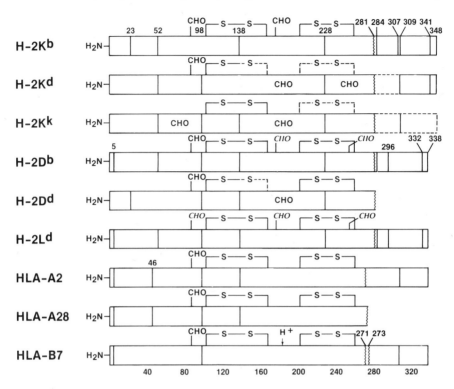

Figure 4. Schematic outlines of structural properties of six H-2 molecules and three HLA molecules. Straight vertical lines indicate positions of methionine residues and thus sites of CNBr cleavage. The irregular vertical lines indicate C-terminal positions of the papain-solubilized molecules as determined for K^b and B7. The presence of dashed lines in the S-S bonds indicates that the exact position of at least one Cys of this bond has not been determined, although it is presumed to be located identically to the Cys residues of H-2K^b. The locations of carbohydrate moieties (CHO) are indicated. Those not in italics are known to exist and those in italics are presumed to exist based on the presence of the appropriate recognition sequence for glycosylation. Other CHOs shown within the rectangles mark known glycopeptides. H$^+$ indicates position of acid cleavage site.

are the Met residues highly conserved, thereby providing the basis for a general sequencing strategy for H-2 molecules, but the size and location of the disulfide loops are apparently identical and the positions of carbohydrate groups are conserved.

Also, as shown in Fig. 4, HLA molecules have overall structural features similar to those of H-2 molecules, thus permitting a similar strategy for sequence analyses. HLA-B7 is somewhat exceptional in that it has fewer methionine residues than other class I molecules that have been studied. Consequently, the initial cleavage strategy for HLA-B7 relied on the presence of an acid cleavage site between residues 183 and 184. Further fragmentation of the acid cleavage products was performed in a manner similar to that mentioned for H-2K^b.

B. Primary Structure of H-2K^b and HLA-B7

Table II details the complete amino acid sequences of H-2K^b and HLA-B7. H-2K^b is 348 residues long whereas HLA-B7 has 339 residues. As indicated in Fig. 4, HLA-B7 and H-2K^b also have identical carbohydrate attachment sites at Asn-86. H-2K^b has a second glycosylation site at Asn-176. Also, both molecules have internal disulfide loops that are identical in size and location. The first disulfide loop encompasses residues 101–164 and the second spans positions 203–259. H-2K^b has two Cys residues that are not involved in disulfide loop formation (position 121 and position 337). There are also two free Cys residues in HLA-B7, both of which occur in the carboxy-terminal portion of the molecule (positions 308 and 325). In both molecules, a hydrophobic region extends approximately from residue 284 to residue 304 and is followed by a cluster of charged, basic residues (positions 308–312). The papain cleavage site, or, more correctly, the position at which papain ceases to further digest the nondenatured molecules, has been identified as Val-281 in H-2K^b (Martinko et al., 1981) and Leu-270/Thr-271 in HLA-B7 (Lopez de Castro et al., 1979). In their studies on pooled HLA molecules, Trägårdh et al. (1980) found Thr-271 to be the C terminus of papain-cleaved molecules.

C. Molecular Organization

The structural information shown in Table II led to the derivation of the schematic model for class I antigens shown in Fig. 5. As depicted, such molecules consist of three regions—an extracellular region (residues 1–283), a hydrophobic, transmembrane region (~residues 284–307), and a hydrophilic, cytoplasmic region (~308 to the carboxy terminus). The extracellular region can be further subdivided into three domains (N, C1, and C2 in the mouse and α1, α2, and α3 for human molecules). Postulation of the existence of such domains was prompted by evidence of primary structural homologies of class I heavy chains and β$_2$M to IgG constant region domains (Orr et al., 1979a,b; Trägårdh et al., 1980). Other evidence that supports the existence of such domains includes (1) the near-identical size and linear arrangement of both disulfide loop domains (C1 and C2), (2) the alignment of carbohydrate moieties in the N and C1 domains, and (3) the statistically significant homology (~30%) between the amino-terminal domain and the first disulfide loop domain (Krangel et al., 1980). An additional observation that lends support to the proposed globular domain structure is the fact that limited digestion with papain occurs between C2 and the transmembrane

Table II. Comparison of the Amino Acid Sequences of H-2K^b and HLA-B7^a

	10	20	30	40	50	60	70	80	90

CHO at position 86 (H-2K^b)

H-2K^b: GPHSLRYFVTAVSRPGLGEPRYMEVGYVDDTETVRFDSDAENPRYEPRARWMEQEGPEYWERETQKAKGNEQSFRVDLRTLLGYYNQSKG

HLA-B7: -S--M---Y-S-----R----FIS-------Q--------AS--E----P-I---------D-N--IY-AQA-TD-ES--N-R------EA (CHO)

	100	110	120	130	140	150	160	170	180

CHO at position 176 (H-2K^b)

H-2K^b: GSHTIQVISGCEVGSDGRLLRGYQQYAYDGCDYIALNEDLKTWTAADMAALITKHKWEQAGEAERLRAYLEGTCVEWLRRYLKNGNATLL

HLA-B7: ----L-SMY--D-P-------HD------K-------RS------T--Q--QR-----A-R---QR------E------E--KDK-E

	190	200	210	220	230	240	250	260	270

H-2K^b: RTDSPKAHVTHHSRPEDKVTLRCWALGFYPADITLTWQLNGEELIQDMELVETRPAGDGTFQKWASVVVPLGKEQYYTCHVYHQGLPEPL

HLA-B7: -A-P--T-----PISDHEA----------E-----RD-DQT--T----------R-E--A----S-E--R-----Q-E---K--

	280	290	300	310	320	330	340

H-2K^b: TLRWEPPPSTVSNMATVAVLVVLGAAIVTGAVVAFVMKRRRNTGGKGGDYALAPGSQTSDLSLPDCKVMVHDPHSLA

HLA-B7: ------SSQSTVP VG VAG AV -VV- ----A--C()--KSS------S-SQ-AC-DSAQG-DVSLTA

^{a}Sequences are given in the single-letter amino acid code. Dashed lines indicate identity to the K^b sequence. CHO indicates position of a glycosyl unit. The parentheses denote a position in the HLA molecule where a deletion must be made in order to achieve maximum alignment to H-2K^b. H-2K^b is from Coligan et al. (1981); corrections were made at positions 196, 263, 268, 275, 276, 313, and 343 according to those derived from the proposed H-2K^b cDNA sequence of Reyes et al. (1982a). Only the original assignments at positions 263, 275, and 276 have been confirmed as errors made during the original protein sequence determination; the other discrepancies have yet to be reinvestigated at the protein sequence level. The C-terminal residues (LA) were also apparently missed during the protein determination (Uehara et al., 1981b), probably owing to premature washout from the sequencer cup. HLA-B7 is from Ploegh et al. (1981b).

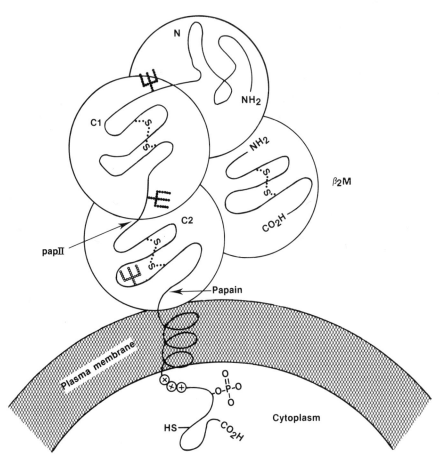

Figure 5. A schematic representation of an H-2 class I molecule in the plasma membrane.

region (Tm) and between C1 and C2 (papII) (Trägårdh *et al.*, 1979; Coligan *et al.*, 1980).

More recent data supporting the organization of class I heavy chains into domains come from studies on the genetic organization of class I genes. As shown in Fig. 6, genomic clones of murine class I heavy chains are organized into eight exons (Steinmetz *et al.*, 1981b) that coincide with the aforementioned domain structure. Exon 1 corresponds to a 21-residue precursor sequence, and exons 2, 3, and 4 correspond to the three extracellular domains. The membrane binding region is encoded in exon 5, and the cytoplasmic segment of H-2 molecules is encoded by three small exons (6, 7, and 8). Current evidence indicates that human class I molecules lack the exon analogous to exon 8 of the mouse and therefore have only seven exons (Malissen *et al.*, 1982).

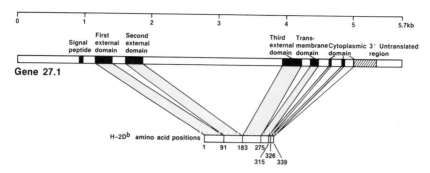

Figure 6. Organization of exons and introns in gene 27.1 compared to the H-2D^b class I antigen, showing the location of intervening sequences with respect to the amino acid positions. Exons 1–8 are designated by black boxes and are aligned with their corresponding protein domains. Compared to the H-2D^b molecule, the third external domain of gene 27.1 is longer by three codons at its 3' end. Adapted from Steinmetz *et al.* (1982) using the H-2D^b sequence provided by Reyes *et al.* (1982b) and Maloy and Coligan (1982).

Figure 5 shows the presence of three carbohydrate moieties on class I heavy chains. HLA molecules that have been studied have only the one in the amino-terminal domain. All H-2 molecules that have been analyzed have glycosyl groups attached to both the N and C1 domains at Asn-86 and Asn-176, respectively. Some H-2 antigens, e.g., H-2K^d and H-2D^b (Kimball *et al.*, 1981a), are known to carry a third carbohydrate group that is attached to Asn-256 in the C2 domain (Maloy and Coligan, 1982).

The membrane-binding region is about 24 residues long in H-2 (Uehara *et al.*, 1981a) and HLA (Robb *et al.*, 1978), approximately spanning residues 284–307. This length of a polypeptide in an α-helix conformation is capable of spanning a lipid bilayer 35 Å deep (Guidotti, 1977). There are no charged or polar amino acids found in this region, similar to analogous regions in other integral proteins (von Heijne, 1981b). That the hydrophobic region penetrates the membrane was proven by Walsh and Crumpton (1977), who showed that HLA heavy chains in inside-out membrane vesicles could be iodinated via lactoperoxidase catalysis.

The cytoplasmic region consists of the carboxy-terminal portion of the molecule and contains a large percentage of hydrophilic residues. At the boundary between the membrane and the cytoplasmic domains there is a cluster of basic amino acids that are thought to anchor the molecule in the lipid bilayer via charge interactions with the negatively charged cytoplasmic surface of the membrane (von Heijne and Blomberg, 1979). Analogous clusters of basic residues have been observed in other membrane-bound molecules (von Heijne, 1981b).

The C-terminal region contains a prosthetic group that in HLA-A2 (Pober *et al.*, 1978) has been shown to be phosphoserine. H-2K^k is also phosphorylated (Rothbard *et al.*, 1980) in this part of the molecule. By analogy to HLA-A2, H-2K^k was also assumed to possess a phosphoserine residue, but Lalanne *et al.*

(1982) among others point out that the threonine residue at position 313 in H-2 (see Table VI) could also serve as a phosphorylation site. The exact role of cytoplasmic region phosphate groups in H-2 and HLA has not been elucidated, but it is possible that class I molecules interact with cytoskeletal elements through conformational changes occurring via such phosphate moieties.

D. Secondary and Tertiary Structure

What little is known about the secondary and tertiary structures of class I molecules has been revealed by circular dichroism (CD) studies. Lancet *et al.* (1979) have shown that HLA and β_2M share common features of secondary structure, especially a high content of β-pleated sheet structure. Calculations on HLA indicate at least 75% β-pleated sheet, approximately 5% α-helix, and 20% random coil structure. CD studies on the acid cleavage fragments of HLA-B40 revealed that the fragments comprising the amino-terminal domain and first disulfide loop domain retained most of their original β-pleated sheet structure (Strominger *et al.*, 1981). The acid cleavage fragment that contained the second disulfide loop, however, lost its native configuration and assumed a predominantly random coil configuration. While this suggests that the structure of this domain is dependent on that of the rest of the molecule, one must be cautious in the interpretation. The cleavage site lies within the α3 domain and therefore such cleavage could disrupt the folding of the second disulfide loop and thus the secondary structure. CD analysis of HLA that was dissociated from β_2M and then allowed to renature in the absence of β_2M also revealed a partial loss of β-pleated sheet structure. This suggests that the native configuration of the heavy chain is also somewhat dependent on quaternary interactions (see Section III).

E. Oligosaccharide Units

As mentioned previously, the number of polysaccharide moieties on class I molecules appears to be variable. All known class I saccharide units are N-linked and thus require the recognition sequence Asn-X-Ser/Thr for attachment (Hubbard and Ivatt, 1981). These saccharide moieties are attached cotranslationally and are initially present as high-mannose-type units (Dobberstein *et al.*, 1979; Ploegh *et al.*, 1979). During the process of transport to the cell surface, which requires 25 to 60 min, the saccharide units are converted from the high-mannose type to complex-type oligosaccharides (Krangel *et al.*, 1979; Ploegh *et al.*, 1981a,b). The approximate structures of the complex saccharide units present on HLA and H-2 alloantigens have been provisionally determined by compositional analyses and susceptibilities to glycosidases (Fig. 7). In the case of H-2,

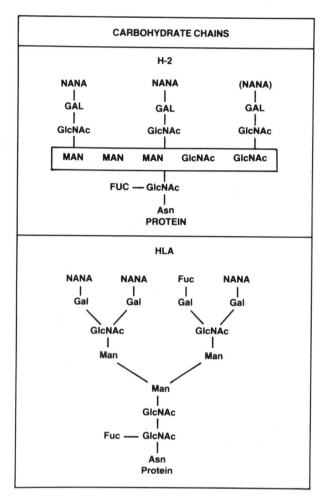

Figure 7. The proposed structures of the saccharide moieties attached to H-2 (Nathenson and Cullen, 1974) (top) and HLA (Strominger *et al.*, 1981) (bottom). Abbreviations: Asn, asparagine; Fuc, Fucose; Gal, galactose; GlcNAc, *N*-acetylglucosamine; Man, mannose; NANA, *N*-acetyl neuraminic acid.

this structure was determined by analyses of the total glycopeptides isolated from H-2^b or H-2^d alloantigens and thus should be regarded as an average structure. Data of Kimball *et al.* (1981a) suggest that the saccharide unit attached to position 256 of the H-2K^d and -D^b alloantigens differs from those attached at positions 86 and 176. Future studies require the determination of the nature of the linkages between the monosaccharide units of the oligosaccharide moieties. Also, aside from microheterogeneity, it is not clear whether all glyco units on a given H-2 molecule have the same structure, or whether the glyco units present on different gene products are the same.

The functional role of the class I saccharide units is poorly understood, as is the case for such moieties on other glycoproteins. Studies on H-2 (Black *et al.*, 1981) and HLA (Ploegh *et al.*, 1981a) employing tunicamycin, an inhibitor of N-linked glycosylation, have shown that the saccharide moieties are not required by these molecules for transport to, or insertion into, the membrane. Furthermore, the lack of carbohydrate does not affect the association of the heavy chain with β_2M. Most studies have also indicated that the saccharide units are not involved in the alloantigenic activity of class I molecules. Enzymatic removal of carbohydrate failed to alter H-2 (Nathenson and Cullen, 1974) or HLA (Parham *et al.*, 1977) alloantigenic activity and isolated H-2 glycopeptides have been shown to be devoid of H-2 activity (Nathenson and Cullen, 1974). Furthermore, cells grown in the presence of tunicamycin express alloantigenically active, carbohydrate-free HLA on their surfaces (Ploegh *et al.*, 1981a). These studies, however, do not rule out the possibility that some of the extensive public and private specificities known to exist on class I molecules (J. Klein, 1975) may be related to carbohydrate structures, as suggested by the work of Sandersen *et al.* (1971).

Black *et al.* (1981) have found that H-2 saccharide units may play a role in the recognition and/or lysis of virally infected cells by H-2 restricted T killer cells. These investigators found that tunicamycin treatment did not inhibit the surface expression of either H-2 or vesicular stomatitis virus (VSV) glycoprotein, but did reduce by about 50% the lysis of VSV-infected cells by VSV-immune, H-2 identical killer cells. On the other hand, lysis of the tunicamycin-treated target cells by alloimmune effector cells was not affected. Similar results (Jackson *et al.*, 1976; Braciale, 1977) for other viruses have been obtained with another inhibitor of glycosylation, 2-deoxy-D-glucose.

The possibility that T cells specifically recognize carbohydrate moieties on H-2 molecules is difficult to reconcile with the allelic-associated variations in amino acid sequence and the ability of CTL to recognize sequence variations in H-2 mutants (see Section IX.B). However, Sherman (1980) has shown that CTL can recognize at least 23 different determinants on H-2 molecules, and it seems likely that some of these determinants are either indirectly (protein conformational determinants) or directly (carbohydrate determinants) affected by the present of carbohydrate.

While the exact role of the carbohydrate moieties in the function of class I molecules remains to be elucidated, it has become increasingly clear that cell-surface carbohydrate moieties play a significant role in many aspects of the cellular interactions that regulate immunity. Lymphoid cells have been shown to have lectinlike activities as integral components of their plasma membranes, some of which are apparently involved in certain types of blastogenesis (Decker,

1980) and the mediation of cytotoxicity reactions (Muchmore *et al.*, 1980). Furthermore, specific cell-surface saccharide moieties have been implicated in the binding of lymphokines to cells (Amsden *et al.*, 1978). The involvement of the class I carbohydrate moieties in these and other processes of the immune system obviously warrants further investigation.

F. Size Heterogeneity

The molecular weight of class I heavy chains has been reported to be approximately 45,000; however, not all the heavy chains of H-2 class I antigens have the same molecular weight. The molecular weight of the H-2K^d antigen has been estimated to be between 46,000 and 48,000, whereas the H-2D^d antigen has an estimated size of 43,000 (Schwartz *et al.*, 1980; Krakauer *et al.*, 1980; Dobberstein *et al.*, 1979; Fox and Weissman, 1979). Krakauer *et al.* (1980) also showed that the H-2D^b molecule has a molecular weight slightly larger (~45,000) than those of H-2K^b and H-2D^d, although smaller than that of H-2K^d. No such molecular weight variations have been reported for HLA heavy chains. Data from recent structural studies indicate that the H-2 size heterogeneity can be attributed to two factors: differences in extent of glycosylation and in length of the protein chains.

As discussed previously, protein sequence studies indicated that H-2K^d and H-2D^b have three saccharide units (attached at positions 86, 176, and 256), whereas H-2K^b and H-2D^d have only two carbohydrate groups (attached at positions 86 and 176). DNA sequence analyses (see Tables III–VI), which reveal the appropriate recognition sites for glycosylation, combined with molecular weight determinations of precipitated protein (Robinson, 1982), indicate that H-2L^d is glycosylated similarly to H-2K^d and H-2D^b.

Examination of recently described amino acid sequences derived from DNA clones of other class I molecules (Tables III–VI) indicates that all known murine class I molecules may be glycosylated at position 86.* Also, except for the protein sequence encoded by the Qa pseudogene 27.1, all murine class I molecules appear to be glycosylated at position 176. Whether this lack of glycosylation is reflective of murine *Tla* region gene products remains to be determined. The gene sequence data support the conclusions drawn from the protein sequence

---

*Even though it is required for N-linked glycosylation to occur, the presence of the recognition sequence Asn-X-Ser/Thr in the primary structure does not necessarily mean that glycosylation does occur. The overall protein conformation appears to control accessibility of the recognition sequence to glycosyl transferases such that only 33% of known recognition sites in eukaryotic proteins are glycosylated, and, of those, some are glycosylated inefficiently (Hubbard and Ivatt, 1981). However, since class I molecules are conformationally related, it is likely that, if glycosylation is known to occur at a site in one molecule, it will occur at identical sites in other molecules.

data in that glycosylation at position 256 appears to be highly variable. Eight of the twelve amino acid sequences listed for murine class I molecules (see Table V) have the appropriate recognition sequence for glycosylation at Asn-256.

Not only do the number of carbohydrate groups on H-2 molecules vary, but, in addition, the size of these groups at particular positions also appears to be variable. The majority of the carbohydrate groups in H-2 antigens have been estimated to contribute approximately 3000 daltons each to the molecular size of H-2 heavy chains (Nathenson and Cullen, 1974), but the glycosyl moiety attached at Asn-256 in H-2K^d and H-2D^b appears to contribute substantially less to the size of these molecules (Kimball *et al.*, 1981a).

The other structural feature that leads to size heterogeneity in murine class I molecules is differences in peptide chain lengths among H-2 molecules (see Table VI). For instance, H-2K^b has 348 amino acids and H-2K^d has 347 residues, whereas H-2D^b and H-2L^d are 338 residues long. This aspect of size heterogeneity, which in extreme cases is about 1000 daltons, is discussed in greater detail in Section V.F.

V. COMPARISON OF PRIMARY STRUCTURES OF MURINE AND HUMAN CLASS I MOLECULES

A major goal of primary structural studies on histocompatibility antigens is to determine, by means of sequence comparisons, regions of diversity and similarity, in hope of determining which portions of the molecules are responsible for various biological reactivities. For such comparisons, extensive primary protein structure information is now available for six H-2 antigens, three HLA antigens, and an HLA antigen pool. In addition, extensive amino acid sequence data have been deduced from cDNA and genomic clones of mouse and human MHC class I antigens. Tables III–VI compare the amino acid sequences of these various H-2 and HLA antigens and amino acid sequences deduced from cDNA and genomic clones of mouse and human class I molecules. These tables of protein sequences and DNA-derived amino acid sequences are organized according to the aforementioned genomic organization reported for mouse (Steinmetz *et al.*, 1981b) and human (Malissen *et al.*, 1982) class I heavy chain molecules.

A. The Precursor Sequence (Exon 1) and Amino Terminal Domain (Exon 2)

Table III compares amino acid sequences in exons 1 and 2. Exon 1 corresponds to the precursor sequence, or signal peptide (Blobel and Dobberstein, 1975) of class I molecules. As might be expected, the two L^d clones have iden-

Table III. Amino Acid Sequence Comparisons of the Precursor Peptides (Exon 1) and First Extracellular Domains (Exon 2) of Murine and Human Class I Molecules[a,b]

EXON 1

```
                       -20           -10            -1
27.5 (Lᵈ)ᶜ,ᵈ           MAPRTLLLLLAAA()WPDSDPR
CH4A (Lᵈ)              -------------()-------
27.1 (Qa)             --LTM----V---LTLIETRA
pHLA 12.4             ----------SGALALTQTWA
```

EXON 2

```
            1         10        20        30        40        50        60        70        80        90
H-2Kᵇ       GPHSLRYFVTAVSRPGLGEPRYMEVGYVDDTEFVRFDSDAENPRYEPRARWMEQEGPEYWERETQKAKGNEQSFRVDLRTLLGYYNQSKG
H-2Kᵈ       ------------------------FIA--------Q------D-A-F----P--------EQ--RV--SD--W----ST--AQR-------
H-2Kᵏ       ---------------H---------K--FI------------V----------------RR----------------------R---
H-2Dᵈ       -S------------------F-------N-------------------I----------RR-------A--R-----A--
H-2Dᵇ       ----M----E------E---IS-----NK----------------P--------------Q--W----S--N-----A--
27.5 (Lᵈ)   ----M----E--------IS-----NK-----------------Q-P---------I--I---Q--W---N-----A--
CH4A (Lᵈ)   ----M----E--------IS-----NK-----------------Q-P---------I--I---Q--W---N-----A--
27.1 (Qa)   -Q--Q--H------------W-IS-----Q--------------M----------------M---H-----GS---AQS------
pH-2III                                                    R--I-------------------R----E-
HLA-B7      -S---M---Y-S-----R----FIS-------Q-------AS--E----P--I----------D-N--IY-AQA-TD-ES--N-R-----EA
HLA-A2      -S---M--F-S-----R----FIA-------Q-------ASQ-M---P-I----D----KV-AHAHTV---G--R-----ZA
HLA-A28     -S---M--Y-S-----R----FIA-------Q-------ASQ-M---P-I----D-N-RNV-AQS-TD---G--R-----EA
HLA-pool    -S---M--Y-S-----R----FIA-----N-Q-------AS--Q---P-I--------D-Q--IY-AHA-TD-ES--N-R-----EA
pHLA 12.4   RS--M---Y-TM----A----FIS-------Q-------DAS--E----P---R--K--D-N--IC-AQA-TEREN--IA-R-----E-
```

[a] Exons are arranged according to Steinmetz et al. (1981b) and Malissen et al. (1982).

[b] H-2Kᵇ sequence was taken from Coligan et al. (1981); H-2Kᵈ, Kimball et al. (1981b); H-2Kᵏ, Rothbard et al. (1980); Mole et al. (1982); H-2Dᵈ, Nairn et al. (1981); H-2Dᵇ, Maloy et al. (1981) and Maloy and Coligan (1982); 27.5, Moore et al. (1982) (corrections of the published sequence were generously provided by L. Hood); CH4A, Evans et al. (1982); 27.1, Steinmetz et al. (1981b); pH-2III, Steinmetz et al. (1981a); pHLA 12.4, Malissen et al. (1982); HLA-B7, Ploegh et al. (1981b); HLA-A2 and HLA-A28, Lopez de Castro et al. (1982); HLA pool, Trägardh et al. (1979). (*) Indicates species-specific residues.

[c] DNA clones that could be assigned to a genetic locus or region have that assignment listed in parentheses.

[d] After transfection into L cells, serological analyses of the product encoded by clones 27.5 (Goodenow et al., 1982) and CH4A (Evans et al., 1982) indicate that they both encode H-2Lᵈ. It seems most likely that the two differences reported in the protein sequence encoded by these clones (positions 208 and 268) (see Table V) are due to DNA sequencing errors.

24

Kimball and Coligan

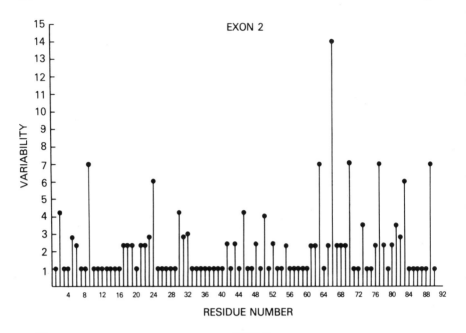

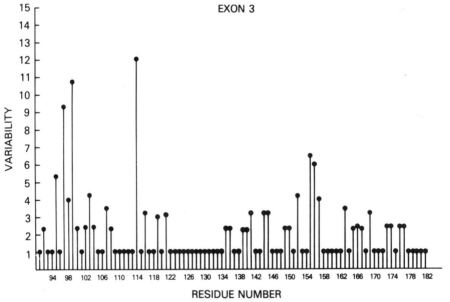

Figure 8. Variability of the amino acid residues in the three extracellular domains of murine class I molecules. Calculated from the data in Tables III, IV, and V according to Wu and Kabat (1970).

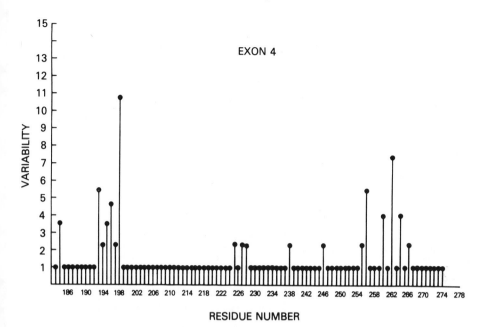

Figure 8. (*Continued*)

tical precursor peptides. Other comparisons reveal that precursor peptides have homologies ranging from 50% to 60%. Despite this relatively low sequence homology, the important property of hydrophobicity (von Heijne, 1981a) has been maintained in all the class I signal peptides.

Exon 2 coincides with the first extracellular domain, positions 1–90, of class I molecules. Homology among H-2 molecules in this domain ranges between 74% and 93%. When HLA molecules are compared, homologies between 86% and 91% are observed. By contrast, comparison of H-2 and HLA results in homologies of 67–73%, which are slightly less than the intraspecies homologies.

As can be seen in Table III and in the variability plot for H-2 molecules (Fig. 8), differences among class I molecules are not randomly distributed but tend to occur in clusters. One region of major diversity occurs between residues 61 and 83. In this region, the percentage homologies among H-2 molecules range from 48% to 83%, while HLA-B7 compared to -A2 or -A28 yields 55% and 65% homology, respectively. HLA-A2 and -A28, two highly cross-reactive molecules, are 75% homologous. Interspecies homologies range from 25% to 57%. In addition to this relatively large section of variability, other scattered sites of variability are found as small clusters in this domain (e.g., positions 30–32) or as single positions of variability (e.g., positions 9 and 89).

Table IV. Amino Acid Sequence Comparisons of the First Disulfide Loop Domains (Exon 3) of Mouse and Human Class I Molecules[a,b]

```
                91        100       110       120       130       140       150       160       170       180
                                                           **             *                                  *
          GSHTIQVISGCEVGSDGRLLRGYQQYAYDGCDYIALNEDLKTWTAADMAALITKHKWEQAGEAERLRAYLEGTCVEWLRRYLKNGNATLLRT
H-2K^b
H-2K^d    ----F-RMF - -  W                                                              -
H-2K^k     -  MYI     K--  -  -              -----------V        -  -  -  -          ---

H-2D^d    ---L-WMA-- - -  ------ W-F-- -- ----
H-2D^b    ---L-QM---DL--W----- L-F--E-R       Q--RR------A---  -  -  -  -          --------

27.5 (L^d) -T--L-WMY--D--------- E-F----R       Q--RR------ S- A--HYK----- E----H
CH4A (L^d) -T--L-WMY--D--------- E-F----R       Q--RR------A-YY----- E----H

27.1 (Qa)  ----L-WMY--DM-------- L-F--E-R        ------------V--- Q--RR------I-KDQ-----  MQS-----  QL-KE------

pH-2II     ------RL---D---W----- E------------------------                         -H------------
pH-2III    -------------------- E-----------------------  A---D---
pH-2^d-1                                        Q--RR------A---D---  E------
pH-2^d-3   --------------------- -------------------  Q--RR------A---D---  E------                          --

HLA-B7     ----L-SMY--D--P------ HD--P---------------K------ RS----T-- Q--QR---A-R---QR----- E-------  E--KDK-E-A

HLA-A2     ----LZRMY-----W F--------------K-----K---          QT-------A-HV--Q-----  --E  E--Q--
HLA-A28    ----- MY-D-------F------R-D-----K--- S------    --- QT-------A-HV--Q----  - E--KE--Q--

HLA-pool   ----L-SMY--D--P------ HD-I-----P--------K------ RS----T-- Q--QR---A-RA--QR----- E-------  E-RKDK-E-A
pHLA 12.4  ----M--MY--D--P--PF----E-H--------K------ RS----- Q--R--A-RR--QR-V----- EF------  E--KE--Q-A
```

[a] See footnotes to Table III.
[b] pH-2II and pH-2III sequences are from Steinmetz et al. (1981a); pH-2^d-1 and pH-2^d-3 are from Kvist et al. (1981).

B. The First Disulfide Loop Domain (Exon 3)

This region extends from residue 91 to residue 182. As shown in Table IV and Fig. 8, mouse class I molecules contain three clusters of notable diversity between residues 95–99, 114–116, and 152–157. Several of the most variable positions in H-2 molecules (positions 97, 99, and 114) occur in these clusters. Similar clusters exist in HLA molecules (Lopez de Castro *et al.*, 1982). Such regions are not as variable in HLA molecules, but this may reflect the limited number of HLA molecules so far available for comparison.

C. The Second Disulfide Loop Domain (Exon 4)

The second disulfide loop domain is the most highly conserved region in class I molecules (Table V and Fig. 8). The sequence homology between residues 200–274 is 95% among H-2 molecules and >98% among HLA molecules. The conservation of primary structure in this region is probably required to preserve a biologically important function. Thus this highly conserved region has been proposed to contain a β_2 M-binding segment of class I molecules, and a recent study by Yokoyama and Nathenson (1983) lends credence to this concept. In that study, H-2K^b was mildly digested with several proteolytic enzymes and subsequently H-2K^b heavy chain peptide fragments still associated with β_2 M were isolated. Sequence analyses revealed that these heavy chain peptides were derived from the second disulfide loop domain, thus indicating that β_2 M binds to this domain.

The third extracellular domain of murine class I molecules (see Table V) has two regions of sequence diversity: between residues 193–198 and residues 255–268. The former shows six different sequences in H-2. HLA molecules, on the other hand, are nearly invariant in this domain.

One other aspect of variability in the fourth exon is that the amino acid sequences deduced from H-2 clones 27.1 (Qa) and pH-2^d-1 contain three residues more than most other H-2 or HLA molecules. The three-residue insert occurs after residue 274. H-2D^d also contains a similar three-residue insert (R. Nairn and J. E. Coligan, unpublished results). Based on that and additional sequence data, pH-2^d-1 is thought to encode a molecule closely related to H-2D^d.

The amino acid sequences of H-2D^b and H-2L^d in this exon warrant further comment. There is at most one difference between these two molecules in exon 4 and, in fact, this is the only difference between positions 158 and 339, compared to 26 differences between D^b and K^b and 30 differences between D^b and the sequence derived from clone pH-2^d-1 (H-2D^d-like). Thus, H-2D^b and H-2L^d have the highest amino acid sequence homology (94%) of any two H-2 molecules for which extensive primary structure is known. In addition to their sequence homology, both D^b and L^d bind β_2 M very poorly (Maloy *et al.*, 1980; Coligan *et al.*, 1980) compared to D^d, and both have three glycosyl units whereas D^d has

Table V. Amino Acid Sequence Comparisons of the Second Disulfide Loop Domains (Exon 4) of Mouse and Human Class I Antigens [a]

```
           183      190       200       210       220       230       240       250       260       270
           *                          *        **  ** **  *                           *    *
H-2Kᵇ       DSPKAHVTHHSRPEDKVTLRCWALGFYPADITLTWQLNGEELIQDMELVETRPAGDGTFQKWASVVPLGKEQYYTCHVVHQGLPEPLTLRW
H-2Kᵈ        - - -                                                                    ---    N - --H-
pH-2ᵈ-4 (Kᵈ)ᵇ ---------PIS-GA------------T------------A----------------------------------N----H-K----------
H-2Kᵏ                                                                                              -I

H-2Dᵈ                                                                                    - K-
H-2Dᵇ       ------------P-SKGE----------T-----------------------------------------------N---R---E-------

27.5 (Lᵈ)   ------------P-SKGE--------A-----------T------------------------------------------N--R---E------
CH4A (Lᵈ)   ------------P-SKGE-----------------T-------------------------------------------N--R---E---H------

27.1 (Qa)   -P---------P-SYGA------------T--T-----------V----------------------------N-----N-E---------GRWᶜ

pH-2II      -P----------R---GD-----------T--------------------------------------------N--R---E------
pH-2ᵈ-1     -P----------R---GD--------------T-E------------------------------------LK---E-E-()-------GKEᶜ
pH-2ᵈ-3     ------------P-S-GE-----------T-------------------------------------------N--R---E-------

HLA-B7      -P--T-------PISDHEA-------------E------RD--DQT--T--------------R-E--A---S-E-R-----Q-E--K-----

HLA-A2      -A--T-H---AVSDHEA-------------E------RD--DQT--T------E---A---S-Q--R-----Q-E--K---
HLA-28      -A--    ---AVSDHEA-------------E------  D--DQT--T---------VA----S-Q--R-----Q-E--K--

HLA-pool    -P--T-------PISDHEA-------------E------RD--NQT--N------R------A------S-E-R-----Q-E--K-----
pHLA 12.4   -P--T-M---PISDHEA-------------E------RD--DQT--T---------A----S-E-R-----Q-E-------
```

[a] See footnotes to Tables III and IV.
[b] pH-2ᵈ-4 is from Lalanne et al. (1982).
[c] Clones 27.1 and pH-2ᵈ-1 have inserts of three amino acid residues after position 274.

only two. Largely because they were the first D-region molecules to be identified in their respective haplotypes, D^d and D^b were presumed to be alleles. However, the biochemical similarities of the $H-2L^d$ and $-D^b$ molecules suggest that the D^b and L^d genes are more likely to be alleles than those for D^b and D^d.

D. The Transmembrane Region (Exon 5) and the Cytoplasmic Domain (Exons 6-8)

Table VI details amino acid sequences of the transmembrane region (exon 5) and the cytoplasmic domain (exons 6-8).

1. Exon 5

Homologies among the murine molecules in the domain corresponding to exon 5 are similar to the homologies found in the extracellular portions of the molecules. They range from 67% (p-2^d-1 versus K^b) to 100% (27.5 versus D^b). The two HLA molecules which can be compared also show high homology (79%), but the interspecies homologies are drastically lower (about 40%) than the extracellular homologies. [The interspecies homology can be increased to 58% by inserting gaps in appropriate places (Uehara et al., 1981a).] These relatively low interspecies homologies probably reflect the function of this portion of the molecule. If its sole function is to anchor the molecule into the membrane, it is probably not necessary to retain particular amino acid residues, but only hydrophobic residues.

In most cases, at the interface of the membrane-binding region and cytoplasmic segment of class I H-2 molecules the sequence Arg-Arg-Arg occurs. The fact that this region of H-2K^d ends with only two basic residues (Arg-Arg) distinguishes it from essentially all other known class I molecules, including those of human origin, which also end with three basic residues (Table VI). The protein sequence derived from the Qa pseudogene 27.1 (Steinmetz et al., 1981b) suggests the possibility that other class I molecules may emulate H-2K^d in this respect. However, 27.1 contains the termination codon TGA at the site that normally encodes the third Arg residue (position 312). A single base change, T to A, yielding AGA, would produce an Arg codon and thus return the sequence encoded by the pseudogene to Arg-Arg-Arg.

HLA molecules have basic residues similar to those in H-2 between positions 308 and 312, but a Lys is substituted for Arg at position 312 in B7 and A2. The HLA cDNA clone, pHLA 12.4, has the sequence Arg-Lys-Lys.

2. Exon 6

Residues encoded in the region corresponding to exon 6 are identical or highly homologous in all H-2 molecules. HLA molecules are also nearly identical to one another, but differ significantly from H-2 molecules in this region. The

Table VI. Amino Acid Sequence Comparisons of the Transmembrane (Exon 5) and Cytoplasmic (Exons 6–8) Domains of Mouse and Human Class I Molecules[a,b]

Position markers along the reference sequence: 275, 280 (Exon 5 start), 290, 300, 310; 320 (Exon 6); 330 (Exon 7); 340, 350 (Exon 8). Asterisks (*) above the H2-K^b reference sequence mark selected positions.

	Exon 5	Exon 6	Exon 7	Exon 8
H2-K^b	EPPPSTVSNMATVAVLVVLGAAIVTGAVVVAFVMKMRRRNT	GGKGGDYALAP	GSQTSDLSLPDCK	VMVHDPHSLA
H2-K^d	KL------TVII------------()----	------VN-----	------------P-	----------
pH-2^d.4 (K^d)	------------()----	------VN-----	-Y-------G---	----------
H2-K^k	----	-		
H2-D^b	-------D-Y-VI----G----MAII------()----	----	---S-EM---R---	A
27.5 (L^d)[c]	----D-Y-VI----G----MAII------()----		---S-EM--R---	A
CH4A (L^d)[d]	----D-Y-VI----G----MAII------()----		---S-EM--R---	A
27.1 (Qa)[e,c]	----Y-------I-V-D----VAII----N()--X--	--Q---C-P--	--XS--R-----G---	A
pH-2I	---		---S--M--------	-
pH-2II	----D-Y-VI----G----MAII-----()----		---S-EM--R---	GDTLGSDWGGAMWT
pH-2^d.1	--S--KT-TVII--P-----VVIL--M-----()----		---S--M-------	-
pH-2^d.3	----F-D-Y-VI----G----MAII------()----		---S-EM------	A
HLA-B7[f]	--SSQSTVP VG VAG AV -VV- ------A--C()--KSS	------S-SQ-A	C-DSAQG-DVSLTA	
HLA-A2	W()--KSS	DR----S-SQ-A	S-DSAZG-DVSLTA	
pHLA 12.4	--SSQPTVP IVGIVAGL--LV-V--------A--W()-KKSS	DR---S-SQ-A	S-NSAQG-DVSLTA	

[a] See footnotes to Tables III and IV.
[b] pH-2I sequence was taken from Steinmetz et al. (1981a).
[c] The exact C-terminal residues (after position 338) of the murine genomic clones are unknown.
[d] Residues at positions 287–316 and 326–339 were provided by G. Evans (personal communication).
[e] An X indicates the position of a noncoding base sequence.
[f] Exon 8 is absent from HLA molecules; instead, exon 7 is one residue longer than in the mouse (Malissen et al., 1982).

fact that this region is so highly conserved suggests that it may be critical to the biological activity of class I molecules.

3. Exons 7 and 8

While most of the murine class I molecules whose protein sequences or nucleotide sequences are known terminate at amino acid position 339, there are exceptions. The deduced amino acid sequence of cDNA clone pH-2II indicates that the protein it encodes terminates at position 352 and has a unique carboxy terminus. Other notable exceptions are H-2K^b, H-2K^d, and pH-2^d-4, whose products terminate at position 348 and which have the identical C-terminal octapeptide, VHDPHSLA, encoded in the eighth exon. The genetic implications of this C-terminal variability in murine class I molecules are discussed in Section V.F. In contrast to H-2 molecules, current evidence indicates that there are only two cytoplasmic exons (6 and 7) in HLA molecules.

Discounting the differences in length, the protein sequence homology among the cytoplasmic portions (positions 307–339) of the murine class I molecules (Table VI) ranges from 81% to 94%. This homology among the C-terminal segments is similar to the approximately 85% homology observed when the extracellular portions of those molecules are compared. The C-terminal portions of HLA molecules also show about 90% homology when compared to each other. However, comparisons of the sequences of the human cytoplasmic segments with those of the murine molecules reveal an approximate homology of 30%, or about 45% if appropriate gaps are introduced (Uehara et al., 1981b). This is in marked contrast to the extracellular homology of murine and human class I molecules, which is about 70%.

E. Structural Correlates of Alleles

Because of their apparent allelism, one would expect to find structural correlates of products of K- and D-locus allotypes. Previous comparisons of peptide maps (Brown et al., 1974) and N-terminal amino acid sequences (Nathenson et al., 1981) have failed to demonstrate evidence for such sequences. However, a search of the more extensive sequence data in Tables III–VI suggests that amino acid sequences unique to allelic gene products may exist.

Analyses of the N-terminal 140 residues reveal little evidence of sequences characteristic of genetic regions (alleles) of class I molecules. However, certain amino acid sequences, shown in Table VII, which occur after residue 140, appear to distinguish products of K-, D-, and Tla-region molecules. Thus, all known K-end molecules have the sequence LITKH between residues 141–145 whereas all known D-end molecules express QITRR at this site. Therefore, on the basis of the apparent K-locus-specific residues extant between residues 141

Table VII. Amino Acid Sequences Characteristic of Products of Different Class I Loci[a]

Antigen or cDNA clone	141–145	296–299	309	329–332	339–352	Locus or region
Mouse						
H-2K^b	LITKH	AIVT	M	TSDL	VMVHDPHSLA	K
H-2K^d			M	TSDL	VMVHDPHSLA	K
pH-2^d-4^b		AIVT	M	TSDL	VMVHDPHSLA	K
H-2K^k	LITKH		M			K
pH-2III	LITKH					K
H-2D^b	QITRR	MAII	()^c	SSEM	A	D_1
H-2L^d	QITRR	MAII	()	SSEM	A	D_1
pH-2^d-3		MAII	()	SSEM	A	D_1
pH-2II		MAII	()	SSEM	GDTLGSDWGGAMWT	D_2
pH-2^d-1^d	QITRR	VVIL	()	SSDM	A	D_3
pH-2I				SSDM	A	D_3
27.1 (Qa)	QITRR	VAII	()	SSDR	A	Qa
Human						
HLA-B7	QITQR	VVVXe	()	SAQG	A	B_1
pHLA-12.4	QITKH	AVVT	()	SAQG	A	B_2
HLA-A2	QTTKH		()	SAZG	A	A
HLA-A28	QTTKH		()			A

[a] See footnotes to Tables III, IV, and VI for sources of data.
[b] Clone pH-2^d-4 is probably H-2K^d.
[c] ( ) indicates deletion based on alignment to H-2K^b.
[d] Clone pH-2^d-1 may be H-2D^d (unpublished amino acid sequence data, R. Nairn and J. E. Coligan).
[e] X indicates that no residue has been assigned for that position.

and 145 one would predict that clone pH-2III is the product of a K-locus gene in the H-2^k haplotype. However, this gene product is not H-2K^k, since the derived protein sequence differs from the known protein sequence of H-2.23 (Table IV). It is noteworthy that O'Neill and Parish (1981) have recently presented data indicating the presence of two K-region molecules in the k haplotype.

K- and D-end molecules are further differentiated by their C-terminal residues. In general, D-end molecules terminate nine residues earlier than K-end molecules and lack the C-terminal nonapeptide -MVHDPHSLA. In addition, the Met at position 309, deleted in D-end molecules, may also be an exclusive property of K-locus products. Because of these apparent K-locus structural features, one would predict that clone pH-2^d-4 also encodes a K-region molecule. In support of this prediction, H-2K^d and pH-2^d-4 differ in only two positions out of 59 available for comparison.

At positions 296–299 and 329–332, other amino acid sequences exist that appear to distinguish *K*-region, *D*-region, and *Qa*-region molecules. Furthermore, the *D*-region molecules can be subdivided into three types based on sequences at these positions and at their C termini. Types D$_1$ and D$_2$ share sequences that differ from D$_3$ at positions 296–299 and 329–332. Type D$_1$ and D$_2$ (pH-2^d-1) are distinguished by differences in their C termini.

The postulated region-specific sequences are obviously based on sparse data. Formal proof of their existence requires sequence information from additional class I molecules. The apparent lack of region-specific residues in the N-terminal 140 amino acid residues of these molecules, as well as the paucity of such sequences overall, may be a reflection of constraints placed on the divergence of these molecules by their similar biological function(s). This may be the result of parallel evolution and/or may reflect the ready exchange of genetic information among class I genes by such mechanisms as gene conversion (Baltimore, 1981).

F. Origin of C-Terminal Heterogeneity

As can be seen in Table VI, current data indicate that H-2 class I molecules vary in their C-terminal residues (positions 339–352), e.g., H-2K^b is 348 residues in length whereas H-2D^b is 338. However, certain data raise the question of whether these C-terminal residues are defined for each molecule or whether a given class I molecule has the option to be expressed with different C termini.

Information from the sequence analyses of genomic H-2 clones (genes 27.1, 27.5, and CH4A) indicates that each class I molecule may have within its gene sequence the information for each type of C terminus. This is illustrated in Fig. 9, in which an abbreviated form of the region encompassing the 3′ coding region

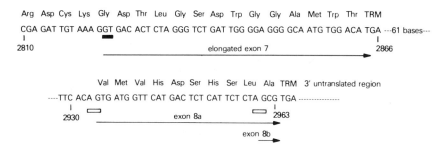

Figure 9. A portion of the 3′ coding region of gene 27.5 showing the optional C-terminal base sequences. Base numbers of the clone are indicated. Solid bar denotes the GT site that potentially begins an intron and open bar denotes AG sites that potentially end introns (Breathnach and Chambon, 1981). TRM signifies a termination codon.

of gene 27.5 is shown. The first type of C terminus (elongated exon 7) is generated in instances where exon 8 is not spliced into the coding sequence. In this
case, the GT donor splice site is apparently overlooked and the coding sequence
reads through exon 7 into the intron, wherein a termination codon is encountered
after 13 codons. The only evidence for the existence of such a C terminus in
H-2 class I molecules is from cDNA clone pH-2II (Steinmetz *et al.*, 1981a). The
protein sequence encoded by this clone does not correlate with any as yet identified protein molecule.

In cases where exon 8 is spliced in, there are two alternative AG acceptor
sites (Fig. 9). One begins at base 2933, which initiates exon 8a, and the other
begins at base 2960, which initiates exon 8b. The cDNA clone pH202 (H-2K^b)
is an example in which exon 7 is spliced to the upstream acceptor site such that
exon 8a is utilized, while cDNA clone pH203 (H-2D^b) is an example where the
downstream acceptor site for exon 8b is used. In both cases, the same termination codon is encountered, followed by the same stretch of 3′ noncoding DNA.

In cases where the C-terminal sequences of cDNA clones or protein molecules are known, the exact C terminus utilized by a particular class I molecule
is known, if only in regard to the source of the material. (A listing of these clones
and molecules is given in Table VIII.) However, in instances where only the
genomic DNA sequence is known, as in the case of clones 27.5 and CH4A, the
C-terminal sequence of the molecules encoded by this gene cannot as yet be
ascertained (Fig. 9). The C termini ascribed to the H-2L^d clones were thus
arbitrarily assigned.

Obviously, as pointed out in Section IV.F, the variability in the C termini
of class I molecules explains some of the observed size heterogeneity among
these molecules. More importantly, the differential splicing patterns at the 3′
end of H-2 class I molecules could have important biological significance in that
antigens with distinct cytoplasmic domains and functions can be produced.
However, it remains to be seen whether each H-2 class I molecule can possess

Table VIII. Characterization of H-2 Class I Molecules According to their C-Terminal Residues[a]

C-terminal configuration	Amino acid sequence	Clone or molecule
	339 340 350	
Elongated exon 7	G D T L G S D W G G A M W T	pH-2II
Exon 8a	VMV HDPHS LA	pH202 (H-2K^b); H-2K^d
Exon 8b	A	pH203 (H-2D^b); pH-2^d-1; pH-2^d-3; pH-21

[a] Data are from: pH-2I and pH-2II, Steinmetz *et al.* (1981a); pH202, Reyes *et al.* (1982a); H-2K^d, Kimball and Coligan (1983); pH203, Reyes *et al.* (1982b); pH-2^d-1 and pH-2^d-3, Kvist *et al.* (1981).

only one of the three possible alternative sequences, or if each class I molecule can express any one of the potential C-terminal sequences, depending on such variables as cell type, metabolic state of cells of origin, or even random chance. Of interest in this regard is that current data indicate that human class I molecules, which apparently have only seven exons, may not have optional C termini.

VI. *Tla*-REGION MOLECULES

There are still only sparse amino acid sequence data for these antigens. The data for Qa antigens that are available reveal homology to transplantation antigens. Table IX compares amino terminal sequences of H-2K^b (Coligan *et al.*, 1981) and Qa-2 (Soloski *et al.*, 1982) and the protein sequence derived from the Qa pseudogene, 27.1 (Steinmetz *et al.*, 1981b). It shows that only 1 out of 15 positions (7%) available for comparison between H-2K^b and Qa-2 are homologous (Table IXA). However, if the Qa-2 assignments after residue 3 are shifted two positions toward the amino terminal (Table IXB), there is concordance at 13 out of 18 positions (72%). Sequence analyses (Soloski *et al.*, 1982) revealed

Table IX. Comparison of Amino Acid Sequences of Qa-2 and H-2 Antigens[a]

```
A                      5        10       15        20
  H-2Kb    G P H S L R Y F V T A V S R P G L G E P
  Qa-2         H     L   Y F     V   R     L

                       25       30       35        40
  H-2Kb    R Y M E V G Y V D D T E F V R F D S D A
  Qa-2         F     V L Y V       F   R F


B                      5        10       15        20
  H-2Kb    G P H S L R Y F V T A V S R P G L G E P
  Qa-2         H   L Xb Y F X     V   R     L
  27.1 (Qa) G Q H S L Q Y F H T A V S R P G L G E P

                       25       30       35        40
  H-2Kb    R Y M E V G Y V D D T E F V R F D S D A
  Qa-2     X F     V L Y V       F   R F
  27.1 (Qa) W F I S V G Y V D D T Q F V R F D S D A
```

[a] Data for Qa-2 taken from Soloski *et al.* (1982). Data for Qa pseudogene 27.1 taken from Steinmetz *et al.* (1981b).
[b] X indicates that the residue at that position is still unassigned but is known to be different from the residue assigned to that position in H-2K^b.

that, in addition to the differences at positions 22 and 26 (Table IXB), Qa-2 is missing Arg residues at positions 6 and 21 and a Val residue at position 9 that are present in H-2K^b. The missing Arg residues are invariant in H-2 and HLA molecules. It is also noteworthy that Qa pseudogene 27.1 could encode a molecule that has 77% homology to H-2K^b without requiring a frameshift, but is similar to Qa-2 in that there are no Arg residues at positions 6 and 21. Instead, Gln and Trp residues are substituted at these positions, respectively. If products similar to the one encoded by the Qa pseudogene exist, then the frameshift differences between such products and the reported sequence of Qa-2 probably reflect differences between molecules encoded at different loci.

There are no amino acid sequence data available for Tla antigens. The fact that attempts at N-terminal sequence analysis have so far met with failure (Cunningham *et al.*, 1977; S. G. Nathenson, personal communication) suggests that these molecules have blocked N termini. Peptide mapping studies, though, have begun to supply information regarding the homology of Tla antigens to other class I molecules. Thus, Tla antigens (Yokoyama *et al.*, 1981) appear to be less homologous to H-2 molecules than are Qa antigens (Soloski *et al.*, 1982). (Tl versus H-2 showed 15–35% peptide homology while Qa versus H-2 showed 20–50% peptide homology.) When Tla antigens from different haplotypes were compared to each other, however, higher peptide homology (70–80%) was noted. Similarly high peptide homologies among Qa antigens were also observed. These peptide mapping data indicate that the Tla-region molecules are more homologous to each other than classical transplantation antigens are to each other. The latter demonstrate only about 35% peptide homology among themselves (Brown *et al.*, 1974). The 80% peptide homology seen among Tla antigens indicates at least 95% amino acid sequence homology. No direct peptide mapping comparisons of Tla and Qa antigens have been performed yet.

VII. CLASS I MOLECULES OF OTHER SPECIES

Class I antigens, analogous to those present in man and mouse, have been detected in all vertebrate species that have been examined (Götze, 1977), and, when analyzed, their biochemical properties have been similar to those reported for the human and murine prototypes, e.g., rat (Blankenhorn *et al.*, 1978), chicken (Vitetta *et al.*, 1977), rabbit (Kimball *et al.*, 1979), and miniature swine (Lunney and Sachs, 1978). Multiple loci encoding class I molecules also appear to exist in most, if not all, of these other species.

However, despite the identification of class I molecules in species other than man and mouse, there has been a paucity of primary structural information about these molecules, for two main reasons. First is the lack of inbred strains, let alone congenic strains, which are important for the development of specific serological reagents useful for detecting class I molecules and which provide a less complex source of material. Second are the difficulties involved in isolation and sequence determinations of molecules available in such small amounts. However, the availability of cross-hybridizing DNA probes, which are specific for highly conserved regions of the class I genome, have made these problems less acute. In this regard, Singer *et al.* (1982) have recently isolated class I genes of the miniature swine, and sequence information should be forthcoming.

Despite the difficulties, limited N-terminal sequences of class I molecules have been obtained for a number of species, and these are compared with all available N-terminal sequences for man and mouse in Fig. 10. As indicated by the bars at the bottom of Fig. 10, there is clear homology among the species. Because of the fragmentary nature of the data, it is difficult to quantitate the levels of interspecies homology for the chicken, rat, and guinea pig. However, Fig. 11 shows interspecies homologies for representative molecules of species where contiguous N-terminal sequence data are available. In general, the interspecies homology, which averages about 80%, is only slightly less than the intraspecies homology, which averages about 88%. While the degrees of homology indicated here represent comparisons of only about 10% of the total primary structure of the class I molecules (~35 out of ~340 residues), comparisons of entire sequences of human and mouse molecules indicate that these N-terminal homologies are likely to be representative of the overall homologies of the extracellular portions of the molecule. The homology shown in Figs. 10 and 11 indicates that the class I genes of the MHC share a common ancestry over the more than 300 million years since the avian and mammalian evolutionary lines diverged from one another.

Further examination of the sequences in Fig. 10 reveals the presence of species-associated residues. These are residues that distinguish all or most of the gene products of a gene family of one species from those of a second species. Not only are such residues present in the amino termini of the class I molecules, but comparison of entire human and murine sequences indicates that such residues occur throughout the length of the class I molecules (Tables III–VI). The genetic implications of these species-associated residues are discussed in Section X.B.

VIII. HOMOLOGY OF CLASS I MOLECULES TO OTHER MOLECULES

A much-discussed issue has been the evolutionary relationship between class I antigens and immunoglobulins. Several years ago $\beta_2 M$ was found to be about 30% homologous to Ig constant region domains and was thus referred to as a free immunoglobulin domain (Peterson *et al.*, 1972). Similarities of the heavy chains of class I molecules to immunoglobulins are suggested by the presence of

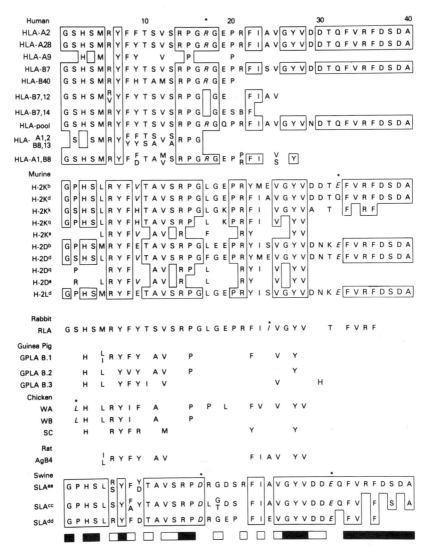

Figure 10. Amino-terminal sequences for class I histocompatibility antigens from several vertebrate species. Boxed residues are those that are constant within a species. Solid bars indicate residues that show no variation among species; open bars indicate positions that show very little variation. Sequence positions that are indicated by asterisks and italics are species-associated residues. HLA sequences are from: A2, Orr et al. (1979b); A28, Lopez de Castro et al. (1982); A9, Allison et al. (1978); B7, Orr et al. (1979b); B40, B7,12, B7,14, Ploegh et al. (1981b); pool, Trägårdh et al. (1980); A1,2, B8,13, Bridgen et al. (1976); A1, B8, Ballou et al. (1976). H-2 sequences are from: K[b], K[d], D[b], D[d], see review of Nathenson et al. (1981); K[k], Mole et al. (1982) and Rothbard et al. (1980); K[q], Cook et al. (1978) and Maizels et al. (1978); K[s], D[q], D[s], Maizels et al. (1978); L[d], Coligan et al. (1980) and Moore et al. (9182). Data for other species are from: rabbit, Wilkinson et al. (1982); guinea pig, Schwartz et al. (1980); chicken, Vitetta et al. (1977) and Huser et al. (1978); rat, Blankenhorn et al. (1978); swine, Metzger et al. (1982).

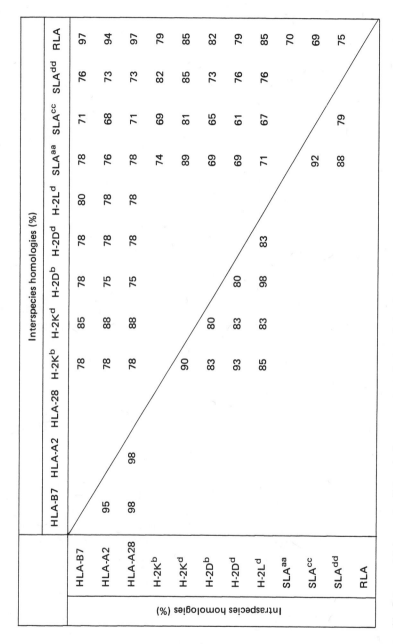

Figure 11. Intra- and interspecies N-terminal sequence homologies of class I antigens. The homologies were calculated from possible comparisons within the N-terminal 40 residues. For positions in SLA where two residues were assigned, if one residue was identical to the compared sequence, 50% identity was credited for that position.

Ig-like domain subregions in H-2K^b and HLA-B7 (Table II, Fig. 5). Comparison of HLA sequences (Orr *et al.*, 1979a; Trägårdh *et al.*, 1980) to immunoglobulin molecules revealed that the second disulfide loop domain (α3) had a low but statistically significant homology to Ig constant region domains, particularly C$_H$3, and to β$_2$M (35% and 30%, respectively) (Orr *et al.*, 1979a; Trägårdh *et al.*, 1980). These data were later supported by a homology search in which greater value was given to matches of the rare amino acids, Cys, Trp, and His (Strominger *et al.*, 1980). A recent analysis (Steinmetz *et al.*, 1981a), which compared the cDNA sequence of H-2^d clone pH-2II to the DNA sequences of the mouse Ig M constant region domains, supported the homology discerned by protein sequence analyses. More importantly, however, this study revealed that the third base positions in the codons of these molecules were highly conserved. This finding strongly suggests that the homologies between transplantation antigens and immunoglobulins arose by divergent rather than convergent evolution, because convergent evolution drives different genes to produce similar sequences without any selective pressures for the conservation of the third base positions in codons. Thus, immunoglobulins and transplantation antigens appear to be members of the same supergene family.

Recent data indicate that not only class I but also class II molecules are members of the Ig supergene family. Protein sequence (Kratzin *et al.*, 1981) and DNA sequence (Larhammar *et al.*, 1981) analyses indicate that the extracellular portion of HLA-DR β chains consists of two disulfide-loop-containing domains. As shown in Fig. 12, the β-chain domain nearest the cell membrane displays homology with the Ig-like (α3) domain of HLA heavy chains, β$_2$M, and Ig light and heavy chain constant domains. The β-chain sequence shows between 22%

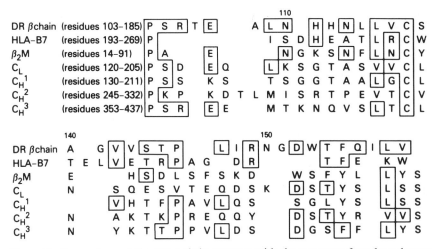

Figure 12. Comparison of the DR β-chain sequence with the sequences from homologous domains of HLA, β$_2$M, kappa light chain (C$_L$), and IgG1 heavy chain (C$_H$1, C$_H$2, and C$_H$3). Adapted from Larhammar *et al.* (1981).

and 40% homology to these other sequences. These levels of homology are at least as strong as the homology among other members of this supergene family (Larhammar *et al.*, 1981).

These homology comparisons indicate that the humoral and cellular branches of the immune system have diverged from a common ancestral gene. However, recent evidence showing that Thy-1 antigen is a member of the same supergene family (A. F. Williams and Gagnon, 1982) suggests that the conserved structure among these molecules has nothing directly to do with the functioning of the immune system, since Thy-1 is found in tissues unrelated to the immune response, e.g., the brain. Also, A. F. Williams and Gagnon (1982) have evidence for the presence of a Thy-1 homolog in the brain of squids. Consequently, Williams and his co-workers have proposed that Thy-1 is one of a set of Ig-related structures that mediate cell recognition in morphogenesis (Cohen *et al.*, 1981). In this hypothesis, the Ig-like domain common to these molecules is considered a stable platform for the display of determinants and thus the Ig domain would serve as a basic recognition unit for cell interactions (Fig. 13).

IX. RECOGNITION SITES ON CLASS I MOLECULES

A. Alloantigenic Determinants

By comparing the available primary structures of class I molecules, it is possible to begin to localize regions of the molecules and particular amino acid

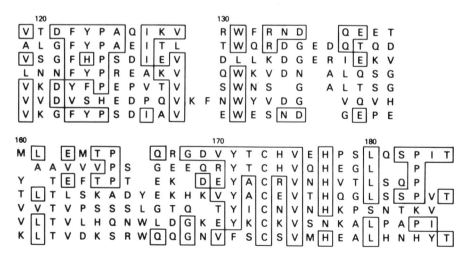

Figure 12. (*Continued*)

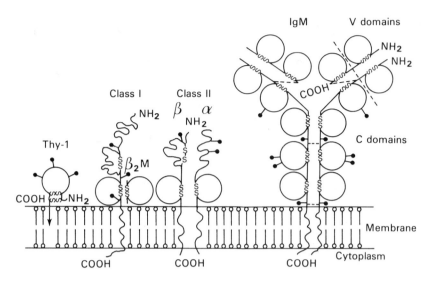

Figure 13. Molecules in the Ig superfamily depicted on the cell surface. Ig domains and their homologous regions in the other molecules are represented by circles. Intrachain disulfide bonds are shown by S-S symbols and interchain bonds in IgM by dashed lines. N-linked carbohydrate structures are shown by the club (♟). It is believed that the class I, class II, and IgM molecules are integrated into the membrane by a hydrophobic protein sequence; but for Thy-1 the evidence indicates that a nonprotein structure is responsible for membrane integration. Adapted from A. F. Williams and Gagnon (1982).

residues that are involved in forming the alloantigenic specificities of these molecules. As mentioned previously, the overall homology among H-2 or HLA class I molecules is about 85%. As indicated in Fig. 8, the variability in protein sequence for H-2 molecules appears to be confined to discrete regions or single positions interspersed with highly conserved regions. The greatest variability is in three regions, residues 62–83, 95–121, and 193–198, while the greatest homology in the sequence occurs between residues 199 and 254. Although fewer data are available, comparison of HLA molecules reveals regions of variability very similar in location to those of H-2 molecules (Fig. 14). At least three clusters of differences are evident: positions 65–80, 105–116, and 177–194. When a fourth region of less extensive variability is included (positions 138–156), it can be calculated that 74% of all the substitutions in the HLA molecules fall within four segments that in total comprise only 25% of the molecule. This further indicates that the variability in class I molecules occurs mainly in the N-terminal portion of the molecule and that it is nonuniformly distributed.

Recently studies by Steinmetz et al. (1982) at the genomic level support the protein structure comparisons. These investigators isolated gene probes from cDNA clones pH-2II and pH-2III (see Table III and VI) specific for 5′ (codons 63–160) and 3′ (codons 183–329) class I gene segments. Hybridization of these

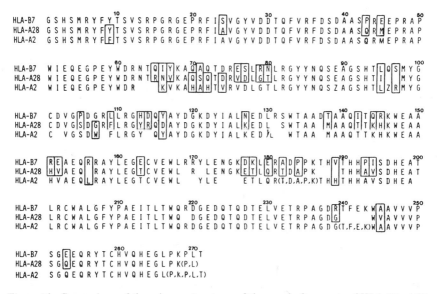

Figure 14. Comparison of the primary structures of the papain fragments of HLA-B7, -A28, and -B7. Boxed residues are those that are different among the proteins being compared. Blanks correspond to nonassigned positions. From Lopez de Castro *et al.* (1982).

clones with isolated cosmid clones revealed that the 3′ probe hybridized to all clones with the same intensity, whereas the 5′ probe gave differences in intensity ranging over two orders of magnitude, thus again indicating that the greatest variability in class I molecules occurs in the N-terminal half.

Comparison of the HLA-2 and -A28 molecules (Fig. 14) is particularly interesting because these molecules are antigenically very similar (Joysen and Wolf, 1978). As might be expected, this similarity is reflected in a high amino acid sequence homology (96%). Therefore, differences in primary structure between these molecules should serve to localize residues involved in alloantigenic sites. Of the 235 comparable positions in thse molecules, only ten positions (9, *66*, *70*, *71*, *72*, *74*, 95, *107*, *116*, and 245) are known to have different amino acid residues (Fig. 14). Seven of these positions (italicized above) are located within the clusters of diversity discussed previously. Furthermore, the three positions of difference (9, 95, 245) that lie outside of these clusters represent conservative amino acid interchanges, which makes it unlikely that they play a role in the alloantigenicity of these molecules. In contrast, three of the other positions (66, 74, and 116) show charge differences and position 107 shows a Gly-Trp interchange, all of which are nonconservative differences.

The data of Lopez de Castro *et al.* (1982) suggest that it may be feasible to achieve a more detailed map of the antigenic determinants on class I molecules by correlating primary structure with serological analyses. A monoclonal antibody, MB40.1, has been observed to react strongly with HLA-B7 and -A28 and weakly with HLA-A2 (Parham and McLean, 1980). This suggests that some of the residues that are identical in HLA-B7 and HLA-A28, but different in HLA-A2, may be primarily involved in the epitope recognized by MB40.1. Only two of five positions with amino acid interchanges (74 and 107) have differences that are nonconservative and only one of these (position 74) involves a charge difference. Thus, it may be tentatively suggested that Asp-74 and/or possibly Gly-107 constitutes an important portion of the antigenic determinant recognized by MB40.1 antibody.

The amino acid differences observed among the various H-2 and HLA molecules are undoubtedly responsible for their antigenic differences. Most likely the regions of amino acid differences are directly involved in forming allodeterminants. However, without knowledge of the three-dimensional structure of histocompatibility antigens, it is not possible to say whether the linear clusters of variability noted above actually constitute multiple allodeterminants or whether some or all of them combine into three-dimensional arrays to comprise larger epitopes. On the other hand, it is possible that some of the amino acid substitutions lead to conformational changes in distal parts of the class I molecules, which then behave as allodeterminants.

B. Sites Recognized by T Cells

Over the years a number of mutations have been detected in murine class I molecules by screening for unexpected graft rejections (reviewed by Nairn *et al.*, 1980b). From these mutant animals, a series of well-characterized mutant strains of mice have been developed. In addition to altered graft rejection responses, these mutant strains show strong histogenic reactivities with the parental inbred strains according to a variety of tests (reviewed by J. Klein, 1978). The mutant molecules have also been shown to affect the associative recognition of membrane-bound structures such as viral components (Zinkernagel and Klein, 1977) and chemically modified proteins (Forman and Klein, 1977) by CTL. Therefore, it was anticipated that the biochemical identification of the structural changes in the mutant molecules would serve to localize the region of the molecule in which polymorphism can serve as a specific and effective signal for recognition by the immune system.

Of the approximately 30 known H-2 mutations, 17 occur in the *H-2K^b* gene. The availability of such a large series of mutants in which altered immunological reactions could be attributed to a particular locus provided the initial impetus for the determination of the structure of the parent H-2K^b molecule.

Mutations sites in the H-2K^b molecules were localized by comparative tryptic peptide mapping (see review by Nairn *et al.*, 1980b). As shown in Fig. 15, amino acid sequence analyses of the tryptic peptides containing mutation sites revealed

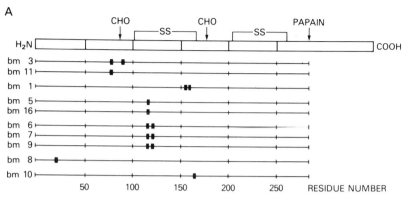

Figure 15. The bm series of mutants at the H-2K locus. (A) A schematic depiction of the position at which mutations occur. (B) Tabulation of the reported amino acid substitutions in the H-2K^{bm} mutants compared to the residues at these positions in H-2L^d and -D^b.

the exact position of the mutations and in many cases the nature of the amino acid interchange. The data indicate that no mutant molecule differs from the parent molecule by more than two amino acid residues and that all the mutation sites occur at positions of known variability among the H-2 class I molecules. Comparative tryptic peptide mapping studies have also been carried out between the mutant and parent K^k and K^f molecules (Ewald et al., 1979). Although no amino acid sequences were determined, the limited number of tryptic peptide differences between the mutant and parent molecules suggest changes in the mutant molecules similar to those reported for the K^b mutants.

While these data clearly indicate that minute differences in the primary structure can give rise to profound alterations in functional properties, recent experiments by Sherman (1982) indicate that the mutant amino acid substitution sites need not be directly involved in the determinants recognized by CTL. In this study the reactivity of C57BL/6 (parent) anti-B6.C-H-2^{bm11} (mutant) CTL clones with other bm mutants (bm1, bm3, bm4, bm8, bm9, bm10) was studied. As expected on the basis of a shared mutation at amino acid position 77 (Fig. 15), the vast majority of bm11-specific clones (83%) also recognized the bm3 target. It was suggested that the antigenic determinants recognized by the 17% of the CTL that did not recognize bm3 are obscured or disrupted on the bm3 molecule as a result of the second mutation at position 89. Most interesting, however, was the observation that the majority of the clones (62%) recognized not only targets that possessed the mutation at position 77, but also at least one of the other K^b mutants, which are identical to the wild-type K^b at position 77. Based on these results, it would seem that different and often distal amino acid substitutions in an H-2 molecule can result in antigenic determinants, which, if not identical, are at least similar enough to permit comparable T-cell recognition as reflected in the comparable degree of lysis of different mutant target cells. Therefore, these results indicate that single amino acid substitutions in H-2 molecules can result in the appearance of new immunogenic determinants that do not include the substituted amino acid responsible for the alteration. However, since the amino acid sequences of mutant K^b molecules have yet to be completely determined, it must be kept in mind that bm3 mutant and the other bm mutants may share as yet undetected amino acid substitutions that could account for at least some of the observed cross-reactivities.

Variant human class I molecules that appear to be analogous to the murine mutant H-2 molecules have been detected using a functional assay based on the recognition of virally infected cells by cytotoxic T cells (Biddison et al., 1980, 1981). In this assay T cells are primed in vitro by stimulation with virally infected, autologous cells. Such CTL are "restricted" to the recognition and lysis of target cells that possess not only the priming virus strain but also the HLA-A or -B antigens of the autologous cells (see Section XII).

Studies on the human viral immune CTL have demonstrated that these cells recognize viral antigens that are highly associated with the serologically defined HLA-A and -B specificities (Misko et al., 1980; Sethi et al., 1980). However, recent studies by Biddison et al. (1980) have indicated that the association between the serologically defined HLA-A2 specificity and the -A2 restriction antigen recognized by CTL is incomplete. CTL restricted to HLA-A2 and influenza virus killed all HLA-A2 flu-infected target cells except for cells from one particular donor, M7. (This A2 variant could also be distinguished from other A-2-positive donors by alloimmune CTL.) Serological analysis of the M7 donor showed that it carried an HLA-A2 molecule that was indistinguishable from the A2 antigen of all other A2-positive donors. Recently, during a screening of a more extensive panel of A2-positive donors (27 individuals), two more variants with distinctive functional and biochemical characteristics were identified (Biddison *et al.*, 1982). Preliminary comparative tryptic peptide mapping studies indicate that the variant A2 heavy chains may each differ from the JY HLA-A2 heavy chain shown in Fig. 13 by only a single tryptic peptide, which contains one or two amino acid substitutions. In the case of M7, the tryptic peptide has been tentatively localized to positions 36–44 of the intact HLA-A2 molecule (Lopez de Castro *et al.*, 1982).

The occurrence of variant HLA molecules is not unique to A2. Studies by Biddison *et al.* (1981) showed that HLA-A3 molecules display similar variation, as do HLA-Bw44 moleucles (Tekolf *et al.*, 1982). As with the A2 molecules, no serological distinctions were evident among the various A3 and Bw44 molecules.

The simplest interpretation of the above studies is that a given HLA antigen, e.g., A2, bears multiple distinct CTL restriction antigens (determinants) and that HLA-A2 molecules from unrelated donors may differ with respect to the possession of some or all of these determinants. Specific T-cell clones that respond to a given foreign antigen, e.g., flu virus, may recognize some but not all of the A2 restriction determinants. The bases for these different restriction determinants most probably are related to differences in primary structure similar to those that have been detailed for the K^b mutants and that have been implicated for the A2 variants. Elucidation of the nature of these structural changes in the human variant molecules should help define a molecular basis for associative recognition of virus-infected cells by CTL.

X. EVOLUTION OF CLASS I GENES

A. Gene Duplication

Accumulating evidence provides strong support for the previously postulated concept (Silver *et al.*, 1976; Bodmer, 1978) that the multiple class I genes have arisen by a series of gene duplication events. Primary evidence for this notion comes from the data, presented previously, that show close structural relationships among the various class I molecules. Recent data from the mouse (discussed subsequently) indicate that many of these duplication events have occurred relatively recently in evolutionary time in that such events appear to be strain-specific. This suggests that the class I duplication events are ongoing and that they occur independently within each species.

Initial evidence supporting the notion of relatively recent class I gene duplications came from the identification of a second gene product (H-2L) encoded in the D region of certain mouse haplotypes (Lemonnier *et al.*, 1975; Hansen *et al.*, 1977). Primary structural data (Coligan *et al.*, 1980) and peptide map comparisons (Sears and Polizzi, 1980) indicated that H-2L^d is no more like -D^d than any other H-2 molecule, indicating that it was probably not the result of a recent duplication of the *H-2D^d* gene. However, peptide map comparisons indicated that the H-2D^q and -L^q are remarkably similar, as are -L^d and -L^q (Rose *et al.*, 1980). The latter two molecules are also serologically indistinguishable (Levy and Hansen, 1980). These results suggest that D^q and L^q might be the result of a recent gene duplication and that the *H-2^d* haplotype could have acquired H-2L from this haplotype or another by recombination. The failure to detect the H-2L molecule in several other haplotypes, e.g., *b*, *s*, and *k*, either by immunoprecipitation (Hansen *et al.*, 1980) or by DNA probes specific for the *L* locus (Steinmetz *et al.*, 1982), suggests that all haplotypes have not acquired the *L* allele or that it has been lost by deletion in some mouse strains.

In addition to the L molecule, recent investigations have indicated the presence of additional class I molecules that appear to be the result of recent gene duplications. Iványi and Démant (1979) and Sears and Polizzi (1980) have described a new molecule (H-2M^d) in the D region that, unlike L^d, is very similar to D^d. A close structural similarity appears to exist between D^d and M^d since their public and private specificities appear to be identical, except that some anti-H-2.28 sera react with H-2D^d but not with H-2M^d. Co-capping experiments (Iványi and Démant, 1981) have also indicated the existence of two H-2D^k molecules (D1^k and D2^k) that are antigenically very similar. Hansen *et al.* (1981) have reported an additional D-region gene product (H-2R) in the *d* and *q* haplotypes that appears to be structurally very closely related to the L^d, D^q, and L^q molecules discussed previously.

Thus, there is extensive evidence that a series of gene duplications has given rise to multiple molecules in the D region of *d*, *q*, and *k* haplotype mice. Other recent studies have indicated that similar gene duplications have occurred in the K region. O'Neill and Parish (1981) and Iványi and Démant (1981) have described the existence of two closely related K^k and K^d molecules, respectively.

In addition to the above phenotypic evidence for gene duplication, the recent study of Steinmetz *et al.* (1982) provides striking evidence at the gene level that the class I genes have undergone a series of relatively recent gene duplications. These investigators cloned DNA from BALB/c (H-2^d) sperm in large fragments (cosmids). Examination of this cosmid library revealed 13 gene clusters, each containing 1–7 class I genes, 36 class I genes in total. Seven genes found in cluster 1 displayed extensive restriction site homology. When examined by restriction mapping, genes at the 3′ end of the cluster and their flanking sequences were found to be almost identical while the class I genes at the 5′ end of the cluster were homologous to one another, but distinctly less homologous to the genes at the 3′ end. This homology strongly suggests that these genes arose by relatively recent and multiple duplications. Examination of the region analogous to cluster 1 in H-2^k and H-2^b mice indicated that in each strain unique gene deletions and genetic reorganization have occurred.

As was indicated by recent studies of the class I gene products, this study of class I genes supports the concept that differences in gene number and organization exist within the regions (or clusters) of class I genes of different strains of mice, presumably due to homologous but unequal crossing-over. Extensive regions of homology that exist in the class I genome probably are instrumental in promoting such crossing-over.

B. Species-Associated Residues

The data discussed above suggest that duplication of class I genes is an on-going process within each species. The extent of this species-specific gene duplication is unknown, i.e., how many class I genes did each species inherit from a common ancestor? The occurrence of species-associated residues in all species for which extensive N-terminal sequence data are available (Fig. 10) suggests that the duplication of all class I genes may have occurred after speciation (Maizels et al., 1978). More extensive comparison of the multiple human and murine molecules indicates that species-associated residues occur throughout their length (Tables III–VI). At 36 positions where all murine class I molecules have the same amino acid residue, a different residue is present in the human class I molecules. Further support for gene duplication after speciation is the fact that while there is significant homology (~70%) between human and mouse class I molecules, there is no evidence of greater structural homology between the gene products of particular HLA and H-2 loci.

Obviously, the evidence for species-associated residues is based on a relatively small amount of sequence data and, thus, sequence data for more class I molecules will be required for formal proof. One must also be aware that alternative genetic mechanisms could explain the existence of such residues. For example, if ancestral D and K genes were present prior to the divergence of mammals, parallel evolution could have occurred within each species, perhaps mediated by some process such as unequal crossing-over or gene conversion (Baltimore, 1981). There is some evidence that such genetic mechanisms have been involved in the evolution of class I molecules (see Section X.C).

C. Generation of Diversity

Subsequent to gene duplication, the accumulation of point mutations is the most probable means of generating polymorphism in class I genes. The large extent of the diversity, which is difficult to explain, may be the result of an inordinately high mutation rate and selective pressures related to function. The mutation rate for the K-locus genes appears to be two to three orders of magnitude higher than that for other mammalian genes (J. Klein, 1978). Nevertheless, one would still expect the existence of structural properties that are unique to the products of alleles (or apparent alleles). In other words, one would expect genes from a given genetic region (or cluster) to be structurally related. However, comparisons of peptide maps (Brown et al., 1974) and N-terminal amino acid sequences (Nathenson et al., 1981) have failed to demonstrate evidence for such sequences. A search of the more extensive data provided by protein and nucleic acid sequences (Table VII) hints that sequences unique to allelic gene products may exist (Section V.E), although not to the extent that would be expected for alleles.

A genetic mechanism that could account for the overall absence of region-specific structural properties (so-called K-ness and D-ness) and that at the same time could account for some of the observed patterns of diversity is gene conversion. This is a nonreciprocal genetic process by which a particular segment of a given gene, A, becomes identical to the corresponding portion of another related but nonidentical gene, B (Baltimore, 1981; Egel, 1981). Such a genetic mechanism would be an advantageous way of maintaining sequence homogeneity in gene families. Although formal proof for gene conversion only exists for fungi and yeasts (see Baltimore, 1981), circumstantial evidence suggests that this mechanism may be operative in the immunoglobulin (Schreirer et al., 1981; Clarke et al., 1982) and hemoglobin (Slightom et al., 1980) gene families. For example, for immunoglobulins it has been shown that two nonallelic murine immunoglobulins, Ig2a[a] and Ig2b[a], share sequence segments that are not present in an apparently allelic product, Ig2a[b], a result that has been interpreted as a strong case for gene conversion (Schreirer et al., 1981).

Certain data indicate that gene conversion is also an operative genetic mechanism in class I gene families. For instance an interesting aspect of the K^b mutant molecules is that, at all positions where K^b-mutant amino acid interchanges occur, differences also occur between K^b and D^b or L^d (Fig. 15). In cases where the mutant amino acid residues are known, they are identical to those present in L^d and, except for position 155, D^b. This indicates that most, if not all, of the mutant K^b molecules contain amino acid sequences that could be derived from other class I genes. Gene conversion could readily account for the generation of the K^b mutant molecules—especially bm1, bm3, bm6, bm7, and bm9, which require more than single point mutations in close proximity—and, in addition, explain their similarity to other class I molecules at the mutation sites.

Obviously, gene conversion of the K^b gene by the D^b gene, the only other b haplotype gene whose sequence is known, could not account for the bm1 and bm10 mutants. However, such events could conceivably involve any of a number of other class I genes that exist in the genome. In this regard, it is interesting to note that, while a Met residue or codon has never been observed at amino acid position 165 in K- or D-region gene products or genes, as is present in the bm10 mutant, a Met codon at this position has been observed in a Tla region gene (Steinmetz *et al.*, 1981b).

A detailed comparison of the HLA-A2, -A28, and -B7 amino acid sequences (Fig. 13) offers further circumstantial evidence of gene conversion in the class I gene family (Lopez de Castro *et al.*, 1982). Only one (position 66) out of 235 positions available for comparison between the three molecules is different in all three antigens. In five out of the ten differences between HLA-A28 and HLA-A2 the corresponding residue in HLA-B7 is identical to HLA-A28 (positions 9, 70, 72, 74, and 107); in four of the remaining five positions HLA-B7 and HLA-A2 are identical. Even more striking is the fact that four out of five amino acid residues spanning positions 70–74 in HLA-A28 are identical to the corresponding segment of HLA-B7, but are different from that of HLA-A2 in four of these positions. Similar examples of restricted variability that could be explained by gene conversion are evident in the H-2 molecules. For example, H-2K^b and -D^b share all residues spanning positions 41–45 (Table III), where K^b and K^d differ in three of those five positions.

Thus, gene conversion appears to be a viable mechanism for explaining the patterns of variability noted in class I molecules. With such a mechanism, point mutations accumulated in one or several genes of a multigene family could be transferred to other genes of the family. Multiple but not identical gene conversion events among members of the family would result in the shuffling of the pool of sequences such that each member could achieve a unique sequence, yet the overall variability of the family would be restricted. Such a mechanism would not only explain the restricted pattern of variability observed in class I molecules, but could also explain the apparent lack or near lack of sequences common to alleles.

XI. GENE NUMBER AND EXPRESSION

Using the technique of Southern blotting, it is possible to estimate the number of genes present in an individual that have homology with a chosen gene probe (Southern, 1975). Analysis of various mouse strains by this technique (Cami *et al.*, 1981; Steinmetz *et al.*, 1981a; Margulies *et al.*, 1982) indicated that approximately 15 genes show homology to class I gene probes. Owing to limitations of the technique, the gene numbers estimated from Southern blots represent minimal estimates. As mentioned previously, Steinmetz *et al.* (1982), employing cosmid gene libraries, have shown that the actual number of class I genes is closer to 36.

It is not easy to reconcile the existence of 36 class I genes with the lower number of class I products that have been observed by serological and protein studies.

There are several explanations for the discrepancy, the first of which concerns the existence of pseudogenes; such genes are not transcribed under normal conditions because they contain defects such as the presence of inappropriate nonsense or stop codons within the normal coding sequence. Other defects such as an error in the splice signals can also prevent a gene that is transcribed from being translated and expressed. Steinmetz *et al.* (1981b) have shown that at least one H-2^d class I gene (27.1) is apparently a pseudogene. In addition, the HLA genomic clone pHLA 12.4 of Malissen *et al.* (1982) may also be a pseudogene, as suggested by the absence of a key Cys residue, which is involved in the formation of the first disulfide bridge, and by the inability of this gene to transfect L cells. The fact that such a high percentage (2 of 4) of the class I genomic clones whose sequences have thus far been determined are pseudogenes suggests that a significant number of those genes yet to be analyzed may also be pseudogenes. (It should be emphasized that even pseudogenes can act as reservoirs for genetic exchange.)

An additional explanation for the large number of genes is the possibility that certain class I products have gone undetected. For class I genes that are known to be expressed, their level of expression and often their tissue specificity are genetically regulated. H-2L and HLA-C (K. A. Williams *et al.*, 1980) molecules are expressed at lower levels than K and D or A and B antigens, respectively, while Tla molecules encoded by the *Tla* region are normally only expressed on certain tissues (Flaherty, 1981). It therefore seems likely that additional, as yet undetected, class I differentiation antigens will account for some of the 36 detected class I genes.

In the class of Tl antigens, viral infection can affect the regulation of expression such that tumor cells of mouse strains that do not normally express given Tl specificities now express them (see Flaherty, 1981). The numerous observations of the loss of native H-2 antigens and/or of the expression of "alien" H-2 specificities (see review Festenstein and Schmidt, 1981) on tumor cells may also indicate that the expression or at least the level of expression of other class I genes is under regulatory control, as originally proposed by Bodmer (1973). Comparison of several tumor cell lines with untransformed cells of the same genotype reveals a high frequency of anomalous H-2 expression, as judged by the reactivity of the tumor cells with anti-H-2 sera non-cross-reactive with the parent cells. Furthermore, if these sera are absorbed with certain untransformed allogenic cells, the reactivity against tumor is lost. These serological differences between normal and tumor cells are taken to reflect the expression of "alien" transplantation antigens, i.e., class I molecules that are normally expressed in other haplotypes. In several instances these observations have trivial explanations, such as the presence of viral antibodies in mouse alloantisera (P. Klein, 1980) or the fact that the strain of origin of the tumor cells was inappropriately assigned. In more bona fide cases of the expression of abnormal H-2 specificities, it would seem most likely that viral infection has altered the gene of a given class I gene cluster that is expressed and/or the level of expression of such a gene. It is likely that these newly expressed molecules, while cross-reactive with "alien" class I molecules, are not identical to them.

A final explanation for the discrepancy between the observed numbers of genes and their gene products may be due to the fact that not all expressed class I molecules are membrane-bound but that some, in fact, may be secreted. These latter molecules may have to date gone largely undetected. Kvist *et al.* (1980) and Ramanathan *et al.* (1982) have reported the existence of 40,000-dalton class I heavy chains in mouse sera that, by the lack of particular allotypic determinants, appeared to be distinguishable from membrane-bound H-2 molecules. A study by Cosman *et al.* (1982a) provides additional support for the concept that some class I genes code for secreted molecules. These investigators, working with cDNA clones from adult mouse liver (*q* haplotype), observed that one cDNA clone, which contained a coding sequence 88% homologous for positions 198–279 of the H-2K^b amino acid sequence, did not contain a coding sequence for the membrane-binding, hydrophobic region. Instead, there were insertions of hydrophilic residues in this clone. The total transcript was 301 amino acids long and thus could represent a shortened, secreted form of a class I molecule. More recently, these investigators (Cosman *et al.*, 1982b) have shown that the expression of this class of *H-2*-related mRNA is tissue-restricted, it is detectable in liver but not in brain, kidneys, testis, or thymus. The existence and function of secreted class I molecules obviously warrant further investigation.

XII. FUNCTION OF CLASS I MOLECULES

As has been discussed, the class I loci are exceedingly polymorphic. The most likely reason for this extraordinary polymorphism is that it is in some way beneficial to the survival of the species.

Zinkernagel and Doherty (see review, 1979) were the first to provide data concerning the natural function of class I molecules. They found that the lysis of virally infected cells by CTL involved a recognition not only of viral antigens on the infected cell surface but also of *H-2K* and *-D* gene products and that these H-2 molecules had to be identical to those of CTL. Thus, CTL "learn" to recognize viral antigens in the context of the H-2K, -D, and -L antigens of the sensitizing (antigen-presenting) cell, a phenomenon referred to as H-2 "restriction." Furthermore, the specificity of such restricted cells is quite exquisite in that virus-immune T cells can distinguish between parent and mutant H-2 alleles (see review, McKenzie *et al.*, 1977) that differ by only one or two amino acid residues (see Section IX.B). The fact that H-2K and -D glycoproteins are expressed on all cells (Klein, 1975) possibly reflects the evolutionary development of a mechanism of viral immunity.

While the ability of CTL to discriminate between self and other H-2 molecules is probably based on structural differences among these molecules, the molecular events involved in the recognition and destruction of virally infected cells remain to be elucidated. Fundamentally, it is not known whether the recognition event occurs via two receptors (one for the viral antigen and another for the H-2 molecule) (the dual recognition model) or via a single receptor that recognizes a complex of the viral antigen and the H-2 molecules (the altered-self model). (In the case of the dual recognition model, it is possible that both receptors are distinctly located on the same molecule.)

While the definitive resolution of this question awaits isolation and characterization of the elusive CTL receptor(s), multiple studies have been directed toward defining the relationship between the H-2 and viral antigens on the target cell. If the single-receptor (altered-self) model is correct, as advocated by a number of investigators (Doherty and Bennink, 1981; Benacerraf, 1981), the H-2 and viral antigens are presumed to exist in close proximity on the surface of the target cells.

Direct physical evidence indicating the association of class I molecules and viral antigens has been obtained using a variety of techniques, including direct binding of H-2 or HLA to viral protein (Helenius $et\ al.$, 1978), co-precipitation of viral and transplantation antigens as high-molecular-weight complexes from detergent extracts of virally infected cells (Kvist $et\ al.$, 1978), and co-capping of H-2 and viral antigens (Schrader and Edelman, 1976; Senik $et\ al.$, 1979; Zarling $et\ al.$, 1980). In addition to a physical relationship, other studies (Bubbers $et\ al.$, 1978; Geiger $et\ al.$, 1979), have demonstrated a functional correlation in the association of viral and H-2 antigens. In the case of Friend virus (FV), Bubbers $et\ al.$ (1978) noted that purification of this virus from the sera of infected animals resulted in co-purification of H-2 activity. This purification was not random in that H-2K^k and H-2D^b were co-purified while H-2D^k and H-2K^b were not. This correlated with their CTL data, since H-2^b and H-2^k anti-FV killer cells recognize FV with H-2D^b or H-2K^k but not with H-2K^b or H-2D^k.

That a physical association exists between viral antigens and H-2 molecules is further suggested by studies which reveal that a hierarchy exists between H-2 antigens and their ability to be recognized in the context of particular viral proteins. For example, the ability of CTL to respond to the SV40 tumor-associated specific antigen (TASA) in association with H-2 molecules is ranked as follows: K^b, D^b > K^k, K^f, D^f, D^q > K^s, D^s > D^d; no response to SV40 TASA is found in association with the H-2K^d, -D^k, and -K^q alleles (Pfizenmaier $et\ al.$, 1980). A hierarchy in CTL responsiveness has also been described for other viruses (Doherty $et\ al.$, 1978; Zinkernagel $et\ al.$, 1978) and for 2, 4, 6-trinitrophenyl-modified cells (Shearer and Schmitt-Verhulst, 1977). These data suggest that the various allelic K- and D-region-encoded molecules have different affinities for SV40 TASA. Alternatively, preferential recognition might reflect different affinities of the T-cell receptors for the various K or D antigenic determinants complexed with SV40 TASA and therefore may be a reflection of the T-cell repertoire.

No matter if these hierarchical associations in CTL responsiveness to *H-2K* and *-D* gene products are due either to differences in affinity of the H-2 gene products for various foreign antigens or to differences in affinity of receptors in the T-cell repertoire, the implication is that the structures of the class I molecules are very important for CTL-generated immunity. In this regard, the ability of certain class I molecules to associate with specific viral membrane proteins may be the driving force in generating genetic polymorphism of class I molecules, i.e., the more class I molecules available, the more likely that one will associate with a given viral protein.

It must be kept in mind that trivial explanations for the observed hierarchy of CTL responsiveness are possible. For example, such a hierarchy could be related to differences in concentration of H-2K and -D molecules on the cell surface or to differences in their rate of synthetic turnover. Table X compares the relative order for magnitude of expression and synthetic turnover of H-2K and -D antigens with the hierarchy of CTL responsiveness to TASA in association with these molecules. Although there is some correlation, especially in the cases of D^k and K^k, there is no strict relationship between CTL responsiveness and either of the other properties. Furthermore, if such a relationship did exist, the hierarchy of CTL responsiveness would be the same for all foreign antigens and this is not true. For example, the D^k molecule acts as a potent restriction antigen in response to alpha viruses (Müllbacher and Blanden, 1978) and H-2K^b is a weak restriction antigen for CTL responses against influenza (Doherty *et al.*, 1978). These are in contrast to the SV40 TASA results.

While the results indicating an association between foreign membrane molecules and class I antigens support the feasibility of the altered-self or single-

Table X. Comparison of the Relative Turnover Rate and Relative Cell-Surface Concentration of H-2K and -D Molecules with the Relative Ability of These Molecules to Be Recognized by CTL in Association with SV40 TASA

Turnover rate[a]	$K^k > K^s = D^s = D^d > K^b = D^b \gg D^k \gg K^d$
Magnitude of expression[b]	$D^b > K^k = K^d = K^b = D^q > D^d > K^q > D^k$
Hierarchy of CTL recognition with SV40 TASA[c]	$K^b = D^b > K^k = K^f = D^f = D^q > K^s = D^s > D^d \ggg K^d, D^k, K^q$

[a] Determined by measuring the rate of shedding of H-2K and -D molecules after ^{125}I labeling with lactoperoxidase. In general, except for D^d, the same results were obtained regardless of genetic background. Turnover of D^d appeared to be controlled by gene mapping to the left of I-A (data of Emerson *et al.*, 1980).

[b] Cell-surface concentration was measured by radioimmunoassay in a number of mouse strains (O'Neill and McKenzie, 1980). Antigen expression was allele-specific and independent of the expression of other K, D, or I antigens. Magnitude of expression in F_1 hybrids was slightly lower but relatively similar (O'Neill, 1980).

[c] Data of Pfizenmaier *et al.* (1980).

receptor model, other studies do not. Numerous investigations, using a variety of techniques, have failed to detect measurable associations between H-2 and viral antigens on the cell surface (Fox and Weissman, 1979; Calafat *et al.*, 1981; Zarling *et al.*, 1982; Cartwright *et al.*, 1982). However, these negative results must be regarded with caution since it is not known how many of these postulated antigenic complexes are required on an antigen-presenting cell in order for T-cell recognition to occur.

One possible explanation for the different results is that some H-2-restricted viral antigens may associate with H-2K/D proteins, whereas others simply may not. Thus, some viruses, such as vaccinia, vesicular stomatitis, and adenovirus (Geiger *et al.*, 1979; Senik *et al.*, 1979; Kvist *et al.*, 1978), may produce viral proteins that bind H-2 molecules, whereas other viruses, such as certain tumor viruses and Sendai viruses, might not (Fox and Weissman, 1979; Zarling *et al.*, 1982; Calafat *et al.*, 1981). Since in the latter cases dual recognition by the CTL would be required, and since it seems unlikely that CTL possess different recognition systems for different viruses, such an explanation supports the concepts that CTL lysis occurs via dual recognition, even in cases where the viral and H-2 antigens are in close contact.

In conclusion, while the ultimate resolution of the debate as to the nature of the molecular moieties recognized by CTL awaits the isolation and definition of the binding properties of T-cell receptors, it is clear that the variability in primary structure of class I molecules plays a key role in the CTL recognition process and that such variability affects host resistance to invading organisms.

XIII. SUMMARY AND PERSPECTIVES

Within the past five years, extensive primary structural information has been accumulated on H-2 and HLA class I antigens by both protein and DNA sequence determination. This information indicates that the extracellular portions of these molecules are likely to be spatially arranged very similarly to the domains of immunoglobulins. The availability of tens-of-milligrams quantities of HLA, SLA, and possibly H-2 should allow confirmation of this model by spectroscopic and X-ray crystallographic studies. The accumulated amino acid sequences have also shown that the extracellular structural polymorphism is nonrandomly distributed, mainly occurring in discrete regions within the N-terminal 140 residues. The regions between residues 61 and 83 and between residues 105 and 116 appear to be particularly involved in the alloantigenic determinants. Further structural comparisons of antigenically related but dissimilar molecules will permit further delineation of allodeterminants. In addition, the examination of peptide fragments of class I molecules for reactivity with monoclonal antibodies may be helpful for localizing allodeterminants.

Structural studies on H-2 mutant molecules indicate that T cells are capable of recognizing apparently subtle changes (one or two amino acid substitutions) in class I structure. The mutant sites are in general located in polymorphic portions of the molecule. Continued studies on the structure of H-2 mutant molecules, as well as HLA variants, should further define the nature of the determinants recognized by T cells, although it must be kept in mind that each class I molecule may have 20 or more such recognition sites. A promising means for defining the portions of class I molecules involved in T-cell recognition as well as the nature of the determinants recognized involves the fact that isolated class I genes capable of being recognized by T cells can be reexpressed in fibroblasts. The effect of defined alterations in these genes on T-cell recognition can thus be examined. This approach should be important not only in defining recognition sites but also in determining how amino acid interchanges affect the associative recognition of class I molecules and foreign cell-surface molecules.

Through the use of recombinant DNA technology, we have not only rapidly accumulated a large amount of sequence information but also gained knowledge of the number and organization of class I genes. In BALB/c mice, 36 distinct class I genes have been identified. It remains to be seen whether other strains of mice have similar numbers of class I genes; this information will help determine whether or not class I genes are in a dynamic state of expansion and contraction. Furthermore, it will be interesting to see whether all of these genes are within the boundaries of the MHC or are even on the murine 17th chromosome (6th chromosome for humans).

Another intriguing question is what fraction of the genes are expressed, or capable of being expressed, and which are pseudogenes. Interesting in this regard is the fact that, of the two H-2 and two HLA genes whose sequences have been thus far determined, one of each is apparently a pseudogene. Continued DNA sequence and gene transfection studies should provide the answer to this question. The existence of multiple, closely related class I genes also raises the possibility that there may be examples, in addition to Qa and Tla, of tissue-specific expression of individual class I genes. In addition, some data indicate that not all class I molecules are membrane-bound.

Finally, an important but unanswered question is what regulates the expression of class I genes. Certainly, the regulation of expression of different members of the family is controlled by tissue-specific factors, e.g., H-2 versus Qa and Tla. Furthermore, it is known that, while class I and antibody gene families appear to be members of a supergene family as reflected by their homology and similar molecular organization, these gene families use at least some distinct regulatory mechanisms. DNA rearrangements and somatic mutation occur in the antibody, but probably not in the class I gene family. However, both gene families appear to use gene conversion as a mechanism for maintaining sequence homogeneity in family members. It will be interesting to determine whether there are still other types of regulatory mechanisms shared by those related gene families.

ACKNOWLEDGMENTS

We would like to thank our colleagues—Bruce Ewenstein, Tom Kindt, W. Lee Maloy, John Martinko, Rod Nairn, Stan Nathenson, and Hiroshi Uehara—for their dedicated participation in the H-2 protein sequence studies reported here. We are also appreciative for helpful discussions of the manuscript with Jim Braatz, Tom Kindt, Eric Lillehoj, W. Lee Maloy, Mary Ann Robinson, and Marie Rose van Schravendijk. It is a particular pleasure to acknowledge the secretarial and editorial assistance of Carol Godlove in the preparation of the chapter.

XIV. REFERENCES

Allison, J. P., Ferrone, S., Walker, L. E., Pellegrino, M. A., Silver, J., and Reisfeld, R. A., 1978, *Transplantation* **26**:451.

Amsden, A., Ewan, V., Yoshida, T., and Cohen, S., 1978, *J. Immunol.* **120**:542.

Arce-Gomez, B., Jones, E. A., Barnstable, C. T., Solomon, E., and Bodmer, W. F., 1978, *Tissue Antigens* **11**:96.

Ballou, B., McKean, D. J., Freedlender, E. F., and Smithies, O., 1976, *Proc. Natl. Acad. Sci. U.S.A.* **73**:4487.

Baltimore, D., 1981, *Cell* **24**:592.

Benacerraf, B., 1981, *Science* **212**:229.

Berggärd, I., and Bearn, A. G., 1968, *J. Biol. Chem.* **243**:4095.

Biddison, W. E., Ward, F. E., Shearer, G. M., and Shaw, S., 1980, *J. Immunol.* **124**:548.

Biddison, W. E., Shearer, G. M., and Shaw, S., 1981, *J. Immunol.* **127**:2231.

Biddison, W. E., Kostyu, D. D., Strominger, J. L., and Krangel, M. S., 1982, *J. Immunol.* **129**:730.

Black, P. L., Vitetta, E. S., Forman, J., Kang, C.-Y., May, R. D., and Uhr, J. W., 1981, *Eur. J. Immunol.* **11**:48.

Blankenhorn, E. P., Cecka, J. M., Goetze, D., and Hood, L., 1978, *Nature (London)* **274**:90.

Blobel, G., and Dobberstein, B., 1975, *J. Cell Biol.* **67**:852.

Bodmer, W. F., 1973, *Transplant. Proc.* **5**:1471.

Bodmer, W. F., 1978, *Harvey Lect.* **72**:91.

Braciale, T. J., 1977, *J. Exp. Med.* **146**:673.

Breathnach, R., and Chambon, P., 1981, *Annu. Rev. Biochem.* **50**:349.

Bridgen, J., Snary, D., Crumpton, M. J., Barnstable, C., Goodfellow, P., and Bodmer, W. F., 1976, *Nature (London)* **261**:200.

Brown, J. L., Kato, K., Silver, J., and Nathenson, S. G., 1974, *Biochemistry* **13**:3174.

Bubbers, J. E., Chen, S., and Lilly, F., 1978, *J. Exp. Med.* **147**:340.

Calafat, J., Démant, P., and Janssen, H., 1981, *Immunogenetics* **14**:203.

Cami, B., Brégégere, F., Abastado, J. P., and Kourilsky, P., 1981, *Nature (London)* **291**:673.

Cartwright, G. S., Smith, L. M., Heinzelmann, E. W., Ruebush, M. J., Parce, J. W., and McConnell, H. M., 1982, *Proc. Natl. Acad. Sci. U.S.A.* **79**:1506.

Cigén, R., Ziffer, J. A., Berggärd, B., Cunningham, B. A., and Berggärd, I., 1978, *Biochemistry* **17**:947.

Clarke, S. H., Claflin, J. L., and Rudikoff, S., 1982, *Proc. Natl. Acad. Sci. U.S.A.* **79**:3280.

Cohen, F. E., Novotný, J., Sternberg, M. J. E., Campbell, D. G., and Williams, A. F., 1981, *Biochem. J.* **195**:31.

Coligan, J. E., and Kindt, T. J., 1981, *J. Immunol. Methods* **37**:287.

Coligan, J. E., Kindt, T. J., Nairn, R., Nathenson, S. G., Sachs, D. H., and Hansen, T. H., 1980, *Proc. Natl. Acad. Sci. U.S.A.* **77**:1134.

Coligan, J. E., Kindt, T. J., Uehara, H., Martinko, J., and Nathenson, S. G., 1981, *Nature (London)* **291**:35.

Coligan, J. E., Gates, F. T., III, Kimball, E. S., and Maloy, W. L., 1983, *Methods Enzymol.* **91**:413.

Cook, R. G., Vitetta, E. S., Uhr, J. W., Klein, J., Wilde, C. E., III, and Capra, J. D., 1978, *J. Immunol.* **121**:1015.

Cosman, D., Khoury, G., and Jay, G., 1982a, *Nature (London)* **295**:73.

Cosman, D., Kress, M., Khoury, G., and Jay, G., 1982b, *Proc. Natl. Acad. Sci. U.S.A.* **79**:4947.

Cunningham, B. A., Wang, J. L., Berggärd, I., and Peterson, P. A., 1973, *Biochemistry* **12**:4811.

Cunningham, B. A., Henning, R., Milner, R. J., Reske, K., Ziffer, J. A., and Edelman, G. M., 1977, *Cold Spring Harbor Symp. Quant. Biol.* **41**:351.

Dawson, J. R., Silver, J., Shepard, L. B., and Amos, D. B., 1974, *J. Immunol.* **112**:1190.

Decker, J., 1980, *Mol. Immunol.* **17**:803.

Dobberstein, B., Garoff, H., Warren, G., and Robinson, P. J., 1979, *Cell* **17**:759.

Doherty, P. C., and Bennink, J. R., 1981, *Fed. Proc.* **40**:218.

Doherty, P. C., Biddison, W. E., Bennink, J. R., and Knowles, B. B., 1978, *J. Exp. Med.* **148**:534.

Duncan, W. R., Wakeland, E. K., and Klein, J., 1979, *Immunogenetics* **9**:261.

Egel, R., 1981, *Nature (London)* **290**:191.

Emerson, S. G., Murphy, D. B., and Cone, R. E., 1980, *J. Exp. Med.* **152**:783.

Evans, G. A., Margulies, D. H., Camerini-Otero, D., Ozato, K., and Seidman, J. G., 1982, *Proc. Natl. Acad. Sci. U.S.A.* **79**:1994.

Ewald, S. J., Klein, J., and Hood, L. E., 1979, *Immunogenetics* **8**:551.

Ewenstein, B. M., Freed, J. H., Mole, L. E., and Nathenson, S. G., 1976, *Proc. Natl. Acad. Sci. U.S.A.* **73**:915.

Festenstein, H., and Schmidt, W., 1981, *Immunol. Rev.* **60**:85.

Flaherty, L., 1981, in *The Role of the Major Histocompatibility Complex in Immunology* (M. Dorf, ed.), pp. 33–55, Garland STPM Press, New York.

Forman, J., and Klein, J., 1977, *Immunogenetics* **4**:183.

Fox, R. I., and Weissman, I. L., 1979, *J. Immunol.* **122**:1697.

Freed, J. H., Sears, D. W., Brown, J. L., and Nathenson, S. G., 1979, *Mol. Immunol.* **16**:9.

Gates, F. T., III, Coligan, J. E., and Kindt, T. J., 1979, *Biochemistry* **18**:2267.

Gates, F. T., III, Coligan, J. E., and Kindt, T. J., 1981, *Proc. Natl. Acad. Sci. U.S.A.* **78**:554.

Geiger, G., Rosenthal, K. L., Klein, J., Zinkernagel, R. M., and Singer, S. J., 1979, *Proc. Natl. Acad. Sci. U.S.A.* **76**:4603.

Goding, J. W., 1981, *J. Immunol.* **126**:1644.

Goodenow, R. S., McMillan, M., Örn, A., Nicolson, M., Davidson, N., Frelinger, J. A., and Hood, L., 1982, *Science* **215**:677.

Gorer, P. A., 1936, *Br. J. Exp. Pathol.* **17**:42.

Götze, D. (ed.), 1977, *The Major Histocompatibility System in Man and Animals*, Springer-Verlag, Berlin, Heidelberg, New York.

Groves, M. L., and Greenberg, R., 1982, *J. Biol. Chem.* **257**:2619.

Guidotti, G., 1977, *J. Supramol. Struct.* **7**:489.

Hansen, T. H., Cullen, S. E., and Sachs, D. H., 1977, *J. Exp. Med.* **145**:438.

Hansen, T. H., Ozato, K., and Sachs, D. H., 1980, *Ann. Immunol. (Paris)* **131c**:327.

Hansen, T. H., Ozato, K., Melino, M. R., Coligan, J. E., Kindt, T. J., Jandinski, J. J., and Sachs, D. H., 1981, *J. Immunol.* **126**:1713.

Helenius, A. Morein, B., Fries, E., Simons, K., Robinson, P., Schirrmacher, V., Terhorst, C., and Strominger, J., 1978, *Proc. Natl. Acad. Sci. U.S.A.* **75**:3846.

Henriksen, O., Robinson, E. A., and Appella, E., 1979, *J. Biol. Chem.* **254**:7651.

Hilgert, I., Kandutsch, A. A., Cherry, M., and Snell, G. D. 1969, *Transplantation* **8**:451.

Hubbard, S. C., and Ivatt, R. J., 1981, *Annu. Rev. Biochem.* **50**:555.

Huser, H., Zeigler, A., Knecht, R., and Pink, J. R. L., 1978, *Immunogenetics* **6**:301.

Hyman, R., and Stallings, V., 1977, *Immunogenetics* **4**:171.

Iványi, D., and Démant, P., 1979, *Immunogenetics* **8**:539.

Iványi, D., and Démant, P., 1981, *Immunogenetics* **12**:397.

Jackson, D. C., Ada, G. L., Hapel, A. J., and Dunlop, M. B. C., 1976, *Scand. J. Immunol.* **5**:1021.

Jones, P. P., Murphy, D. B., Hewgill, D., and McDevitt, H. O., 1978, *Immunochemistry* **16**:51.

Joysen, V. C., and Wolf, E., 1978, *Br. Med. Bull.* **34**:217.

Kimball, E. S., and Coligan, J. E., 1983, *Mol. Immunol.* **20**:11.

Kimball, E. S., Coligan, J. E., and Kindt, T. J., 1979, *Immunogenetics* **8**:201.

Kimball, E. S., Maloy, W. L., and Coligan, J. E., 1981a, *Mol. Immunol.* **18**:677.

Kimball, E. S., Nathenson, S. G., and Coligan, J. E., 1981b, *Biochemistry* **20**:3301.

Klein, J., 1975, *Biology of the Mouse Histocompatibility-2 Complex*, Springer-Verlag, New York.

Klein, J., 1978, *Adv. Immunol.* **26**:44.

Klein, J., 1979, *Science* **203**:516.

Klein, J., 1981, *Immunology Today* **10**:Centerfold.

Klein, J., Juretic, A., Baxevanis, C. N., and Nagy, Z. A., 1981, *Nature (London)* **291**:455.

Klein, P., 1980, *Transplant. Proc.* **12**:16.

Krakauer, T., Hansen, T. H., Camerini-Otero, R. D., and Sachs, D. H., 1980, *J. Immunol.* **124**:2149.

Krangel, M. S., Orr, H. T., and Strominger, J. L., 1979, *Cell* **18**:979.

Krangel, M. S., Orr, H. T., and Strominger, J. L., 1980, *Scand. J. Immunol.* **11**:561.

Kratzin, H., Yang, C.-Y., Götz, H., Pauly, E., Kölbel, S., Egert, G., Thinnes, F. P., Wernet, P., Altevogt, P., and Hilschmann, N., 1981, *Hoppe-Seyler's Z. Physiol. Chem.* **362**:1665.

Kvist, S., Östberg, L. Persson, H., Philipson, L., and Peterson, P., 1978, *Proc. Natl. Acad. Sci. U.S.A.* **75**:5674.

Kvist, S., Klein, J., and Peterson, P. A., 1980, *Immunogenetics* **10**:499.

Kvist, S., Bregegere, F., Rask, L., Cami, B., Garoff, H., Daniel, F., Wiman, K., Larhammar, D., Abastado, J. P., Gachelin, G., Peterson, P. A., Dobberstein, B., and Kourilsky, P., 1981, *Proc. Natl. Acad. Sci. U.S.A.* **78**:2772.

Lalanne, J. L., Brégégere, F., Delarbre, C., Abastado, J. P., Gachelin, G., and Kourilsky, P., 1982, *Nucleic Acids Res.* **10**:1039.

Lancet, D., Parham, P., and Strominger, J. L., 1979, *Proc. Natl. Acad. Sci. U.S.A.* **76**:3844.

Larhammar, D., Wiman, K., Schenning, L., Claesson, L., Gustafsson, K., Peterson, P. A., and Rask, L., 1981, *Scand. J. Immunol.* **14**:617.

Lemonnier, F., Neauport-Sautes, C., Kourilsky, F. M., and Démant, P., 1975, *Immunogenetics* **2**:517.

Levy, R. B., and Hansen, T. H., 1980, *Immunogenetics* **10**:7.

Lopez de Castro, J. A., Orr, H. T., Robb, R. J., Kostyk, T. G., Mann, D. L., and Strominger, J. L., 1979, *Biochemistry* **18**:5704.

Lopez de Castro, J. A., Strominger, J. L., Strong, D. M., and Orr, H. T., 1982, *Proc. Natl. Acad. Sci. U.S.A.* **79**:3813.

Lunney, J., and Sachs, D., 1978, *J. Immunol.* **120**:607.

McCune, J. N., Humphreys, R. E., Yocum, R. R., and Strominger, J. L., 1975, *Proc. Natl. Acad. Sci. U.S.A.* **72**:3206.

McKenzie, I. F. C., Pang, T., and Blanden, R. V., 1977, *Immunol. Rev.* **35**:181.

Maizels, R. M., Frelinger, J. A., and Hood, L., 1978, *Immunogenetics* **7**:425.

Malissen, M., Malissen, B., and Jordan, B. R., 1982, *Proc. Natl. Acad. Sci. U.S.A.* **79**:898.

Maloy, W. L., and Coligan, J. E., 1982, *Immunogenetics* **16**:11.

Maloy, W. L., Hämmerling, G., Nathenson, S. G., and Coligan, J. E., 1980, *J. Immunol. Methods* **37**:287.

Maloy, W. L., Nathenson, S. G., and Coligan, J. E., 1981, *J. Biol. Chem.* **256**:2863.

Margulies, D. H., Evans, G. A., Flaherty, L., and Seidman, J. G., 1982, *Nature (London)* **295**:168.

Martinko, J. M., Uehara, H., Ewenstein, B. M., Kindt, T. J., Coligan, J. E., and Natheson, S. G., 1981, *Biochemistry* **19**:688.

Metzger, J.-J., Lunney, J. K., Sachs, D. H., and Rudikoff, S., 1982, *J. Immunol.* **129**:716.

Michaelson, J., 1981, *Immunogenetics* **13**:167.

Michaelson, J., Rothenberg, E., and Boyse, E. A., 1980, *Immunogenetics* **11**:93.

Misko, I. S., Moss, D. J., and Pope, J. H., 1980, *Proc. Natl. Acad. Sci. U.S.A.* **77**:4247.

Mole, J. E., Hunter, F., Paslay, J. W., Bhown, A. S., and Bennett, J. C., 1982, *Mol. Immunol.* **19**:1.

Moore, K. W., Sher, B. T., Sam, Y. H., Eakle, K. A., and Hood, L., 1982, *Science* **215**:679.

Moosic, J. P., Nilson, A., Hämmerling, G. J., and McKean, D. J., 1980, *J. Immunol.* **125**:1463.

Muchmore, A., Decker, J., and Blaese, R., 1980, *J. Immunol.* **125**:1306.

Müllbacher, A., and Blanden, R. V., 1978, *Immunogenet.* **7**:551.

Nairn, R., Nathenson, S. G., and Coligan, J. E., 1980a, *Eur. J. Immunol.* **10**:495.

Nairn, R., Yamaga, K., and Nathenson, S. G., 1980b, *Annu. Rev. Genet.* **14**:241.

Nairn, R., Nathenson, S. G., and Coligan, J. E., 1981, *Biochemistry* **20**:4739.

Nakamuro, K., Tanigaki, N., and Pressman, D., 1973, *Proc. Natl. Acad. Sci. U.S.A.* **70**:2863.

Nathenson, S. G., and Cullen, S. E., 1974, *Biochim. Biophys. Acta* **344**:1.

Nathenson, S. G., and Davies, D. A. L., 1966, *Proc. Natl. Acad. Sci. U.S.A.* **56**:467.

Nathenson, S. G., Uehara, H., Ewenstein, B. M., Kindt, T. J., and Coligan, J. E., 1981, *Annu. Rev. Biochem.* **50**:1025.

O'Neill, H. C., 1980, *Immunogenetics* **11**:241.

O'Neill, H. C., and McKenzie, I. F. C., 1980, *Immunogenetics* **11**:225.

O'Neill, H. C., and Parish, C. R., 1981, *Mol. Immunol.* **18**:713.

Orr, H. T., Lancet, D., Robb, R. J., Lopez de Castro, J. A., and Strominger, J. L., 1979a, *Nature (London)* **282**:266.

Orr, H. T., Lopez de Castro, J. A., Parham, P., Pleogh, H. L., and Strominger, J. L., 1979b, *Proc. Natl. Acad. Sci. U.S.A.* **76**:4395.

Parham, P., 1979, *J. Biol. Chem.* **254**:8709.

Parham, P., and McLean, J., 1980, *Hum. Immunol.* **1**:131.

Parham, P., Alpert, B. N., Orr, H. T., and Strominger, J. L., 1977, *J. Biol. Chem.* **252**:7555.

Parnes, J. R., and Seidman, J., 1982, *Cell* **29**:661.

Parnes, J. R., Velan, B., Felsenfeld, A., Ramanathan, L., Ferrini, U., Appella, E., and Seidman, J. G., 1981, *Proc. Natl. Acad. Sci. U.S.A.* **78**:2253.

Peterson, P. A., Cunningham, B. A., Berggärd, I., and Edelman, G. M., 1972, *Proc. Natl. Acad. Sci. U.S.A.* **69**:1697.

Pfizenmaier, K., Pan, S.-H., and Knowles, B. B., 1980, *J. Immunol.* **124**:1888.

Ploegh, H. L., Cannon, L. E., and Strominger, J. L., 1979, *Proc. Natl. Acad. Sci. U.S.A.* **76**:2273.

Ploegh, H. L., Orr, H. T., and Strominger, J. L., 1980, *Proc. Natl. Acad. Sci. U.S.A.* **77**:6081.

Ploegh, H. L., Orr, H. T., and Strominger, J. L., 1981a, *J. Immunol.* **126**:270.

Ploegh, H. L., Orr, H. T., and Strominger, J. L., 1981b, *Cell* **24**:287.

Pober, J. S., Guild, B. C., and Strominger, J. L., 1978, *Proc. Natl. Acad. Sci. U.S.A.* **75**:6002.

Ramanathan, L., Rogers, M. J., Robinson, E. A., Hearing, V. T., Tanigaki, N., and Appella, E., 1982, *Mol. Immunol.* **19**:1075.

Reyes, A. A., Schold, M., Itakura, K., and Wallace, R. B., 1982a, *Proc. Natl. Acad. Sci. U.S.A.* **79**:3270.

Reyes, A. A., Schold, M., and Wallace, R. B., 1982b, *Immunogenetics* **16**:1.

Robb, R. J., Terhorst, C., and Strominger, J. L., 1978, *J. Biol. Chem.* **253**:5319.

Robinson, P. J., 1982, *Immunogenetics* **15**:333.

Robinson, P. J., Lundin, L., Sege, K., Graf, L., Wigzell, H., and Peterson, P. A., 1981, *Immunogenetics* **14**:449.

Rogers, M. J., Robinson, E. A., and Appella, E., 1979, *J. Biol. Chem.* **254**:11126.

Rose, S. M., Hansen, T. H., and Cullen, S. E., 1980, *J. Immunol.* **125**:2044.

Rothbard, J. B., Hopp, T. P., Edelman, G. M., and Cunningham, B. A., 1980, *Proc. Natl. Acad. Sci. U.S.A.* **77**:4239.

Sanderson, A. R., Cresswell, P., and Welsh, K. I., 1971, *Transplant. Proc.* **3**:220.

Schrader, J. W., and Edelman, G. M., 1976, *J. Exp. Med.* **143**:601.

Schreirer, P. H., Bothwell, A. L. M., Mueller-Hill, B., and Baltimore, D., 1981, *Proc. Natl. Acad. Sci. U.S.A.* **78**:4495.

Schwartz, B. D., and Nathenson, S. G., 1971, *J. Immunol.* **107**:1363.

Schwartz, B. D., McMillan, M., Shevach, E., Hahn, Y., Rose, S. M., and Hood, L., 1980, *J. Immunol.* **125**:1055.

Sears, D. W., and Polizzi, C. M., 1980, *Immunogenetics* **10**:67.

Senik, A., Démant, P., and Neauport-Sautes, C., 1979, *J. Immunol.* **12**:1461.

Sethi, K. K., Stroehmann, I., and Brandis, H., 1980, *Nature (London)* **286**:718.

Shearer, G. M., and Schmitt-Verhulst, A., 1977, *Adv. Immunol.* **25**:55.

Sherman, L., 1980, *J. Exp. Med.* **151**:1386.

Sherman, L., 1982, *Nature (London)* **297**:511.

Shimada, A., and Nathenson, S. G., 1969, *Biochemistry* **8**:4048.

Silver, J., Cecka, J. M., McMillan, M., and Hood, L., 1976, *Cold Spring Harbor Symp. Quant. Biol.* **41**:369.

Singer, D. S., Camerini-Otero, R. D., Satz, M. L., Osborne, B., Sachs, D., and Rudikoff, S., 1982, *Proc. Natl. Acad. Sci. U.S.A.* **79**:1403.

Slightom, J. L., Blechl, A. E., and Smithies, O., 1980, *Cell* **21**:627.

Snary, D., Goodfellow, P., Hayman, M. J., Bodmer, W. F., and Crumpton, M. J., 1974, *Nature (London)* **247**:457.

Soloski, M. J., Uhr, J. W., and Vitetta, E. S., 1982, *Nature (London)* **296**:759.

Sood, A., Pereira, D., and Weissman, S. M., 1981, *Proc. Natl. Acad. Sci. U.S.A.* **78**:616.

Southern, E. M., 1975, *J. Mol. Biol.* **8**:503.

Stallcup, K. C., Springer, T. A., and Mescher, M. F., 1981, *J. Immunol.* **127**:923.

Steinmetz, M., Frelinger, J. G., Fisher, D., Hunkapiller, T., Pereira, D., Weissman, S. M., Uehara, H., Nathenson, S. G., and Hood, L., 1981a, *Cell* **24**:125.

Steinmetz, M., Moore, K. W., Frelinger, J. G., Sher, B. T., Shen, F. W., Boyse, E. A., and Hood, L., 1981b, *Cell* **25**:683.

Steinmetz, M., Winoto, A., Minard, K., and Hood, L., 1982, *Cell* **28**:489.

Strominger, J. L., Orr, H. T., Parham, P., Ploegh, H. L., Mann, D. L., Bilotsky, H., Sarott, H. A., Wu, T. T., and Kabat, E. A., 1980, *Scand. J. Immunol.* **11**:573.

Strominger, J. L., Engelhard, V. H., Fuks, A., Guild, B. C., Hyafil, F., Kaufman, J. F., Korman, A. J., Kostyk, T. G., Krangel, M. S., Lancet, D., Lopez de Castro, J. A., Mann, D. L., Orr, M. T., Parham, P. R., Parker, K. C., Ploegh, H. L., Pober, J. S., Robb, R. J., and Shackelford, D. A., 1981, in *The Role of the Major Histocompatibility Complex in Immunology* (M. Dorf, ed.), pp. 115–172, Garland STPM Press, New York.

Suggs, S. V., Wallace, R. B., Hirose, T., Kawashima, E. H., and Itakura, K., 1981, *Proc. Natl. Acad. Sci.* **78**:6613.

Tekolf, W. A., Biddison, W. E., Aster, R. D., and Shaw, S. L., 1982, *J. Immunol.* **129**:1974.

Trägårdh, L., Wiman, K., Rask, L., and Peterson, P., 1979, *Biochemistry* **18**:1322.

Trägårdh, L., Rask, L., Wiman, K., Fohlman, J., and Peterson, P. A., 1980, *Proc. Natl. Acad. Sci. U.S.A.* **77**:1129.

Uehara, H., Coligan, J. E., and Nathenson, S. G., 1981a, *Biochemistry* **29**:5936.

Uehara, H., Coligan, J. E., and Nathenson, S. G., 1981b, *Biochemistry* **20**:5940.

Van Someren, H., Westerveld, A., Hagemaijer, A., Mees, J. R., Meera Khan, P., and Zaalberg, O. B., 1974, *Proc. Natl. Acad. Sci. U.S.A.* **71**:962.

Vitetta, E. S., and Capra, J. D., 1978, *Adv. Immunol.* **26**:147.

Vitetta, E. S., Uhr, J. W., Klein, J., Pazderka, F., Moticka, E. J., Ruth, R. F., and Capra, J. D., 1977, *Nature (London)* **270**:535.

von Heijne, G., 1981a, *Eur. J. Biochem.* **116**:419.

von Heijne, G., 1981b, *Eur. J. Biochem.* **120**:275.

von Heijne, G., and Blomberg, C., 1979, *Eur. J. Biochem.* **97**:175.

Walsh, F. S., and Crumpton, M. J., 1977, *Nature (London)* **269**:307.

Wilkinson, J. M., Tykocinski, M. L., Coligan, J. E., Kimball, E. S., and Kindt, T. J., 1982, *Mol. Immunol.* **19**:1441.

Williams, A. F., and Gagnon, J., 1982, *Science* **216**:696.

Williams, K. A., Hart, D. N.-J., Fabre, J. W., and Morris, P.-J., 1980, *Transplantation* **29**:274.

Wolfe, P. B., and Cebra, J. J., 1980, *Mol. Immunol.* **17**:1493.

Wu, T. T., and Kabat, E. A., 1970, *J. Exp. Med.* **132**:211.

Yokoyama, K., and Nathenson, S. G., 1983, *J. Immunol.* (in press).

Yokoyama, K., Stockert, E., Old, L. J., and Nathenson, S. G., 1981, *Proc. Natl. Acad. Sci. U.S.A.* **78**:7078.

Zarling, D. A., Keshet, I., Watson, A., and Bach, F., 1980, *Scand. J. Immunol.* **8**:497.

Zarling, D. A., Miskimen, J. A., Fan, D. P., Fujimoto, E. K., and Smith, P. K., 1982, *J. Immunol.* **128**:251.

Zinkernagel, R. M., and Doherty, P. C., 1979, *Adv. Immunol.* **27**:51.

Zinkernagel, R., and Klein, J., 1977, *Immunogenetics* **4**:581.

Zinkernagel, R. M., Althage, A., Cooper, S., Kreeb, G., Klein, P. A., Sefton, B., Flaherty, L., Stimpfling, J., Shreffler, D., and Klein, J., 1978, *J. Exp. Med.* **148**:592.

HLA-DR and Renal Transplantation

Peter J. Morris and Alan Ting

Nuffield Department of Surgery
University of Oxford
John Radcliffe Hospital
Oxford OX3 9DU, United Kingdom

I. INTRODUCTION

The serological detection of leukocyte antigens in man began some 20 years ago. Their subsequent recognition as histocompatibility antigens led to immediate interest in the possible application of leukocyte typing and matching to improve renal allograft survival. In the late 1960s it became apparent that these leukocyte antigens could be grouped into two series of allelic antigens. The two series of the major histocompatibility complex (MHC) in man (designated HLA-A and -B) were shown to be genetically controlled by two loci on chromosome 6.

The outcome of intrafamilial renal allografts is very much in accord with the genetic disparity for HLA between donor and recipient. There has been considerable controversy about the influence of matching for HLA-AB in cadaver transplantation, but there is now some degree of consensus, namely that grafts well matched for HLA-AB show about a 10–20% better graft survival at 1 year than poorly matched grafts (Morris *et al.*, 1978a).

In the early 1970s it was recognized that the reactivity of lymphocytes from two individuals in culture [mixed lymphocyte reaction (MLR)] was not determined by differences in HLA-AB between the cell donors but by differences at a separate locus within the HLA complex, subsequently named HLA-D (Yunis and Amos, 1971). This finding provided an explanation for the strong reactivity often seen in MLR between cells identical for HLA-AB. Furthermore, the MLR resulted in the generation of cytotoxic T lymphocytes, whose activity was directed at the lymphocytes that stimulated the responder population in the

65

first place. Thus it seemed that this was an *in vitro* model of the *in vivo* immune response to a tissue allograft, and also an explanation for the not infrequent rejection of HLA-AB-identical renal allografts in unrelated recipients.

Using homozygous typing cells in one-way MLR, a number of determinants of the HLA-D system were defined. Subsequently antisera were found that detected the same determinants or very closely linked antigens, and hence these were called HLA-DR (D-related) antigens (Bodmer *et al.*, 1978). The typing of donors and recipients of cadaver renal allografts for HLA-D using typing cells homozygous for HLA-D was not applied clinically, first because the result of the test could not be obtained prospectively (since the test takes 7 days to perform), and second because HLA-DR was defined soon after HLA-D. In general each HLA-D antigen could be detected serologically, and therefore the numerical designation of each DR antigen paralleled that of the D determinants. There is a good correlation between the designation of HLA-D and HLA-DR in the same individual for most antigens, HLA-Dw6/DRw6 and HLA-Dw4/DR4 being notable exceptions (Bodmer *et al.*, 1978). Convincing evidence for D and DR being separate but yet closely linked loci is still lacking.

Thus if the MLR is accepted as the *in vitro* model of the immune response to an allograft *in vivo* it can be seen why matching for HLA-D/DR rather than matching for HLA-AB is conceptually so attractive: It is directed at the induction phase of the immune response, whereas matching for HLA-AB is directed at the effector arm of the response to the graft. In the presence of immunosuppressive therapy the former might be expected to be more effective.

II. THE SEROLOGY OF HLA-DR

The D/DR determinants are expressed on B but not most T cells (activated T cells express DR antigens). Sera from parous women that reacted with B but not with T lymphocytes were first detected in 1975 by Winchester *et al*. Most of the early studies only indicated that B-cell-reactive antibodies could be found, but the specificity of the reactivity was not determined. However, van Rood *et al.* (1975) did show that the specificities detected in their experiments corresponded to the human MLR determinants, although only three determinants were detected with four antisera.

Within the next two years many sera were found that reacted exclusively with B lymphocytes. Most of these sera had to be absorbed with platelets to remove HLA-ABC antibodies. Using such sera, allelic systems of antigens were defined by multiple serum samples (van Rood *et al.*, 1975; Ting *et al.*, 1976). Some laboratories claimed to be able to distinguish two separate loci coding for the B-cell antigens (Mann *et al.*, 1976). However, it was not until the Seventh

International Collaborative Histocompatibility Workshop held in 1977 (Bodmer *et al.*, 1978) that the relationship of B-cell antigens was convincingly defined. By cluster analysis and other tests for similarity of serological reactions a number of well-defined antigens were recognized.

These antigens were designated DRw1, 2, 3, 4, 5, 6, and 7 and corresponded to the already defined MLR determinants Dw1–7. Furthermore, it was shown by family studies that these DR antigens were coded for by genes belonging to one locus within the HLA system. Study of recombinant families showed that the DR locus was situated next to the HLA-B locus but on the centromeric side of the B locus.

During the Eighth Histocompatibility Workshop (1980), the DR antigens were further characterized, and as a result the provisional designation (w) was removed from DR1, 2, 3, 4, 5, and 7 (Terasaki, 1980). At the present time 10 antigens are recognized and these 10 antigens account for about 95% of the genes of the DR locus (Table I). The DR system appears to be considerably less polymorphic than the HLA-A and -B systems. But there is now evidence that some of the DR antigens may be split into smaller components as has happened extensively with the A and B antigens. However, the splitting of the DR antigens may not be very extensive, as, in the three years between the seventh and eighth workshops, the definition of DR1, 2, 3, 4, 5, and 7 has remained essentially unchanged. There have been some isolated reports that DR4 (Colombe *et al.*, 1980) and DR5 (Curtoni *et al.*, 1980) may be split, but these data have not been confirmed by other laboratories. In 1977 the DRw6 antigen was recognized as being difficult to define, and this still applied at the eighth workshop. In this workshop there was some evidence that DRw6 could be split into three components

Table I. The Frequency of HLA-DR Antigens in a Caucasoid Oxford Population[a]

Antigen	Frequency	Gene frequency
DR1	15.9	0.08
DR2	34.1	0.18
DR3	20.6	0.11
DR4	29.4	0.16
DR5	8.7	0.04
DRw6	33.3	0.18
DR7	27.0	0.15
DRw8	3.2	0.02
DRw9	5.6	0.03
DRw10	NT	—
	TOTAL	0.95

[a] N = 126. NT, not tested.

(Duquesnoy *et al.*, 1980). But the sera used to define DRw6 also reacted with cells having DR1 and 2 or DR3, 5, and 8. At the present time then there are no monospecific DRw6 antisera available.

The existence of other B-cell antigen systems within HLA has been postulated. One such system is the MT system (Park *et al.*, 1980), which consists of three supertypic specificities, MT1, MT2, and MT3. Each supertypic specificity includes different DR antigens: MT1 includes the antigens DR1, 2, and 10 and part of DRw6; MT2 includes DR3, 5, and 8 and part of DRw6; MT3 includes DR4 and 7 and DRw9. Duquesnoy *et al.* (1979) have described another supertypic system comprising MB1, MB2, and MB3. MB1 was shown to be similar if not identical to MT1; MB2 includes DR4 and 5, DRw8, and DRw9; and MB3 and 7 (Table II). The question arises as to the relationship between the DR system and these supertypic systems. There appear to be two possibilities: First, they may represent separate allelic systems, or second, that the supertypic systems may reflect the complex nature of the DR determinants. This very problem has been seen with the HLA-B system and the supertypic antigens 4a and 4b (now referred to as DRw4 and w6). Tosi and his colleagues (Tosi *et al.*, 1978; Corte *et al.*, 1982) have shown that the supertypic antigen DC1 (which is equivalent to MT1 and MB1) and DRw6 reside on separate subsets of molecules on the Daudi cell line, indicating that separate loci control these antigens. More recently Shaw and his colleagues (1980) have produced evidence for a third locus in the DR region situated between D/DR and the GLO locus, which they have called the SB locus.

In our laboratories we have examined two monomorphic monoclonal antibodies to HLA-DR (NFK1 and NFK2) by two-dimensional gel electrophoresis; both antibodies detect products of two loci in addition to that of HLA-DR (Makgoba *et al.*, 1983). One of these products is probably DC1 and one may be a product of the SB locus, but this point is yet to be clarified. Thus there seems little doubt there are several loci in the D/DR region of the chromosome apart from the locus controlling DR, although they must be closely linked to it.

Table II. The DR Antigens Associated with the Allegedly Supertypic Specificities of the MT and MB Series[a]

MT1 = DR1 and 2 and DRw6 and w10
MT2 = DR3 and 5 and DRw8
MT3 = DR4 and 7 and DRw9

MB1 = DR1 and 2 and DRw6 and w10
MB2 = DR4 and 5 and DRw8 and w9
MB3 = DR3 and 7

DC1 = DR1 and 2 and DRw6 and w10

[a]MT1 = MB1 = DC1.

III. THE TISSUE DISTRIBUTION OF HLA-DR

Large amounts of HLA-DR are expressed in the kidney. The precise localization of HLA-DR was determined by using two monoclonal antibodies (NFK1 and NFK2) recognizing monomorphic determinants on the HLA-DR molecule. Both antibodies purify a two-chain molecule of 28,000 and 33,000 daltons on sodium dodecylsulfate–polyacrylamide gel electrophoresis, which has a typical pattern of HLA-DR on two-dimensional gel electrophoresis (Fuggle et al., 1982). Other monoclonal antibodies—to HLA-ABC, both monomorphic [PA2.6 (Brodsky et al., 1979)] and polymorphic [MA2.1 (McMichael et al., 1980)]; leukocyte common antigen (L-C) (Dalchau et al., 1980); human Thy-1 (McKenzie and Fabre, 1981b); and dog Thy-1 (McKenzie and Fabre, 1981a)—were used to study the distribution of HLA-ABC or used as positive and negative controls. Although we have used both immunofluorescence and immunoperoxidase staining of tissues, the latter has proved far more satisfactory, since there is no background staining and the fixed preparations allow comparisons to be made between sections. The technique has been described in detail elsewhere (Fuggle et al., 1982), but we may note briefly that the monoclonal antibody in saturating concentrations is incubated with the cryostat tissue sections, followed by a second layer of a sheep antimouse serum together with heat-inactivated normal human AB serum. Then a third layer, comprising a monoclonal mouse anti-horseradish-peroxidase antibody plus horseradish peroxidase enzyme, is added before development with diaminobenzidene and counterstaining with hematoxylin.

A. Kidney

The localization of HLA-DR in biopsies from 46 kidneys used for transplantation was compatible with our previous absorption and immunofluorescent studies showing that HLA-DR was present in considerable amounts (Williams et al., 1980a; Hart et al., 1981). In the glomeruli HLA-DR was present on endothelium and also mesangium, but not on epithelium. Intertubular capillaries stained intensely in all kidneys, a result that has been noted by others (Hayry et al., 1980; Koyama et al., 1979; Natali et al., 1981; Scott et al., 1981). The endothelium of large vessels showed considerable variation in the staining for HLA-DR, not only between kidneys but also within the same kidney, in some cases being weakly positive and in others, negative (Table III).

In addition to the intertubular capillaries, other intertubular structures stained intensely with HLA-DR and L-C antibodies. These cells were considered to be dendritic cells. They did not stain with nonspecific esterase, had large nuclei and long dendritic processes, and were found mostly between tubules

Table III. Some Examples of the Distribution of HLA-ABC and
HLA-DR in Several Tissues, Including Kidney as Determined by
Immunoperoxidase Staining[a]

Tissue	Cells	HLA-ABC	HLA-DR
Kidney	Glomerulus		
	Endothelium	Present	Present
	Epithelium	Present	Absent
	Mesangium	Present	Present
	Intertubular capillaries	Present	Present
	Dendritic cells	Present	Present
	Tubules		
	Proximal	Present	Variable
	Distal	Present	Absent
	Endothelium of large vessels	Present	Variable
Heart	Muscle	Present	Absent
	Dendritic cells	Present	Present
	Endothelium	Present	Present
Pancreas	Exocrine cells	Absent	Absent
	Endocrine cells	Present	Absent
	Endothelium	Present	Present
	Dendritic cells	Present	Present
Liver	Hepatocytes	Variable[b]	Absent
	Kupffer cells	Present	Present
	Endothelium	Present	Absent
Adrenal	Endocrine cells	Present	Absent
	Endothelium	Present	Present
	Dendritic cells	Present	Present

[a] Adapted from Daar et al. (1983).
[b] Hepatocytes have proved to be definitely positive on some samples obtained from cadaver donors but negative on some samples obtained from needle liver biopsies, the difference perhaps being explained by the method of fixation.

and in some glomeruli. There did not appear to be any quantitative difference in the number of such cells among kidneys tested.

The most interesting finding in this series of kidney biopsies (and one not described previously) was the distribution of HLA-DR in tubules, which varied within and between kidneys. Tubular staining was present in 60% of the kidneys examined but was not present in all tubules. The tubular staining was intracellular and extended throughout the cytoplasm, although it was more dense at the base of the tubule. The staining appeared to be confined to the proximal tubules, and the tubules not staining for HLA-DR were probably distal tubules. However, in 40% of the kidneys examined either tubules did not stain for DR at all or an occasional tubule was very weakly positive, although in these kidneys other structures such as intertubular capillaries and glomeruli stained strongly. Thus there appeared to be considerable heterogeneity of staining of HLA-DR in tubules of the kidney. In contrast, no such heterogeneity was seen in the staining for HLA-ABC or Thy-1, the latter having been shown in our laboratories to be present uniformly throughout the cytoplasm of tubular epithelium.

B. Other Tissues

Extensive distribution studies of HLA-ABC and DR in most tissues of the body have been performed (Daar *et al.*, 1983). Some examples of the distribution of staining for HLA-ABC and HLA-DR are shown in Table III. On the whole HLA-DR appears to be confined to endothelium and the putative dendritic cell in most nonlymphoid tissues, the Kupffer cell staining intensely in the liver. One observation of interest in nonlymphoid tissues is that colonic epithelium, which is normally negative for HLA-DR, does express HLA-DR in some instances where the epithelium has undergone malignant change (Daar *et al.*, 1982).

However, a word of caution about these results is necessary, because, as noted above, the monomorphic monoclonal antibodies used to determine the distribution of HLA-DR do detect the products of two other loci in this D region of the chromosome. Until these investigations have been repeated with appropriate polymorphic monoclonal antibodies to HLA-DR, the conclusions concerning the expression of HLA-DR must be regarded as tentative. The absence of HLA-DR is not affected by this caveat.

C. Relevance of the Distribution of HLA-DR to Transplantation

Subject to the proviso expressed above, the relatively large amount of HLA-DR found in kidney and its pattern of distribution within the kidney are particularly relevant to the induction of an immune response to histocompatibility antigens in a renal allograft and also support our demonstration of the influence of matching for HLA-DR in renal transplantation (which will be discussed in the next section). This assumes that incompatible HLA-DR expressed on nonlymphoid cells can produce the initial proliferative response of T_H cells to the MHC. In support of this assumption is the previous demonstration that dispersed kidney cells in the rat and the pig (Mashimo *et al.*, 1976; Daniel and Edwards, 1975) and endothelial cells from umbilical vein (Hirschberg *et al.*, 1975) will produce proliferation of allogeneic lymphocytes in a mixed-cell reaction. These findings would be compatible with our localization of HLA-DR on renal tubular cells and endothelium, respectively. Nevertheless the recent demonstrations in the mouse and the rat show that a very few dendritic cells in the stimulating population of an MLR are responsible for the proliferative response (Steinman and Witmer, 1978; Mason *et al.*, 1981), which means that the response of lymphocytes in an MLR to dispersed kidney and endothelial cells might be explained by contamination with mononuclear cells of the dendritic lineage, rather than Ia-like antigens expressed on the surface of kidney parenchymal and endothelial cells. However, this appears less likely in the case of the endothelial cell experiments of Thorsby and his colleagues (Hirschberg *et al.*, 1975).

If the proliferation of T_H cells in the allogeneic MLR represents the recognition phase of the *in vivo* response to incompatible MHC antigens, then the dendritic cell might provide the major stimulus *in vivo* for the immune response to an allogeneic kidney. Batchelor and colleagues (1978) have already provided evidence in the rat that purified MHC antigens are poor immunogens and need to be expressed on the surface of a viable mononuclear cell of the lymphoid series for a primary alloimmune response to occur. We have shown in our laboratories that dendritic cells are present in the rat kidney (Hart and Fabre, 1981a) and are probably the putative passenger leukocyte (Hart and Fabre, 1981b). Lechler and Batchelor (1982) have presented convincing *in vivo* evidence in the rat that the dendritic cell in the donor kidney provides the major immunogenic stimulus resulting in rejection of a renal allograft. They were able to show that as few as 10^5 dendritic cells of donor type were able to produce a first set rejection of an established renal allograft after retransplantation into a naive host, whereas 100-fold more T or B lymphocytes had little effect. Thus in the rat the role of incompatible dendritic cells in the donor kidney would seem to be a major one in the induction of the immune response leading to rejection of a renal allograft.

But assuming that HLA-DR rather than HLA-ABC antigens in the human also play a major role in the induction of the immune response to a renal allograft, there may well be additional stimulating cells in the human kidney compared to the rat kidney. For although we have shown in our laboratories that Ia-like antigens are not expressed on rat endothelium, in contrast, in the human kidney, HLA-DR is expressed on the endothelium of intertubular capillaries and glomeruli and to a variable extent on that of large vessels. If endotherlial HLA-DR in the kidney can truly induce T_H-cell proliferation in addition to that expressed on the dendritic cell, matching for HLA-DR in renal transplantation assumes considerable importance.

Of course attributing the induction of the immune response to an allogeneic kidney primarily to DR incompatibility of the dendritic cells and perhaps endothelial cells in the kidney does not mean that other incompatible MHC antigens, such as HLA-ABC, do not induce an immune response against the graft by more conventional pathways involving host macrophage/dendritic cell interaction with antigen and subsequent presentation to T_H cells. This response may be a weaker one and easier to suppress (Lechler and Batchelor, 1982). We have also shown previously in the rat that venous allografts, which probably do not contain dendritic cells and do not express Ia on endothelial cells, were not rejected, but that the recipients did produce a good cytotoxic antibody response directed against class I antigens (Prendergast *et al.*, 1978). Furthermore, in the mouse both skin and cornea can be rejected vigorously across a major histocompatibility barrier in the absence of donor Langerhans cells, which belong to the dendritic lineage (Streilein *et al.*, 1979; Steinmuller, 1981).

Whatever the role of HLA-DR on endothelium in the induction of the immune response, it should be remembered that incompatibility for HLA-DR, as expressed on intertubular capillaries and glomerular endothclium and variably on large vessels, can assume considerable importance if a renal allograft is placed in a recipient specifically sensitized against donor HLA-DR as a result of prior transfusions, pregnancy, or a previous graft. (This subject is further discussed in Section V.)

How can we explain the localization of HLA-DR in the tubules of some 60% of kidneys and in the mesangium of the glomeruli as well as on endothelium? Ia-like antigens on the macrophage, and also no doubt on the dendritic cell, serve to present antigen as altered self to the T_H cell in the induction of an immune response to an antigen (Erb *et al.*, 1976; Puri and Lonai, 1980). Presumably this is the role of the dendritic cell in the kidney, but it seems unlikely that the DR on tubules would serve this purpose. However, Hirschberg *et al.* (1980) have presented evidence that endothelial cells, through the agency of HLA-DR, can present antigen to T_H cells in place of the macrophage. Regardless of whether or not endothelium can present antigen to T_H cells, we would suggest that the distribution of DR in the kidney in some way controls the passage of dendritic cells through the kidney, directing them to sites where antigen or complexes may be deposited. (However, the absence of DR in the tubules of some kidneys is difficult to reconcile with this suggestion.) This could explain the density of DR found on intertubular capillaries, perhaps proximal tubules (not normally considered such a site), and glomerular endothelium and mesangium. The attraction of this hypothesis is that it proposes that the expression of HLA-DR on a cell surface serves the same general purpose in nonlymphoid tissues as in lymphoid tissues, namely that of cellular recognition, and perhaps this is primarily intended to direct the traffic of macrophage and dendritic cells through tissues.

IV. MATCHING FOR HLA-DR IN RENAL TRANSPLANTATION

After the definition of HLA-DR antigens at the Oxford Workshop in 1977 (Bodmer *et al.*, 1978), we were able to type retrospectively most cadaver donors and recipients transplanted in the two years before that time using frozen spleen and blood lymphocytes. The results suggested that matching for DR may influence graft survival (Ting and Morris 1978b). Based on this encouraging correlation, a prospective study of HLA-DR matching in cadaver transplantation was begun. During this time the definition of the HLA-DR antigens, HLA-DR1–7, has remained virtually unchanged. Most problems of definition have been confined to DRw6, for which no operationally monospecific antibody exists (hence it retains the w prefix). In our studies DRw6 was defined by a positive reaction for five antisera in the absence of DR1 and 2. Donors and recipients were selected primarily on the basis of DR matching and the cross-match test, and only minimal attention was paid to HLA-ABC typing. We have also examined our data excluding donor and recipient pairs where DRw6 was involved in the matching, because of this poor definition of DRw6.

Very few donors and recipients could not be typed for HLA-DR in the overall series, and data on 270 cadaver transplants are available (out of a total of 289 cadaver transplants performed since the unit was established in 1975). Immunosuppression has not been constant throughout the study. Patients initially received azathioprine and high doses of steroids (Morris et al., 1978b). This policy was changed to azathioprine and low doses of steroids (Chan et al., 1980), and recently cyclosporin A has been used in some patients in a prospective controlled trial of this drug (Morris et al., 1982). The pregraft transfusion status of patients varies in that patients are not transfused before transplantation unless there is a medical indication. Patients who have not been transfused before transplantation are given a peroperative transfusion on the basis of a controlled trial suggesting that peroperative transfusions also produced the transfusion effect (Williams et al., 1980b). Thus there is a considerably heterogeneity in some of the variables that might influence graft survival, apart from DR matching.

A. DR Incompatibility and Graft Survival

Significantly better graft survival was seen in recipients who received a DR-compatible kidney than in recipients who received a kidney incompatible for one or two DR antigens (Table IV). This is in accord with our earlier analyses

Table IV. Graft Survival Rates in Patients Who Received a Cadaver Kidney Mismatched for 0, 1, or 2 DR Antigens[a]

No. of DR incompatibilities	N	Graft survival (%) at			
		3 months	6 months	12 months	24 months
0	84	78	77	72	70
1	130	73	69	64	56
2	56	64	62	59	49

[a]Actuarial graft survival curves were generated according to the method of Peto et al. (1976). 0 versus 1 and 2: $p = 0.03$.

Table V. Graft Survival Rates in Patients Who Received a Cadaver Kidney
Mismatched for 0, 1, or 2 DR Antigens, but Excluding All Pairs Where
HLA-DRw6 Was Present in Donor or Recipient[a]

No. of DR		Graft survival (%) at			
incompatibilities	N	3 months	6 months	12 months	24 months
0	75	80	80	78	73
1	95	70	68	63	58
2	44	65	63	58	50

[a]0 versus 1 and 2: $p < 0.005$.

(Ting and Morris, 1978b, 1980) and those of several other groups (Thorsby
et al., 1981; van Rood *et al.*, 1981; Goeken *et al.*, 1981; Ayoub and Terasaki,
1982).

Exclusion from the analysis of all 56 pairs where DRw6 was involved in the
matching resulted in an even more significant difference in graft survival between
patients receiving a DR-compatible graft and those receiving an incompatible
graft (Table V).

B. Influence of HLA-ABC

Although minimal attention was paid to matching for HLA-ABC in allocat-
ing kidneys, it was possible that donor–recipient pairs well matched for DR
might also be well matched for ABC because of the known linkage disequilib-
rium between certain B and DR antigens and, in turn, A and B antigens. However, a careful analysis of our data failed to show any influence of HLA-ABC
on the result of matching for HLA-DR. There was no suggestion that combined
matching for HLA-ABC and HLA-DR produced even better graft survival than
matching for HLA-DR alone, as has been suggested by the Eurotransplant data
(van Rood *et al.*, 1981).

C. Blood Transfusions and DR Matching

It is generally accepted that transfusions before transplantation improve the
survival of the subsequent graft; therefore we have examined our data for a joint
effect of transfusions and DR matching. The results suggest that graft survival in
a nontransfused patient is excellent if the graft is matched for HLA-DR (Table
VI), and there is an indication that the graft survival is even better in transfused
patients who receive a DR-compatible kidney. The worst survival rate was seen
in nontransfused patients receiving a DR-mismatched kidney. Our results have

Table VI. The Influence of Blood Transfusions before Transplantation
and Matching for HLA-DR in Cadaveric Renal Transplantation

Transfusions before transplant	No. of DR incompatibilities	N	Graft survival (%) at			
			3 months	6 months	12 months	24 months
None	0	29	76	76	72	67
>1	0	39	84	84	84	77
>1	1, 2	88	85	81	75	64
None	1, 2	69	51	49	48	45

been confirmed by other studies (Opelz and Terasaki, 1980; Goeken et al.,
1981; Ayoub and Terasaki, 1982).

D. HLA-DR and the Mixed Lymphocyte Reaction

We have not been able to show a better correlation between HLA-DR matching and graft survival based on the number of shared HLA-DR antigens between
donor and recipient rather than on the basis of DR incompatibilities. This does
suggest that we are identifying most of the relevant DR antigens, as suggested
by the total gene frequencies shown in Table I. Although in the past we were
unable to show a correlation between the MLR response of the recipient against
the cadaver donor graft outcome (Cullen et al., 1977), we have now gathered
some MLR data between donor and recipients where DR typing was also available (Cullen et al., 1983). This has enabled us to examine the degree of responsiveness against donor lymphocytes in the MLR of some recipients who received
either a DR-compatible or a DR-incompatible kidney. Data for one way MLRs
between recipient (responder) and donor (stimulator) and DR typing were
available in 59 pairs. There was quite a good correlation between DR compatibility and a low responsiveness in the MLR between donor and recipient (Table
VII), which we also found in a study in healthy volunteers (Cullen et al., 1979).
It is of interest that graft failure occurred in 11 of 33 patients followed for 12
months where there was both DR incompatibility and a positive MLR, compared with only 1 of 11 where there was no DR incompatibility and a negative
MLR. The numbers are too low to draw any definite conclusions, but, bearing
in mind the serological inadequacies of the definition of DRw6 and DRw4 and
the technical problems of the MLR in cadaver transplantation, it does appear
that the serological matching of donor and recipient for the DR antigens defined
in 1977 has in general reflected the reactivity in the MLR of recipient lymphocytes to donor lymphocytes. This provides additional support for the relevance
of matching for HLA-DR in renal transplantation.

Table VII. The Association between HLA-DR
Compatibility and MLR Reactivity in 59 Cadaver
Donors and Recipients[a]

No. of DR incompatibilities	MLR responses	
	High	Low
0	4	14
1	22	6
2	12	1

[a]From Cullen et al. (1983).

E. Matching for Supertypic Specificities

As we have discussed earlier, several broadly reactive antigens of the D region (MT1, 2, 3; MB1, 2, 3; DC1) have been defined on B lymphocytes that segregate with HLA, and that may well represent products of separate D-region loci. Duquesnoy has reported that matching for the MB series of antigens, which he first defined (Duquesnoy et al., 1979), is related to better graft survival in one-haplotype-identical living related donors and recipients (Duquesnoy, 1980). Although we have not typed specifically for these antigens, we have reanalyzed our data on the basis of the cross-reacting specificities included in the broad supertypic MB specificities (MB1 = DC1 = DR1, 2, w6; MB2 = DR3, 7; MB3 = DR4, 5). However, we have not been able to show any correlation between compatibility for the MB cross-reacting groups and graft survival. Obviously prospective studies are required with the appropriate antisera that define these supertypic specificities before any firm decision about their importance in matching can be made.

F. The Renal Tubular Expression of HLA-DR and Matching for HLA-DR

We have described in Section III.A the widespread distribution of HLA-DR on human kidneys, and in particular the different patterns of expression of HLA-DR on proximal tubules, HLA-DR being expressed on proximal tubules in some kidneys but not in others. This finding led us to examine the possibility that this quantitative difference in expression of HLA-DR on the renal parenchyma might influence the analysis of matching for HLA-DR and graft survival.

We thus analyzed graft survival in those patients who received a DR-incompatible kidney where the expression of HLA-DR on tubules might have increased the immunogenic stimulus of the graft. However, no evidence in support of this hypothesis was seen in our data (Fuggle et al., 1982).

G. Conclusions

Our own data and a growing body of evidence from other laboratories suggest that matching for HLA-DR alone strongly influences cadaveric renal allograft survival. Further support for this observation is obtained by the relatively low reactivity in the one-way MLR between donor and recipient seen in unrelated DR-compatible people. Nevertheless it should be borne in mind that, although the DR antigens originally defined in 1977 have on the whole remained unchanged, with the exception of DRw6, there is increasing evidence that there are several loci in the D region apart from HLA-DR. This would obviously be relevant to DR matching in transplantation, but to what extent this would alter the present observations is uncertain. Both the I-A and I-E molecules of the mouse MHC may induce cell-mediated lysis and skin allograft rejection in the mouse (Klein *et al.*, 1981). As HLA-DR is considered the homologue of the I-E product, it is possible that matching for other products of the D/DR region may also influence graft survival.

The potentially attractive feature of matching for DR rather than ABC is the apparently limited polymorphism of these antigens, each with a relatively high frequency that makes matching with a moderate-sized pool relatively easy. Lamm (1980) has calculated that if DR compatibility is to be achieved in 95% of donors and recipients then a pool size of approximately 100 patients on dialysis is sufficient. This is a mathematical prediction that does not take into account ABO compatibility and sensitization of recipients causing a positive cross-match and so presents a rather too optimistic picture of the ease of applying DR matching to cadaveric renal transplantation. Nevertheless matching for HLA-DR presents a much simpler problem than matching for HLA-AB and does allow DR matching to be brought within the orbit of transplants of single organs, such as the heart and the pancreas.

V. SENSITIZATION TO HLA-DR

The association between a positive cross-match (antibodies in the recipient's serum reacting with the donor's lymphocytes) and immediate renal allograft failure (hyperacute rejection) was first reported in 1966 by Kissmeyer-Nielsen and his colleagues. Studies over the next three years by other laboratories soon confirmed this initial report (Williams *et al.*, 1968; Patel and Terasaki, 1969). Since then the cross-match test before transplantation has been deemed mandatory, and it has been accepted dogma that renal transplantation is contraindicated in the presence of a positive cross-match.

It was initially believed that all lymphocytotoxic antibodies were directed at HLA-A and -B antigens, but it is now evident that this is not so. Furthermore it is apparent that antibodies to some of these antigens are not associated with rapid graft destruction, i.e., transplantation can be carried out successfully in the presence of a positive lymphocyte cytotoxic cross-match in certain situations.

It is generally accepted that a recipient of a renal allograft with donor-specific HLA-AB antibodies will in most instances hyperacutely reject the graft. However, the effect of donor-specific HLA-DR antibodies on renal allografts is not completely known. Most of the early studies assumed that all antibodies reacting with B lymphocytes were directed at HLA-DR determinants. We now know that this is not true, and B-lymphocyte reactivity resulting in a positive cross-match of recipient serum with donor lymphocytes may be due to antibodies other than anti-DR. Thus at the present time it is impossible to discuss the role of sensitization to HLA-DR without considering the whole spectrum of B-lymphocyte antibodies in patients given a renal transplant.

A. Antibodies Reacting with B Lymphocytes and Their Detection

Three techniques have been used to detect B-lymphocyte-reactive antibodies. First, autoreactive and nonautoreactive B-cell antibodies have been separated by testing the patients' sera in a standard lymphocytotoxicity test against their own lymphocytes in addition to allogeneic lymphocytes. Second, "cold" (?autoreactive) and "warm" (?HLA-DR) antibodies have been separated, generally by alterations of the temperature of the first incubation step in the lymphocytotoxicity test. Third, B-lymphocyte antibodies (?HLA-DR) have been detected by the inhibition of erythrocyte–antibody rosette formation to B lymphocytes (EAI).

B. The B-Lymphocyte Positive Cross-Match in Renal Transplantation

From 1976 to 1978 a number of reports were published showing that transplantation could be successful in the presence of a donor-specific B-cell positive cross-match (Ettenger et al., 1976; Morris et al., 1977; Lobo et al., 1977; Myburgh et al., 1977). In these studies no attempt was made to characterize the antibody other than to note that it reacted with B but not T lymphocytes. Reports indicated that the short-term success rate, and also the long-term outcome, were just as good in B-cell positive cross-match transplants as in negative cross-match pairs.

d'Apice and Tait (1979) have even suggested that donor-specific B-cell antibodies may have an enhancing effect, since they found a 90% one-year graft survival rate in patients receiving a B-cell positive cross-match graft compared with 35% in the grafts with a negative cross-match graft. Support is given to their findings by the previous demonstration in the rat that (1) passive administration of donor-specific antibody to a recipient of a renal allograft led to suppression of rejection rather than antibody-mediated damage of the graft (French and Batchelor, 1969; Stuart *et al.*, 1968; Fabre and Morris, 1972), (2) the major target of the antibody in most antisera was donor Ia (McKenzie *et al.*, 1980), and (3) anti-Ia serum in the presence of heterologous guinea pig complement did not produce hyperacute rejection of a renal allograft (Winearls *et al.*, 1980). These experimental findings in the rat reinforced the general feeling that a renal transplant could be performed safely in the presence of a positive B-cell cross-match. However it was not known at the time that Ia is not expressed on endo-thelium in the kidney in the rat, whereas it is in the human, as we have described in Section III.A.

Our current analysis of the outcome of 52 grafts performed in the presence of a B-cell positive cross-match confirms our earlier data that the overall graft survival is not inferior to that of grafts performed in the presence of a negative cross-match (Table VIII). However, this does disguise the fact that a significant number of grafts in this group either had delayed function or never functioned. As discussed in Section V.F, this greater frequency of delayed function or non-function might be attributed to antibodies against donor DR. There have been other reports of hyperacute rejection of renal allografts in the presence of a positive B-cell cross-match considered to be due to antibodies directed at DR (Berg and Möller, 1980; Mohanakumar *et al.*, 1981). As noted previously, HLA-DR is present on endothelium in the human kidney, in contrast to that of the rat. Therefore it would not be unexpected to see antibody-mediated damage in some instances of a transplant performed in the presence of a positive B-cell cross-match, if the antibody is directed at HLA-DR. But, as already discussed, these B-lymphocyte antibodies are not all anti-DR, which might explain the rather unpredictable outcome of grafts performed in the presence of a positive B-cell cross-match. And even where they are directed at DR the variation that we have observed in expression of DR on large-vessel endothelium in kidneys may vary the effect of donor-specific DR antibody on a particular graft.

Table VIII. The Outcome of Transplantation since 1976 in the Presence of a Negative or a Positive Cross-Match against Donor B Lymphocytes or Donor T and B Lymphocytes

Cross-match	N	Delayed function (%)	Never functioned (%)	Graft survival (%) after		
				3 months	6 months	12 months
Negative	185	35	3.8	75	72	70
B positive	52	58	13.5	70	68	63
B and T positive	18	75	27.8	72	65	65

C. Autoreactive and Nonautoreactive Antibodies

Autoreactive antibodies react with both allogeneic and autologous lymphocytes. They can react with B cells alone or with both T and B cells. Both types of autoreactive antibodies are thought to be directed at non-HLA antigens, since reactivity was demonstrated with the cells from HLA-identical siblings (Stastny and Austin, 1976) and they are negative or weakly reactive with chronic lymphocytic leukemia (CLL) cells that express HLA antigens (Ting and Morris, 1978a).

The main features that distinguish this type of antibody from other (HLA-DR) antibodies are (1) nonreactivity with CLL cells, (2) IgM rather than IgG, (3) occurrence in nontransfused patients without previous pregnancies or transplants, i.e., occurrence in the absence of previous immunization against histocompatibility antigens, and (4) killing of less than 100% of the target cells.

Autoreactive B-lymphocyte antibodies are found in 10–25% of patients on dialysis. The immunizing antigen is unknown since many of the patients studied had never been pregnant or transfused. Furthermore, Park et al. (1977) found auto-B-lymphocyte antibodies in the sera of about 20% of normal subjects.

Transplantation with a B-cell positive cross-match due to autoreactive antibodies is extremely successful (Reekers et al., 1977; Ting and Morris, 1977). Our current analyses show that those transplanted in the presence of a B-cell positive cross-match due to autoantibodies have a significantly better survival rate than those with a B-cell positive cross-match due to alloantibodies, particularly in recipients of first grafts (Table IX). These findings have been confirmed by others (Jeannet et al., 1981; Ettenger et al., 1982). The mechanism by which this apparent improved graft survival is produced is unknown, but it may be related to suppression of the immune response to the graft histocompatibility antigens, possibly through antiidiotype activity of these antibodies.

Successful transplantations with a positive T- and B-cell cross-match due to

Table IX. The Outcome of Transplantation since 1976 in the Presence of a
Positive Cross-Match against Donor B or Donor B and T Lymphocytes
where the Reactivity Can Be Attributed Definitely to Either
Autoantibody or Alloantibody

Cross-match	Autoantibody	N	Never functioned	Graft survival (%)		
				3 months	6 months	12 months
B positive	Yes	18	2	83	78	78
	No	19	3	63	58	53
B and T positive	Yes	16	3	81	75	75
	No	2	2	0	0	0

Table X. Details of the MLR, Pregraft Transfusions, and Reactivity of
Patients' Sera with Donor Lymphocytes and Self Lymphocytes in
Three Patients Each Given a Kidney from a Relative in the Presence
of a Positive Cross-Match[a]

| | | | Percent target cell death | | | |
| | | | Donor | | Self | |
Donor	MLR	No. of pregraft transfusions	T	B	T	B
HLA-identical brother	–	6	25	90	40	44
Father	–	116	90	70	40	70
HLA-identical brother	–	14	90	90	90	NT

[a]NT, not tested. The three grafts are functioning between 12 and 52 months after transplantation.

autoreactive antibodies have also been reported (Cross et al., 1976; Morris and Ting, 1981). We have now transplanted 18 T- and B-cell positive cross-match grafts, and the results are shown in Tables VIII and IX. There were two immediate failures, which were due, in retrospect, to alloantibodies against HLA-AB. Of the 16 transplants where the cross-match almost certainly was due to autoantibodies, one failure was probably technical while the other two are unexplained. It is possible that antibodies to HLA-AB were also present in the sera, but it is also possible that some of these autoantibodies might have caused vascular damage to the cooled allograft (Lobo et al., 1980).

Living related donor transplants have also been successfully performed with a positive autoreactive T- and B-cell cross-match (Stastny and Austin, 1976). We have performed three such transplants; two were from HLA-identical siblings and the other was from the father. The relevant cross-match data and graft outcomes are shown in Table X.

D. "Cold" and "Warm" Antibodies

Iwaki et al. (1978) separated B cold and warm antibodies by performing the incubation step before the addition of complement at either 5°C (cold) or 37°C (warm), but the postcomplement incubation step was always at 25°C. These cold antibodies were autoreactive (Park et al., 1977), were IgM, and subsequently were shown to be directed at cell-surface IgM (Cicciarelli et al., 1980; Takahashi et al., 1980). Takahashi et al. (1981) further showed that the reactivity of these antibodies was inhibited by F(ab')$_2$ but not by Fc and postulated that they may be analogous to antiidiotype antibodies.

B cold antibodies are extremely common in dialysis patients, being found in 67% of 341 patients studied (Takahashi et al., 1981). Lobo (1981) found that

42% of sera from chronic haemodialysis patients had cold-reacting autoreactive antibodies. The B warm antibodies were said not to be autoreactive, and were perhaps directed at HLA-DR antigens (Ayoub *et al.*, 1980).

Ayoub *et al.* (1980) showed that those grafts performed in the presence of a B cold positive cross-match had a better one-year survival rate (58%) than those with B warm (42%) or no (38%) antibodies. These differences, however, were not significantly different. Coxe-Gilliland and Cross (1981) found that donor-specific B warm antibodies were not associated with rapid graft loss but they could only find two patients with B cold antibodies. d'Apice and Tait (1979), in their series of 30 patients with a B-cell positive cross-match, found no indication that the beneficial effect of donor-specific antibodies was related to the optimal temperature of reactivity of the serum. Lobo *et al.* (1978) could not find a correlation between graft rejection and warm or cold antibodies, and similarly our own data do not show any difference in graft outcome based on this temperature-dependent separation of antibody reactivity.

Thus—although we believe that antibodies that react only in the cold are probably autoantibodies and certainly non-HLA antibodies, and that a cross-match due to such antibodies is not a contraindication to transplantation—we do not believe that the converse is true, for not all antibodies reacting in the warm are anti-DR, and they may still be autoreactive. For this reason, in our opinion temperature-dependent cross-matches are of limited value.

E. Inhibition of B-Lymphocyte Rosette Formation with Sensitized Erythrocytes

Using the EAI assay, antibodies reacting with B lymphocytes have been found in dialysis patients. These antibodies have been claimed to be directed to HLA-DR antigens by some authors (Suthanthiran *et al.*, 1978; Soulillou *et al.*, 1978) but not by others (MacLeod *et al.*, 1982). Where the same sera have been studied with both the EAI assay and the lymphocytotoxicity test, no correlation has been seen between the reactions of the two tests. It seems unlikely to us that the EAI test could be expected to have any greater specificity for HLA-DR than the lymphocytotoxicity assay.

Suthanthiran *et al.* (1978) found an excellent correlation between the presence of EAI antibodies and poor graft outcome. Six out of seven grafts performed in the presence of EAI antibodies suffered accelerated graft loss, while only one out of eight recipients with stable graft function had these antibodies before transplantation. These authors postulated that the EAI antibody was directed at HLA-DR antigens, based on their experiments with this type of antibody in the rat. Soullilou *et al.* (1978) could not confirm these findings, and in fact found that patients with EAI factors had a slightly better graft function than those without the inhibitory factor. MacLeod *et al.* (1982) found 85% (11/13) one-year survival of grafts in patients with donor-specific EAI antibodies, compared to 30% (6/20) in patients without EAI antibodies. Thus the presence of EAI antibodies is a good prognostic sign. MacLeod and her colleagues have provided evidence that the specificity of these antibodies is not HLA-DR. It seems to us that autoantibodies would produce a positive EAI assay and hence explain the contradictory results produced by different groups.

F. Antibodies to Donor HLA-DR

We have already discussed how initially it was thought that all B-cell antibodies were directed at HLA-DR. Certainly there is now ample evidence showing that this is not so. Indeed d'Apice and Tait (1980) have suggested that most positive B-cell cross-matches are not caused by HLA-DR antibodies. This conclusion was arrived at after studying the reactivity of 34 sera (from 34 patients who had received a B-cell positive cross-match graft) against B lymphocytes from families. Only 14 of the sera showed reaction patterns that segregated with HLA-DR in these families.

Apart from family studies it is difficult to be certain that a B-cell antibody is anti-HLA-DR. We have defined B-cell antibodies as autoreactive or nonautoreactive and postulated that the latter are anti-DR (Morris and Ting, 1981). The possibility remains that these nonautoreactive antibodies also contain HLA-ABC antibodies, since we have not done platelet absorption studies on the sera. However, if our definition of nonautoreactive antibodies is correct, then we must conclude that donor-specific DR antibodies will be associated with a poorer graft survival rate (see Table IX).

Ayoub et al. (1980) have suggested that the B warm antibodies are directed at HLA-DR, since they are not removed by platelet absorption. In their study patients with this type of antibody did no worse than those with no antibodies, but, if only those patients with high-titer B warm antibodies were analyzed, a poor outcome was seen (22% at one year). The authors conclude that the DR antibody is weaker than the ABC antibodies, but if the DR antibodies are strong then they certainly can cause irreversible graft damage.

Another factor that might help to produce a variable outcome of a transplant, even in the face of a positive cross-match against donor DR, is the differing intensity of expression of DR on the endothelium of the human kidney, which we have described in Section III.A. This further adds to the complexity of the final outcome of a transplant performed in the presence of a donor-specific B-cell positive cross-match.

G. Conclusions

Many different types of antibodies that react with lymphocyte cell-surface antigens can be found in the serum of patients on dialysis. Those directed at

HLA-ABC antigens are a major cause of hyperacute rejection if they are donor-specific. HLA-DR antibodies are rather difficult to define with certainty, but the evidence from our own laboratory and the work of others suggests that donor-specific anti-DR antibodies may cause early graft failure or delayed function. Autoreactive (or cold) antibodies do not damage renal allografts, whether they be reactive with B or with B and T lymphocytes, and there is some evidence that they may be associated with improved graft survival.

The recognition of the different antibodies that produce a positive cross-match has most important clinical implications, for it allows many patients to receive transplants who might otherwise never receive a kidney because of their apparently very broad sensitization against MHC antigens. For example, in our unit 85% of the 70 patients transplanted in the face of a positive cross-match reacted with more than 85% of the random screening panel and would have been considered virtually impossible to transplant if a negative cross-match was a prerequisite for transplantation. Thus, continuing dissection of the specificity of the different antibodies that may cause a positive cross-match is an important advance in the management of the ever-increasing number of highly sensitized patients awaiting transplantation.

ACKNOWLEDGMENTS

This work was supported by grants from the Medical Research Council of the United Kingdom and the National Kidney Research Fund.

VI. REFERENCES

Ayoub, G., and Terasaki, P. I., 1982, *Transplantation* **33**:515.
Ayoub, G., Park, M. S., Terasaki, P. I., Iwaki, Y., and Opelz, G., 1980, *Transplantation* **29**:227.
Batchelor, J. R., Welsh, K. I., and Burgos, H., 1978, *Nature (London)* **273**:54.
Berg, B., and Möller, E., 1980, *Scand. J. Urol. Nephrol. Suppl.* **54**:36.
Bodmer, W. F., Batchelor, J. R., Bodmer, J. G., Festenstein, H., and Morris, P. J. (eds.), 1978, *Histocompatibility Testing 1977*, Munksgaard, Copenhagen.
Brodsky, F. M., Parham, P., Barnstable, C. J., Crumpton, M. J., and Bodmer, W. F., 1979, *Immunol. Rev.* **47**:3.
Chan, L., French, M., Beare, J., Oliver, D. O., and Morris, P. J., 1980, *Transplant. Proc.* **12**:323.
Cicciarelli, J. C., Chia, D., Terasaki, P. I., Barnett, E. V., and Shirahama, S., 1980, *Tissue Antigens* **15**:275.
Colombe, G., Pask, S., and Payne, R., 1980, in: *Histocompatibility Testing 1980* (P. I. Terasaki, ed.), p. 802, UCLA Tissue Typing Laboratory, Los Angeles, California.
Corte, G., Calabi, F., Damiani, G., Bargellesi, A., Tosi, R., and Sorrentino, R., 1982, *Nature (London)* **292**:357.
Coxe-Gilliland, R., and Cross, D. E., 1981, *Transplant. Proc.* **13**:945.

86   Morris and Ting

Cross, D. E., Greiner, R., and Whittier, F. C., 1976, *Transplantation* **21**:307.
Cullen, P. R., Lester, S., Rouch, J., and Morris, P. J., 1977, *Clin. Exp. Immunol.* **28**:218.
Cullen, P. R., Ting, A., and Morris, P. J., 1979, *Transplant. Proc.* **11**:756.
Cullen, P. R., Ting, A., and Morris, P. J., 1983, in preparation.
Curtoni, E. S., Borelli, I., Cornaglia, M., and Olivetti, E., 1980, in: *Histocompatibility Testing 1980* (P. I. Terasaki, ed.), p. 805, UCLA Tissue Typing Laboratory, Los Angeles.
Daar, A. S., Fuggle, S., Ting, A., and Fabre, J. W., 1982, *J. Immunol.* **129**:447.
Daar, A., Fuggle, S., Fabre, J., Ting, A., and Morris, P. J., 1983, in preparation.
Dalchau, R., Kirkley, J., and Fabre, J. W., 1980, *Eur. J. Immunol.* **10**:737.
Daniel, M. R., and Edwards, M. J., 1975, *Br. J. Exp. Pathol.* **56**:349.
d'Apice, A. J. F., and Tait, B. D., 1979, *Transplantation* **27**:324.
d'Apice, A. J. F., and Tait, B. D., 1980, *Transplantation* **30**:382.
Duquesnoy, R., 1980, in: *Histocompatibility Testing 1980* (P. I. Terasaki, ed.), p. 817, UCLA Tissue Typing Laboratory, Los Angeles.
Duquesnoy, R. J., Marrari, M. M., and Annen, K., 1979, *Transplant. Proc.* **11**:1757.
Duquesnoy, R. J., Annen, K. B., Marrari, M. M., and Kauffman, H. M., 1980, *N. Engl. J. Med.* **302**:821.
Erb, P., Feldmann, M., and Hogg, N., 1976, *Eur. J. Immunol.* **6**:365.
Ettenger, R. B., Terasaki, P. I., Opelz, G., Melekzadeh, M., Pennisi, A. J., Uittenbogaart, C., and Fine, R., 1976, *Lancet* **2**:56.
Ettenger, R. B., Jordan, S. C., and Fine, R. N., 1982, *Transplantation* (in press).
Fabre, J. W., and Morris, P. J., 1972, *Transplantation* **13**:604.
French, M. E., and Batchelor, J. R., 1969, *Lancet* **2**:1103.
Fuggle, S., Errasti, P., Daar, A. S., Fabre, J. W., Ting, A., and Morris, P. J., 1982, *Transplantation* (in press).
Goeken, W. E., Thompson, J. S., and Corry, R. J., 1981, *Transplantation* **32**:522.
Hart, D. N., Fuggle, S. V., Williams, K. A., Fabre, J. W., Ting, A., and Morris, P.J., 1981, *Transplantation* **31**:428.
Hart, D. N., and Fabre, J. W., 1981, *Transplantation* **31**:318.
Hart, D. N., and Fabre, J. W., 1981, *Transplant. Proc.* **13**:954.
Hayry, P., von Willebrand, E., and Anderson, L. C., 1980, *Scand. J. Immunol.* **11**:303.
Hirschberg, H., Evensen, S. A., Henricksen, T., and Thorsby, E., 1975, *Transplantation* **19**:495.
Hirschberg, H., Bergh, O. J., and Thorsby, E., 1980, *J. Exp. Med.* **152**:249.
Iwaki, Y., Terasaki, P. I., Park, M. S., and Billing, R., 1978, *Lancet* **1**:1228.
Jeannet, M., Benzonana, G., and Arni, I., 1981, *Transplantation* **231**:160.
Kissmeyer-Nielsen, F., Olsen, S., Petersen, V. P., and Fjeldborg, O., 1966, *Lancet* **1**:662.
Klein, J., Juretic, A., Baxevanis, C. N., and Nagy, Z. A., 1981, *Nature (London)* **291**:455.
Koyama, K., Fukunishi, T., Barcos, M., Tanigaki, N., and Pressman, D., 1979, *Immunology* **38**:333.
Lamm, L. U., 1980, *Lancet* **2**:755.
Lechler, R. I., and Batchelor, J. R., 1982, *J. Exp. Med.* **155**:31.
Lobo, P. I., 1981, *Transplantation* **32**:233.
Lobo, P. I., Westervelt, F. B., and Rudolf, L. E., 1977, *Lancet* **1**:925.
Lobo, P. I., Westervelt, F. B., and Rudolf, L. E., 1978, *Transplantation* **26**:84.
Lobo, P. I., Westervelt, F. B., White, C., and Rudolf, L. E., 1980, *Lancet* **2**:879.
McKenzie, J. L., and Fabre, J. W., 1981a, *Transplantation* **31**:275.
McKenzie, J. L., and Fabre, J. W., 1981b, *J. Immunol.* **126**:843.
McKenzie, J. L., Fabre, J. W., and Morris, P. J., 1980, *Transplantation* **29**:337.
MacLeod, A. M., Mason, R. J., Steward, K. N., Power, D. A., Shewan, W. G., Edward, N., and Catto, G. R. D., 1982, *Transplantation* **34**:273.
McMichael, A. J., Parham, P., Rust, N., and Brodsky, F., 1980, *Hum. Immunol.* **1**:121.
Makgoba, M. W., Fuggle, S., McMichael, A., and Morris, P. J., 1983, *Nature (London)* (in press).
Mann, D. L., Abelson, L., Harris, S., and Amos, D. B., 1976, *Nature (London)* **259**:145.
Mashimo, S., Sakai, A., Ochiai, T., Kountz, S. L., 1976, *Tissue Antigens* **7**:291.

Mason, D. W., Pugh, C. W., and Webb, M., 1981, *Immunology* **44**:75.
Mohanakumar, T., Rhodes, C., Mendez-Picon, G., Goldman, M., Moncure, C., and Lee, H., 1981, *Transplantation* **31**:93.
Morris, P. J., and Ting, A., 1981, *Tissue Antigens* **17**:75.
Morris, P. J., Ting, A., Oliver, D. O., Bishop, M., Williams, K., and Dunnill, M. S., 1977, *Lancet* **1**:1288.
Morris, P. J., Batchelor, J. R., and Festenstein, H., 1978a, *Br. Med. Bull.* **34**:259.
Morris, P. J., Oliver, D. O., Bishop, M., Cullen, P., Fellows, G., French, M., Ledingham, J. C., Smith, J. C., Tiong, A., and Williams, K., 1978b, *Lancet* **2**:1153.
Morris, P. J., French, M. E., Ting, A., Frostick, S., and Hunnisett, A., 1982, in: *International Symposium on Cyclosporin A* (D. White, ed.), p. 355, Elsevier Biomedical, Amsterdam.
Myburgh, J. A., Smit, J. A., Maier, G., and Shapiro, M., 1977, *Lancet* **2**:241.
Natali, P. G., Martino, C., Quaranta, V., Nicotra, M. R., Frezza, F., Pellegrino, M. A., and Ferrone, S., 1981, *Transplantation* **31**:75.
Opelz, G., and Terasaki, P. I., 1980, in: *Histocompatibility Testing 1980* (P. I. Terasaki, ed.), p. 592, UCLA Tissue Typing Laboratory, Los Angeles.
Park, M. S., Terasaki, P. I., and Bernocco, D., 1977, *Lancet* **2**:465.
Park, M. S., Terasaki, P. I., Nakata, S., and Aoki, D., 1980, in: *Histocompatibility Testing 1980* (P. I. Terasaki, ed.), p. 854, UCLA Tissue Typing Laboratory, Los Angeles.
Patel, R., and Terasaki, P. I., 1969, *N. Engl. J. Med.* **280**:735.
Peto, R., Pike, M. C., Armitage, P., Breslow, N. E., Cox, D. R., Howard, M. V., Mantel, N., McPherson, K., Peto, J., and Smith, B. G., 1976, *Br. J. Cancer* **35**:1.
Prendergast, F. J., McGerachie, J. K., Fabre, J. W., Winearls, C. G., and Morris, P. J., 1978, *Transplantation* **27**:49.
Puri, J., and Lonai, P., 1980, *Eur. J. Immunol.* **10**:273.
Reekers, P., Lucassen-Hermans, R., Koene, R. A. P., and Kunst, V. A. J. M., 1977, *Lancet* **1**:1063.
Scott, H., Brandtzaeg, P., Hirschberg, H., Solheim, B. G., and Thorsby, E., 1981, *Tissue Antigens* **18**:195.
Shaw, S., Johnson, A. H., and Shearer, G. M., 1980, *J. Exp. Med.* **152**:565.
Soulillou, J. P., Peyrat, M. A., and Guenel, J., 1978, *Transplant. Proc.* **10**:475.
Stastny, P., and Austin, C. L., 1976, *Transplantation* **21**:399.
Steinman, R. M., and Witmer, M. C., 1978, *Proc. Natl. Acad. Sci. U.S.A.* **75**:5132.
Strenmuller, D., 1981, *Transplant. Proc.* **13**:1094.
Streilein, J. W., Toews, G. B., and Bergstresser, P. R., 1979, *Nature (London)* **282**:326.
Stuart, F. P., Siatoh, R., and Fitch, F. W., 1968, *Science* **160**:463.
Suthanthiran, M., Gailiunas, P., Person, A., Fagan, G., Strom, T. B., Carpenter, C. B., and Garovoy, M. R., 1978, *Transplant. Proc.* **10**:471.
Takahashi, H., Terasaki, P. I., Iwaki, Y., and Nakata, S., 1980, *Tissue Antigens* **16**:176.
Takahashi, H., Terasaki, P. I., Cicciarelli, J. C., Iwaki, Y., Nasu, H., and Slyker, T., 1981, *Tissue Antigens* **17**:67.
Terasaki, P. I. (ed.), 1980, *Histocompatibility Testing 1980*, UCLA Tissue Typing Laboratory, Los Angeles.
Thorsby, E., Moen, T., Solheim, B. G., Albrechtsen, D., Jakobsen, A., Jervell, J., Halvorsen, S., and Flatmark, A., 1981, *Tissue Antigens* **17**:83.
Ting, A., and Morris, P. J., 1977, *Lancet* **2**:1095.
Ting, A., and Morris, P. J., 1978a, *Transplantation* **25**:31.
Ting, A., and Morris, P. J., 1978b, *Lancet* **1**:575.
Ting, A., and Morris, P. J., 1980, *Lancet* **2**:282.
Ting, A., Mickey, M. R., and Terasaki, P. I., 1976, *J. Exp. Med.* **143**:981.
Tosi, R., Tanigaki, N., Centis, D., Ferrara, G. B., and Pressman, D., 1978, *J. Exp. Med.* **148**:1592.
van Rood, J. J., van Leeuwen, A., Keuning, J. J., and Blusse van Oud Alblas, A., 1975, *Tissue Antigens* **5**:73.
van Rood, J. J., Persijn, G. G., Paul, L. C., Cohen, B., Lansbergen, Q., Goulmy, E., Glaas, F. H. J., Baldwin, W., and van Es, L. A., 1981, in: *Proceedings of the Eighth Interna-*

tional Congress of Nephrology (W. Zurukzoglu, M. Papadimitriou, M. Pyrpasopoulos, M. Sion, and C. Zamboulis, eds.), p. 489, University Studio, Thessaloniki.

Williams, K. A., Hart, D. N., Fabre, J. W., and Morris, P. J., 1980a, *Transplantation* **29**:274.

Williams, K. A., Ting, A., French, M. E., Oliver, D., and Morris, P. J., 1980b, *Lancet* **1**:1104.

Williams, G. M., Hume, D. M., Hudson, R. P., Morris, P. J., Kano, K., and Milgrom, F., 1968, *N. Engl. J. Med.* **279**:611.

Winchester, R. J., Fu, S. M., Wernet, P., Kunkel, H. G., Dupont, B., and Jersild, C., 1975, *J. Exp. Med.* **141**:924.

Winearls, C. G., Fabre, J. W., Hart, D. N., Millard, P. R., and Morris, P. J., 1980, *Transplantation* **29**:462.

Yunis, E. J., and Amos, D. B., 1971, *Proc. Natl. Acad. Sci. U.S.A.* **68**:3031.

Changes in T-Lymphocyte Glycoprotein Structures Associated with Differentiation

J. R. L. Pink

Basel Institute for Immunology
CH-4005 Basel, Switzerland

I. INTRODUCTION

The problem to be discussed in this chapter is whether changes in the structure of lymphocyte surface glycoproteins—particularly changes in their carbohydrate portions—occur during normal lymphoid differentiation. A positive answer would argue against suggestions (reviewed in Gahmberg, 1981) that the principal role for glycoprotein carbohydrate is a general one, such as stabilizing protein structure, protecting polypeptide chains from proteolysis, or allowing transport of membrane glycoproteins to the cell surface. Information bearing on the problem is available for only a handful of proteins, of which three are major glycoprotein constituents of rodent thymocyte membranes. I will first discuss the identification and properties of these three proteins and then deal with the addition of sialic acid to these and other glycoproteins during T-lymphocyte differentiation; finally, these results will be compared to those obtained by workers studying glycoproteins from erythrocytes (the only other eukaryotic cell type for which comparable information on developmental changes in glycoprotein structure is available).

II. MAJOR THYMOCYTE GLYCOPROTEINS

A lymphocyte plasma membrane contains between 2 and 5% of the total cellular protein, and, of this fraction, about 10–15% is glycoprotein (Crumpton

89

and Snary, 1974; Standring and Williams, 1978). The major glycoproteins of lymphocyte membranes have been identified by four different methods: large-scale purification of membrane fractions (Crumpton and Snary, 1974; Standring and Williams, 1978); [^{3}H] borohydride-mediated reduction of cell-surface glyco-proteins (following oxidation by either sodium periodate or galactose oxidase) (Gahmberg *et al.*, 1976; Gahmberg and Andersson, 1977); selection of glycopro-teins by various lectins (Lotan and Nicolson, 1979); and lactoperoxidase-cata-lyzed radioiodination of cell-surface polypeptides (Morrison and Schonbaum, 1976), all, or almost all, of which are thought to be glycosylated (Gahmberg 1981).

The results of applying these techniques to rat thymocytes have been re-viewed elsewhere (Williams, 1982) and can be summarized as follows: In rat thymocyte *membrane fractions*, prepared from cells disrupted by shearing or by treatment with Tween-40, only three major bands are detected by periodic acid–Schiff staining after fractionation of the membrane proteins by electro-phoresis in sodium-dodecyl-sulfate-containing polyacrylamide gels (SDS–PAGE) (Standring and Williams, 1978). Table I lists the properties of these three glyco-proteins, which are the Thy-1 antigen, a heavily glycosylated leukocyte sialog-lycoprotein (LSGP) called W3/13,* and a high-molecular-weight glycoprotein called the leukocyte-common antigen (L-CA).

Tritiated *borohydride labeling* of rat thymocytes leads to a similar conclu-sion—the Thy-1, LSGP, and L-CA proteins [plus an unidentified band of apparent molecular weight (AMW) 50,000 (50K)] are the major tritium-labeled species detected by this method (Standring *et al.*, 1978), although at least four other protein bands are labeled less heavily. Borohydride labeling of mouse (Gahmberg *et al.*, 1976; Gahmberg and Andersson, 1977; Standring *et al.*, 1978; Kimura and Wigzell, 1978) and human (Axelsson *et al.*, 1978) thymocytes gives comparable results: The major labeled bands in these species are high-molecular-weight anti-gens corresponding to the L-CA and heavily labeled sialoglycoproteins probably corresponding to the rat LSGP. The mouse Thy-1 antigen is also labeled (Gahm-berg *et al.*, 1976; Standring *et al.*, 1978), although less strongly than the rat homolog. A strong band of AMW 50K and other fainter bands, including one of AMW about 25K, are also labeled on human thymocytes; whether the latter corresponds to the human Thy-1 (known to be present only in low amounts on thymocytes) (Dalchau and Fabre, 1979) or to another (possibly homologous?) protein is not known.

Several groups have used *lectins* to characterize major thymocyte glycopro-teins, following the demonstration by Hayman and Crumpton (1972) that the majority of pig lymphocyte surface glycoproteins (about 80% by weight) bind to

---

*Only about 50% of the rat LSGP band reacts with the W3/13 monoclonal antibody, for reasons still unknown. The term *LSGP* will be used to refer to the totality of the band, and *W3/13 antigen*, to the antigenically active material (Brown *et al.*, 1981; Williams, 1982).

Table I. Major Glycoproteins of Rat Thymocyte Membranes[a]

Protein	AMW (kD)[b]	Percent carbohydrate	Abundance[c]	Also expressed on
Thy-1	25	32	10^6	Neuronal cells, fibroblasts, connective tissue, myoblasts, immature B cells, hemopoietic stem cells
LSGP	95	60	10^5	Neutrophils, plasma cells, brain
L-CA	170	25	7×10^4	Most nucleated hemopoietic cells but no other tissues.

[a] Adapted from Williams (1982).
[b] Apparent molecular weight as derived from SDS–PAGE. Only for Thy-1 is the true molecular weight known (in this case 17.5 kD).
[c] Approximate number of molecules per cell, as measured by antibody binding to the cell surface.

concanavalin A (Con A) or lentil lectin. The L-CA and Thy-1 antigens are the major lentil-lectin-binding proteins of rat thymocytes (Standring and Williams, 1978); the observations of these authors that the LSGP does not bind to lentil lectin illustrates an obvious problem associated with this approach. Similarly, the major labeled proteins selected by Con A from lysates of radioiodinated mouse thymocytes have AMWs of about 200K and 25K and are homologous to the rat L-CA and Thy-1, respectively (Trowbridge et al., 1977; Kamarck and Gottlieb, 1980). In the case of biosynthetically labeled mouse thymocytes, however, the H-2D and -K antigens are the major labeled Con A-binding species (Nilsson and Waxdal, 1976). This apparently anomalous result is probably due to selective incorporation of biosynthetic label ($[^3H]$leucine) into a small proportion of actively metabolizing H-2-rich cells, since H-2 antigens are known not to be abundant on most thymocytes.

Radioiodination of rat or mouse thymocytes, without lectin selection, gives a somewhat more complex pattern of surface proteins (Trowbridge et al., 1977; Standring et al., 1978; Hoessli et al., 1980a) (see Fig. 4e), among which the L-CA and Thy-1 antigens are the most prominent, but the LSGP-type proteins are only weakly labeled. The likely reason for the poor ^{125}I-labeling of the LSGP can be deduced from the amino acid composition of the W3/13 antigen (Brown et al., 1981), which has only 0.5 tyrosine residue per 100 amino acids, as opposed to 3.8 and 2.1 tyrosines per 100 residues for the L-CA and Thy-1 antigens, respectively.

Clearly if there existed membrane proteins that were exposed at the cell surface but that lacked or were poor in tyrosine and carbohydrate (particularly sialic acid, galactose, and galactosamine), they could go undetected by the radioiodination procedure as well as by periodic acid–Schiff staining or borohydride reduction. The C-145 glycoprotein of mouse spleen cells (Pink et al., 1983), for example, is a poorly iodinatable asialoglycoprotein that may nevertheless be an abundant constituent of the cell membrane. Rough calculations suggest, however, that the three heavily glycosylated proteins already described (Thy-1, L-CA, and LSGP) may indeed account for a substantial proportion of the protein, as well as most of the protein-associated carbohydrate, exposed at the surface of rat thymocytes. According to Hayman and Crumpton (1972), glycoproteins constitute about 15% by weight of total membrane protein. Given a membrane protein yield of about 2.8 mg per 10^{10} thymocytes (Standring and Williams, 1978) and the data in Table I (and assuming a molecular weight of 75K for the W3/13 antigen; see page 99), one can estimate that the Thy-1, L-CA, and W3/13 proteins account for approximately 50% of the membrane glycoprotein. In addition, these three proteins account together for about 10^7 sialic acid residues (Brown *et al.*, 1981), a value comparable to the total number of acid-hydrolyzable sialic acid residues on the cell [if the figures given by Despont *et al.* (1975) for the sialic acid content of mouse thymocytes also apply to rat thymocytes]. While such calculations are only approximate, they do accord with the idea that the molecules listed in Table I, plus, possibly, a similar quantity of less heavily glycosylated species, make up most of the protein exposed at the surface of rodent thymocytes.

How far these results apply to lymphocytes from other organs, or from other species, is not clear. Thy-1 is not a major component of mouse peripheral T cells, and it is not detectable on peripheral T cells from various other species. The absence of 10^6 Thy-1 molecules from those cells, however, could be approximately balanced by the presence of major histocompatibility antigens (2×10^5 molecules per peripheral lymphocyte; much less on most thymocytes), which contain about 12% carbohydrate (Williams, 1982). Mature B cells from rodents lack both Thy-1 and LSGP-type antigens but express immunoglobulin and Ia antigens at levels of about 10^5 molecules per cell—again approximately sufficient to compensate for the absence of the T-cell-specific proteins. The phylogenetic question is less easily answered since Thy-1, although a major component of rodent thymocytes, is present at very low levels or not detectable on thymocytes from various other species (humans, dogs, chickens) (Williams and Gagnon, 1982; Williams, 1982). These species may have other major thymocyte glycoproteins. Possible candidates are proteins of AMW 55–65K. The major iodinatable protein of avian thymocytes has an apparent molecular weight of about 65K (Pink *et al.*, 1981), for example, and a major Con A-binding protein from rabbit thymocytes (Schmidt-Ullrich *et al.*, 1978) has an AMW of about 55K.

III. DIFFERENTIATION-ASSOCIATED CHANGES IN THYMOCYTE GLYCOPROTEIN STRUCTURES

In this section, I will discuss the evidence that the structures of the glycoproteins listed in Table I change when a thymocyte differentiates into a mature, peripheral T cell. Such evidence comes mainly from comparisons of molecules isolated from these two cell types. If any difference is found, one is entitled to say that the change is associated with thymocyte maturation only if most peripheral T cells are in fact derived from typical thymocytes and not from some minor unusual thymocyte subpopulation. I make this assumption for the purposes of this review, but one should note that the question of the origin of peripheral T cells is still controversial (see Stutman, 1978; Sharon, 1983).

A. Thy-1

1. Structure and Heterogeneity

Thy-1 antigens have been purified from rat, mouse, dog, and human tissues, and the relatedness of these antigens has been confirmed by serological cross-reaction (Dalchau and Fabre, 1979; Ades et al., 1980). Thy-1-like molecules have also been isolated from the brains of chicken and squid (see Williams and Gagnon, 1982). As mentioned in Section II, the tissue distributions of Thy-1-like proteins differ in different species: The distributions suggest that Thy-1 is a nervous tissue component in all vertebrates (and perhaps in invertebrates too) but that its presence on lymphoid cells is species-dependent.

The Thy-1 antigen as isolated from rat brain and thymus is a protein of molecular weight about 17K, consisting of 111 amino acids and about 30% by weight carbohydrate (Barclay et al., 1976) (Table I). Its amino acid sequence shows a surprising homology of about 20% to immunoglobulin domain sequences (Campbell et al., 1981; Cohen et al., 1981) and is also unusual in that an unidentified substance (possibly lipid or glycolipid) is attached to the protein's carboxy terminus; the unidentified material is presumably responsible for the hydrophobic properties of the molecule (Campbell et al., 1981). Rat brain Thy-1 contains three N-linked oligosaccharide chains, each of which includes two or three glucosamine residues (presumably N-acylated) but no galactosamine. The overall carbohydrate compositions of the brain and thymic Thy-1 molecules are given in Table II (Barclay et al., 1976). These compositions, and studies on the biosynthesis of Thy-1 in a mouse T lymphoma line and various mutants derived from it (Trowbridge et al., 1978), suggest that (as discussed in the next section) Thy-1 molecules from different sources can contain both high-mannose and complex oligosaccharides (Fig. 1). The properties of the mutant cell lines also suggest that alterations in the carbohydrate structure of Thy-1 can prevent its expression at the cell surface (Trowbridge et al., 1978).

The Thy-1 protein sequence (at least in rodents) is almost certainly the product of a single gene, since there is no evidence of amino acid sequence heterogeneity in the rat or mouse Thy-1 structures, and, more importantly, the Thy-1 genetic polymorphism in mice has been correlated with a single amino acid substitution: the Thy-1.1 and Thy-1.2 molecules have arginine or glutamine, respectively, at position 89 of the protein chain (Williams and Gagnon, 1982).

Table II. Carbohydrate Compositions of Glycoproteins Listed in Table I[a]

Protein	Source	Carbohydrate residues per 100 amino acids or (per molecule)[b]						
		Fucose	Mannose	Galactose	Glucosamine[c]	Galactosamine[c]	Sialic acid	Sialic acid[d]
Thy-1	Brain	1.8 (2.0)	11.9 (13.2)	1.8 (2.0)	8.3 (9.1)	1.0 (1.1)	0.2 (0.2)	0.3 (0.3)
	Thymus (lentil-lectin-binding)	1.0 (1.1)	10.6 (11.7)	5.5 (6.0)	9.4 (10.3)	0 (0)	1.8 (2.0)	2.1 (2.3)
	Thymus (not lectin-bound)	0.9 (1.0)	9.4 (10.3)	6.9 (7.6)	11.7 (12.9)	0 (0)	2.2 (2.4)	2.9 (3.2)
LSGP	Thymus	0	0	22.3	0	20.1	27.5	27.2
L-CA	Thymus	0.9	4.4	3.6	5.7	1.1	5.4	2.9

[a] Adapted from Barclay et al. (1976) and Brown et al. (1981).
[b] Determined by gas–liquid chromatography after methanolysis and trimethylsialylation.
[c] Assumed to be N-acetylated.
[d] Determined fluorimetrically.

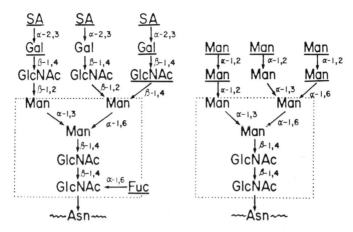

Figure 1. Structures of representative complex (left) and high-mannose (right) oligosaccharides. The common core structure is outlined. Many variants of these representative structures have been found in different glycoproteins; some or all of the underlined residues are missing in typical variants. Adapted from Hubbard and Ivatt (1981).

This polymorphism is expressed by brain as well as lymphoid Thy-1 molecules (Letarte and Meghji, 1978).

Nevertheless, mouse thymocyte Thy-1 preparations subjected to two-dimensional electrophoresis show extensive heterogeneity both in charge and in AMW (Fig. 2a). Almost all of the charge heterogeneity disappears after neuraminidase treatment, and it is presumably due to variation in the number of sialic acid residues per Thy-1 molecule (Ledbetter and Herzenberg, 1979; Hoessli et al., 1980b; Carlsson and Stigbrand, 1982). The AMW heterogeneity is not reduced by neuraminidase treatment and is presumably due to variation in content of neutral sugars. The observations that lentil or pea lectins bind only to Thy-1 molecules of lower AMW (Trowbridge et al., 1977; Standring and Williams, 1978; Ledbetter and Herzenberg, 1979), together with the carbohydrate compositions of lectin-binding and nonbinding forms (Table II), suggest that variations in number of mannose residues and in type of substituent attached to these residues both contribute to Thy-1 heterogeneity.

2. Differences among Thy-1 from Different Cell Types

Thy-1 antigens from rat *brain and thymus* have indistinguishable amino acid compositions but very different carbohydrate residues (Barclay et al., 1976). The carbohydrate compositions of Thy-1 from brain and of the lentil-lectin-binding and nonbinding thymic Thy-1 species are given in Table II. These preparations are presumably all heterogeneous, as discussed above; nevertheless the results show clearly that thymic Thy-1 has less mannose and fucose, and more

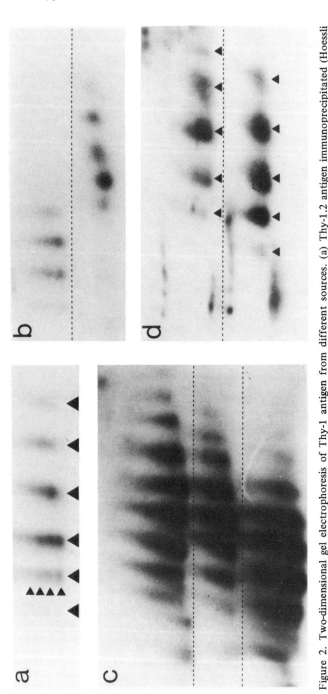

Figure 2. Two-dimensional gel electrophoresis of Thy-1 antigen from different sources. (a) Thy-1.2 antigen immunoprecipitated (Hoessli *et al.*, 1980b) from radioiodinated AKR.Cum mouse *thymocytes*. The immunoprecipitated material was analyzed by nonequilibrium pH gradient electrophoresis from right (acidic) to left (basic) for 1800 V-hr, followed by SDS–PAGE in a 12.5% polyacrylamide gel (from top to bottom). The dried gel was exposed for autoradiography in contact with an intensifying screen for 9 days; only a part of the autoradiogram is shown. Note heterogeneity in both charge (▲) and molecular weight (▲) of Thy-1. The pattern given by the Thy-1.1 antigen is similar to that of Thy-1.2 but is shifted to the left by one charge unit (Hoessli *et al.*, 1980b). (b) Thy-1.1 antigen immunoprecipitated from radioiodinated AKR mouse *thymocytes* (top) and *lymph node cells* (bottom), analyzed as above. The figure shows a montage of portions of the two autoradiograms, arranged so that proteins with the same pI would be vertically aligned. Lymph node Thy-1 is more acidic than thymic Thy-1. (c) Montage of three autoradiograms, aligned as in (b), showing Thy-1.2 antigen immunoprecipitated from radioiodinated Con A-stimulated *blasts* (top), blasts stimulated in a primary one-way mixed leukocyte reaction (middle), and *thymocytes* (bottom). Thy-1 from blasts is slightly more acidic than thymocyte Thy-1. Blasts were prepared according to Irlé *et al.* (1978) from C57Bl/6 mice (irradiated cells from DBA/2 mice were used to stimulate in the mixed leukocyte reaction). (d) Montage of two autoradiograms, aligned as in (b), showing Thy-1.2 (▲) in total lysates of radioiodinated PI798 T *lymphoma* cells (top) and BALB/c *thymocytes* (bottom). Lysates were prepared for electrophoresis as in Hoessli *et al.* (1980b).

glucosamine, galactose, and sialic acid, than brain Thy-1. Analyses of human, rat, or mouse Thy-1 by one- or two-dimensional electrophoresis (Barclay *et al.*, 1976; Cotmore *et al.*, 1981; Hooghe-Peters and Hooghe, 1982) suggest that *fibroblast* and nervous tissue Thy-1 have similar structures, both being less heterogeneous in charge and in AMW than thymic Thy-1.

All these results are consistent in a general way with the replacement of typical high-mannose carbohydrate chains (in brain or fibroblasts) by typical complex oligosaccharides (in thymus) (see Fig. 1). The compositions in Table II also suggest, however, that brain Thy-1 oligosaccharides cannot be entirely high-mannose (since they contain fucose and galactose) and that their thymic counterparts cannot be entirely typical complex oligosaccharides (since these would contain only three mannose residues per chain or nine per Thy-1 molecule).

It is possible that brain and thymic Thy-1 molecules differ not only in the structure of their N-linked oligosaccharide chains but also in the structure of the unidentified material attached to the carboxy terminus of the chain: Rat thymic Thy-1 contains no galactosamine, whereas the carboxy-terminal peptide of brain Thy-1 contains a single galactosamine residue not present in a conventional N- or O-linked carbohydrate chain (Campbell *et al.*, 1981). This interesting possibility deserves further exploration.

A difference between Thy-1 molecules from mouse *thymic and peripheral T cells* was observed by Hoessli *et al.* (1980b), who showed that peripheral Thy-1 was more acidic than thymic Thy-1 (Fig. 2b). This charge difference was entirely due to the presence of extra sialic acid residues on the lymph-node-derived molecules. The average number of extra residues per peripheral Thy-1 can be estimated as about four, if it is assumed that a single charge difference is responsible for the pI differences between adjacent Thy-1 spots in Fig. 2. This estimate is consistent with the addition of one to two sialic acid residues (plus, possibly, neutral sugars as well) to each of the molecule's three complex oligosaccharide chains. In peripheral Thy-1, but not thymic Thy-1, the molecules of highest AMW have the highest sialic acid content, suggesting that Thy-1 carries two classes of sialic acid addition site: a class where sialic acid addition does not result in an observable increase in AMW and a class, occupied only in peripheral Thy-1 molecules, where sialic acid addition is correlated with increased AMW. The fact that sialic acid residues in different environments can have different effects on the mobility of a glycoprotein (glycophorin) in gel electrophoresis has been documented by Gahmberg and Andersson (1982).

Thy-1 from T-lymphoma *cell lines* (Trowbridge *et al.*, 1977; Ledbetter and Herzenberg, 1979) or cloned cytotoxic or helper T-cell lines (Sarmiento *et al.*, 1981) is, at least for some lines, less heterogeneous than thymic Thy-1. Sarmiento *et al.* (1981) also noted small differences (in one-dimensional electrophoretic analysis) between Thy-1 immunoprecipitated from different cell lines or from subsets of thymocytes sorted according to their Thy-1 content. In addition, Thy-1 from at least some T-lymphoma lines or from peripheral *T-cell blasts* (stimulated by Con A or in a mixed leukocyte reaction) is intermediate in average charge between thymic and T-lymphocyte Thy-1 (Fig. 2c, d).

These observations that a given cell type makes a characteristic range of Thy-1 structures (each with, presumably, a characteristic sialic acid content) have not led, however, to any useful correlation between cell *function* and Thy-1 type. Indeed, although total cellular sialic acid content (and thus sialylation of Thy-1) may be related to the ability of the cell to circulate *in vivo* (see Section IV), it is unlikely that Thy-1, given its tissue distribution in different species, has any specific function in lymphoid cells (Williams, 1982).

3. Antigenic Properties of Thy-1 from Different Cell Types

Structurally different Thy-1 molecules might conceivably also differ antigenically. Thomas *et al.* (1978) prepared antisera (in rats) that reacted with mouse brain and thymic tissue and with peripheral T cells from adult, but not 1- or 2-week-old, mice; they suggested that the sera might react with mature as opposed to immature Thy-1. However, it is obvious that studies on tissue distribution alone are insufficient to substantiate such a claim. Stronger evidence for antigenically distinct forms of Thy-1 is that of Auchincloss *et al.* (1982), who describe a monoclonal antibody cytotoxic for thymocytes carrying Thy-1.1 or Thy-1.2 alleles and for peripheral T cells carrying the Thy-1.2 but not the Thy-1.1 allele. The antibody did not react with brain homogenates of either Thy-1 type. Although the authors suggest that the Thy-1.1 antigen may undergo modification during T-cell development, this conjecture must still be considered as not proven, as other explanations of their results are possible. For example, the antibody might react preferentially with complexes or dimers of Thy-1, these being formed more readily with Thy-1.2 than Thy-1.1 molecules and more readily on thymocytes than on peripheral T cells, where Thy-1 concentrations are low.

Further evidence that there might exist antigenically different forms of Thy-1 is that of Sidman *et al.* (1980), who prepared a monoclonal antibody reactive with mouse Thy-1.1 or Thy-1.2 thymocytes, but not peripheral T cells, in immunofluorescence and immunoprecipitation, as well as cytotoxicity assays. The antibody clearly precipitated the Thy-1 antigen from lysates of ^{125}I-labeled thymocytes; however, a previously undescribed 17K polypeptide was also present in these precipitates. These results are unusual, since such coprecipitation of Thy-1 with other proteins has not consistently been observed by any previous workers (Trowbridge *et al.*, 1975; Barclay *et al.*, 1976; Ledbetter and Herzenberg, 1979; Hoessli *et al.*, 1980b). Thus the specificity of the antibody in question is not yet clearly defined; it is possible, for example, that the antibody's target is in fact the 17K polypeptide, and that complexes of this polypeptide with the Thy-1 antigen were present in the conditions of immunoprecipitation used by Sidman *et al.* (1980). In view of this possibility, the question of whether there exist antigenic differences between Thy-1 molecules from different tissues still remains open.

B. W3/13 and Related Lymphocyte Sialoglycoproteins

1. Structure

The W3/13 antigen has been purified (by passage over a monoclonal antibody column) from rat thymocytes (Brown et al., 1981). It is a heavily glycosylated protein (about 60% carbohydrate by weight) whose apparent molecular weight is 95K. Its true molecular weight may be nearer 75K, in view of the fact that glycophorin, which has a rather similar chemical composition to W3/13 (Brown et al., 1981), has an AMW of 39K and a true molecular weight of 31K (see Gahmberg and Andersson, 1982). The carbohydrate composition of the W3/13 antigen (Table 2) suggests that it contains a large number (about 20 per 100 amino acids) of short O-linked carbohydrate chains, possibly of the structure (see Kornfeld and Kornfeld, 1980)

$$\pm \text{Sialic acid} \xrightarrow{\alpha 2-3} \text{Gal} \xrightarrow{\beta 1-3} \text{GalNAc} \rightarrow \text{Ser/Thr}$$
$$\uparrow \alpha 2-6$$
$$\text{Sialic acid}$$

As previously mentioned, proteins that are probably homologous to W3/13 have been described on mouse and human thymocytes. These proteins, called LSGPs (Williams, 1982), have slightly different AMWs (Table III) but share the properties of being present on T but not B cells, of being major borohydride-labeled glycoproteins on thymocytes of each species, and of having their mobilities in SDS–PAGE reduced by neuraminidase treatment. This last property is unusual; for example, neuraminidase treatment of H-2, IgM or IgD, T-200, or Thy-1 chains increases their mobilities in SDS–PAGE, although glycophorin (Gahmberg and Andersson, 1982) behaves like the W3/13 antigen.

The lectin-binding properties of these major borohydride-labeled thymocyte proteins are also unusual. First, the rat and mouse LSGPs are the major peanut agglutinin (PNA)-binding proteins on native (non-enzyme-treated) thymocytes, although not all of the LSGP molecules (from either species) bind the lectin (Brown and Williams, 1982). This lectin reacts strongly with terminal β1-3-linked galactose residues, consistent with the idea that the lectin binds to the less sialylated forms of the O-linked structure illustrated previously. A comparison of the number of PNA-binding sites on mouse thymocytes (about 10^6) (Sharon, 1980) with the number of LSGP molecules per rat thymocyte (about 10^5) (Brown et al., 1981) suggests that many lectin molecules may bind to one LSGP. This is possible, given that the W3/13 molecule has one oligosaccharide chain for every five amino acids, but it seems unlikely that a single W3/13 glycoprotein

Table III. Apparent Molecular Weight ($\times 10^{-3}$) and Lectin-Binding
Specificities[a] of Major Borohydride-Labeled LSGPs from Different
Sources before and after Neuraminidase Treatment[b]

Source	Rat		Mouse		Human	
	Before	After	Before	After	Before	After
Thymus	95	110	100	130	105	120
	(PNA+)	(PNA+)	(HP+,PNA+)	(HP+)		
Peripheral	95	110	100	130	105	120
T cells	(PNA−)	(PNA+)	(HP−,PNA−)	(HP+,VV−)	(HP−)	(HP+,VV−)
Activated	Not done		135	145	120	130
T cells			(VV+,HP−)		(VV+,HP−)	(VV+,HP−)

[a] PNA, peanut agglutinin; HP, *Helix pomatia* lectin; VV, *Vicia villosa* lectin. (+) Indicates
binding to some or all of the relevant glycoprotein molecules; (−) indicates absence of
binding.
[b] References: Rat: Brown and Williams (1982). Mouse: Axelsson *et al.* (1978), Gahmberg
and Andersson (1977), Kimura and Wigzell (1978), Conzelmann *et al.* (1980), Brown and
Williams (1982). Human: Andersson *et al.* (1978), Axelsson *et al.* (1978), Gahmberg and
Andersson (1977), Dalchau *et al.* (1980).

could bind ten or more lectin molecules, and it may be that the lectin, when
bound to whole cells, interacts with glycolipids as well as the LSGP glycoproteins.

Second, the LSGPs from mouse and human thymocytes are the major *Helix
pomatia* (HP) lectin-binding proteins on these cells (the rat LSGP has not been
tested for HP binding) (Axelsson *et al.*, 1978). Again, neuraminidase treatment is
not required for binding to occur. These results, at first sight, suggest that thymic
LSGP molecules carry terminal N-acetylgalactosamine residues, since the HP
lectin exhibits at least tenfold higher affinity for this residue than for galactose.
However, HP lectin does bind weakly to terminal galactose residues (Goldstein
and Hayes, 1978), and it is possible that it binds to the same terminal galactose
residues as does PNA.

2. Differences among LSGPs from Different Cell Types

Axelsson *et al.* (1978) compared the LSGPs of human *thymocytes and
peripheral T cells* and showed that LSGPs from neuraminidase-treated cells of
both types, and from untreated thymocytes, bound HP lectin; however, the
LSGPs from untreated peripheral cells did not bind to the lectin (Hellström
et al., 1976). Similarly, Brown and Williams (1982) showed that PNA would
bind to rat thymocyte LSGP but not peripheral T-cell LSGP, in the absence of
neuraminidase treatment of the cells. These results strongly suggest that LSGPs,
like Thy-1, have sialic acid acceptor sites that are occupied only in peripheral
T cells. Whether the presence of extra sialic acid is the only difference between
thymic and peripheral LSGP is not clear: Rat thymic LSGP contains no glucos-

amine (Table II), but the presence of N-acetylglucosamine on human peripheral lymphocyte LSGP is suggested by the reaction of this molecule with a cold agglutinin antibody with specificity for $Gal \xrightarrow{\beta 1-4} GlcNAc$ β1-6 structures (Childs and Feizi, 1981).

Andersson *et al.* (1978) and Kimura and Wigzell (1978) compared the boro-hydride-labeled proteins of *cytotoxic T-cell* populations (obtained from mixed leukocyte reactions or Con A-stimulated T-cell cultures) with the labeled proteins from thymocytes or peripheral T cells. They found, for both mouse and human lymphocytes, that the most heavily labeled band in the cytotoxic T-cell populations had a higher AMW than that in the unstimulated cells (Table III) and that this band (which, in the case of mouse cells, was called T-145) no longer bound HP lectin, but was instead the major *Vicia villosa* (VV) lectin-binding protein on the cytotoxic T-cell surface. The most straightforward interpretation of these results (Conzelmann *et al.*, 1980) is that the "cytotoxic T-cell specific" T-145 protein is a modified form of the resting T-cell LSGP. The admittedly indirect evidence for a relationship between the two can be summarized as follows:

- Both proteins (like W3/13) are very acidic and are heavily labeled by boro-hydride reduction techniques but not by lactoperoxidase-catalyzed radio-iodination of whole cells.
- The mobilities of both proteins in SDS–PAGE are decreased by neurami-nidase treatment.
- The HP and VV lectins bound by LSGP and T-145 respectively have related but not identical specificities. Both bind to terminal N-acetylgalactosamine residues, VV showing a strong preference for α1-3-linked termini. How-ever, the binding of VV is not simply to this residue, since, for example, fucosylation on the galactose of the blood-group-substance-derived oligo-saccharide GalNAc $\rightarrow$ Gal $\rightarrow$ GlcNAc strikingly reduces its ability to bind to VV, but not to HP (Kaladas *et al.*, 1981). The weak affinity of both lectins for terminal galactose is of similar magnitude. On the basis of present knowledge, it is difficult to explain why VV, but not HP, should bind T-145, since none of the mono- or oligosaccharides tested for bind-ing to VV and HP has shown a strong preference for the former (Kaladas *et al.*, 1981; Hammarström, 1972).
- There is evidence for the existence of proteins intermediate in structure between LSGP and T-145. The postulated intermediate forms bind both HP and VV lectins, although the resting T-cell LSGP binds only HP lectin and the T-145 from Con A-stimulated blasts was defined as binding only VV.

In the original studies on mouse and human LSGP, it was reported that all mouse *T-lymphoma lines*, or human T leukemia cells, expressed this protein (Axelsson *et al.*, 1978). No variations in AMW between LSGPs from one species but of different cellular origin were observed, and all the LSGP proteins bound HP lectin, but not VV, after neuraminidase treatment. In contrast, all the *cytotoxic T-cell lines* (of mouse origin) studied by Conzelmann *et al.* (1980) expressed a T-145-like protein, believed to be a modified form of the normal T-cell LSGP. After neuraminidase treatment, this protein bound both HP and VV lectins and therefore seemed likely to be a form intermediate between the resting T-cell LSGP and the Con A-blast-derived T-145. However, an alternative possibility— that the protein was a mixture of HP- and VV-binding species—was not excluded.

Altevogt *et al.* (1982) obtained somewhat similar results in analyses of a mouse T-cell lymphoma, which expressed the HP-binding LSGP typical of normal T cells, and of its more metastatic variants. Some of these variants instead expressed a T-145-like VV-binding protein, and this protein also bound HP, again consistent with the idea that there exist intermediate forms between the resting T-cell LSGP and the T-145 protein obtained from Con A blasts.

Purification of an LSGP-like protein from a human T-cell line has provided further evidence for variation in LSGP oligosaccharide structures (Saito *et al.*, 1978; Saito and Osawa, 1980). Analysis of this material shows that it contains less total carbohydrates but more mannose, fucose, and glucosamine than rat thymocyte W3/13. Although it is possible that some of these differences are due to impurities in the human LSGP preparation, this material bound strongly to PNA (after neuraminidase treatment) and gave rise, on alkaline hydrolysis, to oligosaccharides with compositions (equimolar sialic acid, galactose, N-acetyl-galactosamine, plus or minus fucose) corresponding closely to the rat LSGP oligosaccharide structure proposed on page 99. The additional fucose in one of the human oligosaccharides could be tissue- or species-specific; alternatively, the W3/13 antigen could represent a nonfucosylated subpopulation of rat thymocyte LSGP (see footnote to page 90).

3. Function

Although it was natural for Kimura and Wigzell (1978) to propose a role in cytotoxicity for the VV-binding T-145 protein obtained from cytotoxic T-cell populations, subsequent results have made this suggestion unlikely. First, MacDonald *et al.* (1981) and Kaufmann and Berke (1981) found no strong correlation between the cytotoxic capacity of various lymphoid cell populations and their expression of VV lectin binding or of T-145. Second, Conzelmann *et al.* (1980) selected for VV-resistant mutants from cytotoxic cell lines and obtained clones that were still cytotoxic, although binding up to 100-fold less VV than the parental line. (However, these lines expressed modified T-145-like proteins, which still bound VV, although their AMWs were higher than that of the parental T-145.) Finally, as mentioned previously, some metastatic clones derived from a T lymphoma without known cytotoxic activity express T-145-like proteins (Altevogt *et al.*, 1982). Thus the roles of the T-145 protein on activated T cells and of the LSGP proteins on resting T cells, neutrophils, and granulocytes remain unknown.

C. High-Molecular-Weight Glycoproteins

1. Structure

L-CA and T-200 are the terms originally used to describe a family of related, high-molecular-weight glycoproteins present on rat (Sunderland et al., 1979) or mouse (Trowbridge et al., 1975; Trowbridge, 1978) lymphocytes, respectively. A homologous protein family has also been described on human lymphocytes (Dalchau et al., 1980; Omary et al., 1980a). In each of these species, antigenically cross-reactive proteins with slightly different AMWs are present on different lymphocyte classes: Proteins of the mouse T-200 family, for example, have AMWs of 180K on thymocytes, 190K and 200 K on peripheral T cells, and 220K on B cells (Trowbridge, 1978; Dunlap et al., 1980; Hoessli and Vassalli, 1980). Peptide mapping of these proteins shows that they have similar structures (Dunlap et al., 1980; Hoessli et al., 1982; Sarmiento et al., 1982). Similar results have been obtained for the corresponding human proteins (Omary et al., 1980a).

The rat L-CA protein has been purified from thymocytes by Sunderland et al. (1979). The L-CA is a glycoprotein containing about 25% carbohydrate by weight; the carbohydrate composition (Table II) is compatible with the idea that the molecule contains several (perhaps 10–15) complex N-linked oligosaccharide chains, and possibly a smaller number of O-linked chains as well (Brown et al., 1981). The L-CA and T-200 proteins are present on thymocytes in amounts of about 5–10 × 10^4 molecules/cell and (like their human homolog) are present on monocytes, granulocytes, and other hemopoietic cells as well as on lymphocytes. Limited tryptic proteolysis of T-200 (Omary and Trowbridge, 1980) splits the molecule approximately in its center and suggests that the molecule consists of a glycosylated extracellular domain and a phosphorylated intracellular domain joined by a membrane-inserted hydrophobic region.

2. Differences among L-CA-like Glycoproteins from Different Cell Types

The basic observation that L-CA-type glycoproteins of different origins have different AMWs but are serologically cross-reactive and biochemically similar could be explained as resulting from (1) postsynthetic modification of a single gene product, (2) variations in nucleic acid rearrangement or processing in different cells, resulting in products sharing some amino-acid sequences of identical genetic origin, or (3) activation of different members of a multigene family in different cell types. None of these possibilities has so far been excluded, but possibility (3) is made less likely by the finding of genetic markers on T-200 and L-CA, coupled with the observation that all forms of T-200 or L-CA, whether on T or B cells or on thymocytes, react with the appropriate alloantisera (Michaelson *et al.*, 1979; Omary *et al.* 1980b; Siadak and Nowinski, 1980; Carter and Sunderland, 1980). The alloantigens involved (Ly-5 in the mouse, ART-1 in the rat) are inherited in a simple Mendelian fashion, a finding clearly consistent with possibilities (1) and (2); however, possibility (3) can be kept alive by postulating either that the various different forms of T-200 or L-CA are encoded by a corresponding number of linked genes, all of which are polymorphic and immunogenic, or that the Ly-5 or ART-1 alloantigens result from similar postsynthetic modifications of related but not identical polypeptides.

The idea that different forms of T-200 differ in carbohydrate content is supported by several observations. Hoessli and Vassalli (1980) demonstrated that the various T-200 species differed in charge but also showed that, after neuraminidase treatment, the *peripheral* T-200 species of lowest AMW was very similar to *thymic* T-200 in two-dimensional gel electrophoretic pattern, suggesting that the native forms of the molecules might differ in their sialic acid content. However, the higher-AMW forms of T-200 could still be distinguished after neuraminidase treatment, so that differential sialylation cannot account completely for T-200 variation.

Differences in lectin-binding properties of different forms of the L-CA and T-200 antigens were reported by Brown and Williams (1982) (Table IV). These authors reported that at least some L-CA molecules from peripheral T or B cells, but no thymocyte L-CA, bound to PNA after neuraminidase treatment, suggesting that oligosaccharides containing sialylated β1-3-linked galactose residues are present in some peripheral, but not thymic, L-CA species. In addition, the B-lymphocyte L-CA was the major soybean-agglutinin-binding protein on these

Table IV. Lectin-Binding Specificities[a] of
High-Molecular-Weight (L-CA or T-200-Related)
Glycoproteins from Different Sources before
or after Neuraminidase Treatment

Source	Rat		Mouse
	Before	After	Before
Thymus	PNA−,SB−	PNA−,SB−	PNA+,SB+?
Peripheral			
T cells	PNA−,SB−	PNA+,SB?	PNA−,SB−
B cells	PNA−,SB+	PNA+,SB+	PNA−,SB+

[a]PNA, peanut agglutinin; SB, soybean lectin. (+) Indicates lectin binding to some or all of the relevant glycoprotein molecules; (−) indicates absence of binding. Data summarized from Brown and Williams (1982). Sidman *et al.* (1980) also show that mouse thymocyte high-molecular-weight glycoproteins, probably including T-200, bind PNA.

cells (either before or after neuraminidase treatment), whereas little or no binding of peripheral T-cell L-CA and none of thymocyte L-CA to the lectin was observed. These findings are good evidence for differences in galactose, and perhaps also *N*-acetylgalactosamine, content of different forms of L-CA.

Childs and Feizi (1981) used antibodies against the blood group antigens I and i to precipitate material carrying I or i specificities from neuraminidase-treated, borohydride-labeled human lymphoid cells. The principal result was that high molecular-weight glycoproteins of B cells (from tonsils or B lymphoma) carried both I and i determinants, whose proposed structures are shown in Fig. 3; however, very little I- or i-positive material with AMW greater than 150K could be precipitated from thymocytes or T-cell lines. The labeled bands precipitated from B lymphocytes had AMWs ranging from 200K to 280K; of these, bands of AMW 200K and 240K reacted with an antibody against structure A of Fig. 3, and bands of AMW 260K and 280K reacted with antibodies against structures B and C of Fig. 3, respectively. Unfortunately it is not clear from these authors' results how many of the labeled bands belong to the L-CA family. The finding of four labeled high-molecular-weight glycoprotein bands in a pure B-cell population is unexpected and is possibly due to the presence of contaminating peripheral T cells in the tonsillar B-cell preparation. If this assumption is correct, the results of Childs and Feizi (1981) suggest that human thymic L-CA carries very little I or i activity, that peripheral B-cell L-CA carries I activity associated with structure C of Fig. 3, and possibly i activity as well; and that peripheral T-cell L-CA may also carry both I and i activity. The authors' observation that L-CA antigen from rat spleen, but not thymus, carries at least the i activity (as measured in an inhibition of binding assay with anti-i antibodies) is consistent

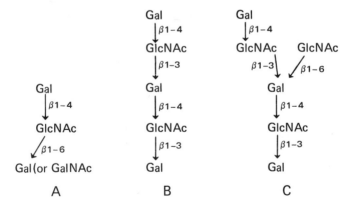

Figure 3. The minimum carbohydrate structures known to react with two different anti-I antibodies (a, c) and one anti-i antibody (b). The i and I determinants are present on linear or branched oligosaccharides, respectively, containing repeating disaccharide (lactosamine) structures. From Childs and Feizi (1981).

with these results and also with the observations of Brown and Williams (1982) that PNA-binding terminal galactose residues are present (after neuraminidase treatment) on peripheral, but not thymic, L-CA molecules.

In agreement with these findings that L-CAs of different origin are antigenically distinct, several groups have observed clearcut (monoclonal-antibody-defined) antigenic differences between L-CA (T-200) molecules present on different types of mouse lymphocytes. Coffman and Weissman (1981a,b) and Kincade *et al.* (1981) prepared monoclonal antibodies that react only with L-CA on B and pre-B cells and on a small proportion of peripheral T cells (including at least some Lyt-2-positive cells). An antibody exhibiting a similar preferential binding to human B-cell L-CA has also been described (Dalchau and Fabre, 1981). However, whether any of these antibodies react with carbohydrate structures on L-CA is not yet clear.

Studies on *tumors and cell lines* of both mouse and human origin show that there is considerable variability in the AMWs of high-molecular-weight glycoproteins from different lines. The main conclusions from these surveys (Judd *et al.*, 1980; Sarmiento *et al.*, 1980; Bach *et al.*, 1981; Glasebrook *et al.*, 1981; Bron *et al.*, 1981; Hoessli *et al.*, 1982) are (1) that variation occurs not only in the L-CA or T-200 protein families, but also in other high-molecular-weight glycoproteins (which will not be discussed further here) (see Fig. 4); (2) that many (at least four to five) different forms of L-CA or T-200 are represented on the cell lines; (3) that one cell line can make two or more different forms of L-CA or T-200 protein; (4) that, at least in human cell lines, the forms of L-CA with higher AMW are richest in sialic acid, but the variations in AMW are not due simply to changes in sialic acid content (Fig. 4) (Morishima *et al.*, 1982); and (5) disappointingly, that the variations have no consistent relationship to the function of the cell line; for example, some but not all cloned cytotoxic T-cell lines express a T-200-like protein (B-220) with the AMW (220K) typical of that for normal B cells (Fig. 4) (Hoessli *et al.*, 1982). Similar observations on human T-cell lines were made by Morishima *et al.* (1982). These studies are all consistent with the notion that variation in AMW of high-molecular-weight glycoproteins is due to variability in their carbohydrate content; however, the variability seems not to be important for growth or function of the cells *in vitro*.

Biosynthesis of T-200 was studied in murine cell lines and mitogen-induced blasts by Watson *et al.* (1981) and Sarmiento *et al.* (1982). The T-cell blasts resulting from stimulation of peripheral lymphocytes (for example, with Con A) have an extra, antigenically distinct T-200 band (T-200A) of higher AMW than the T-200 form on resting T cells (Dunlap *et al.*, 1978; Sarmiento *et al.*, 1982). Precursors of T-200 in a T-cell line and in B-cell blasts were characterized by Dunlap *et al.* (1980); the precursors had different AMWs (of about 170K for the 190K and 200K T-cell molecules and 190K for the B-220 molecule), but since these precursors were already glycosylated no conclusion about the nature of the difference between them could be drawn. Tunicamycin, an inhibitor of N-linked glycosylation, prevents maturation of human L-CA in various cell lines

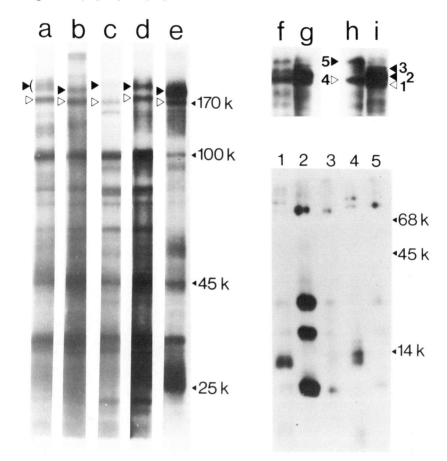

Figure 4. One-dimensional SDS–PAGE and peptide mapping of high-molecular-weight glycoproteins from mouse T-cell lines. (a–i) Cells were radioiodinated and lysed in 0.5% NP-40 (Hoessli *et al.*, 1980b). Nuclei were removed by centrifugation and an aliquot (about 10^5 cpm) of the lysate was taken for analysis by SDS–PAGE in a 7.5% polyacrylamide gel, which was exposed for autoradiography to an intensifying screen for 6 days after the electrophoresis. Only the upper portions of tracks (f–i) are shown. The cells (von Boehmer and Haas, 1981; Schreier *et al.*, 1980) were (a–d) cytotoxic T-cell clones C.SP.2, CB.F1.1, D.F1.1, and D.F1.2; (e) BALB/c mouse thymocytes; (f) cytotoxic T-cell clone B6.1, (g) helper T-cell clone DO3; (h, i) same as (f, g) but the cells were treated with neuraminidase before iodination according to Hoessli *et al.* (1980b). Note that neuraminidase treatment does not eliminate the differences between high-molecular-weight glycoproteins on different lines. Molecular weights of marker proteins are indicated in kilodaltons (k). Note variation in the T-200 family (◄,►) and also in an unrelated family of proteins of AMW about 170K (◁, ▷); the two families can be distinguished serologically (Hoessli and Vassalli, 1980) and by peptide mapping (Dunlap *et al.*, 1980), here carried out as described by Hoessli *et al.* (1982). For peptide mapping, bands 1–5 (AMWs between 170K and 220K) from gels (h, i) were cut out and subjected to SDS–PAGE (17.5% polyacrylamide) in the presence of V8 protease. Autoradiography of the gel (bottom right) shows similarity of T-200-derived bands 2, 3, and 5.

(Judd *et al.*, 1980), but so far these experiments have not led to the characterization of distinct polypeptide precursors for different forms of L-CA or T-200.

IV. SIALYLATION

Since the major T-cell glycoproteins Thy-1, LSGP, and L-CA each bear more sialic acid on peripheral T cells than on thymocytes, one might ask whether every thymocyte surface protein becomes more sialylated when the cell leaves the thymus. Hoessli *et al.* (1980a) identified nine ^{125}I-labeled proteins present on both thymocytes and peripheral lymphocytes from mice. Of these, two were not sialoglycoproteins (as judged by their lack of sensitivity to neuraminidase treatment), four (T-200, Thy-1, and proteins with AMWs 170K and 100K) were more sialylated on peripheral than on thymic cells, and three, including H-2D and -K, were not more sialylated. However, since the H-2 antigens are present in good quantity on only a small population of mature thymocytes, it remains quite possible that every sialoglycoprotein present on immature thymocytes, as well as on peripheral T cells, carries more sialic acid on the latter cell type.

In accord with this idea are the observations of increased sialyl transferase activity and increased sialic acid content of mouse peripheral T cells as opposed to thymocytes (Despont *et al.*, 1975). The increase per cell, about 5×10^7 sialic acid residues, is too large to be accounted for solely by addition of sialic acid to Thy-1, LSGP, L-CA, and H-2 antigens (assuming addition of five residues to each of 2×10^5 Thy-1 molecules; 50 residues to each of 10^5 LSGP molecules; 20 residues to each of 10^5 T-200 molecules; and five residues to each of 5×10^5 H-2 antigens), suggesting either that unidentified cell-surface proteins carry substantial amounts of sialic acid on peripheral T cells, or that the true sialic acid content of peripheral T cells is not as high as suggested by Despont *et al.* (1975), but is nearer the value of about 2×10^7 residues/cell that can be derived from the data of Allan and Crumpton (1970) for pig peripheral lymphocytes.

Since thymocytes divide more rapidly than peripheral T lymphocytes, their levels of sialyl transferase activity (which is known to be correlated with the degree of sialylation in various cell types) (Despont *et al.*, 1975; Atkinson and Hakimi, 1980) might be related to cell cycle time. The observation that Thy-1 molecules from T-cell blasts are less sialylated than on peripheral T cells (Fig. 2c) is consistent with this idea. However, studies on human and mouse fibroblast cultures (see Atkinson and Hakimi, 1980) suggest that glycopeptides from rapidly growing normal cells or transformed cells have unchanged or increased sialic acid levels when compared to glycopeptides from resting cells. In addition, there is not a good correlation between mitotic activity and PNA binding (used as a marker for less sialylated cells) in various lymphoid populations (see Rose and Malchiodi, 1981), so that there is unlikely to be any general, simple correlation between cell division rate and sialic acid content.

Alternatively, the amount of sialic acid on peripheral cells may reflect their degree of maturity (Sharon, 1980) or their ability to circulate without being trapped in the liver by a receptor protein specific for terminal galactose residues (Neufeld and Ashwell, 1980), which are exposed by neuraminidase treatment of peripheral lymphocytes. Such enzyme-treated lymphocytes, like untreated thymocytes, cannot home to lymphoid organs when injected intravenously, but travel to the liver and stay there for at least 24 hr (de Sousa, 1981), presumably until they have either died or regenerated their original sialic acid content. The hypothesis of a relationship between cell-surface carbohydrate structure and circulatory behavior is supported by various lines of indirect evidence [for example, the correlation between metastatic potential and sialic acid content of tumor cell lines reported by Yogeeswaram and Salk (1981), or the greater sialic acid content of mouse Ia antigens derived from splenic B cells, as opposed to adherent cells (Cullen et al., 1981)] and is also discussed by Rose (1982).

V. COMPARISONS AND CONCLUSIONS

It is interesting to compare the changes in the lymphocyte glycoproteins discussed in this chapter with those occurring during red blood cell differentiation (Fukuda and Fukuda, 1981). It has been known for twenty years that a human fetal erythrocyte antigen, i, is replaced by the I antigen typical of adult cells during erythroid development. This change is now known to result from the addition of Gal-GlcNAc($1 \rightarrow 6$) branches to linear polymers of lactosamine, as illustrated schematically in Fig. 3. The major carrier of the I antigen on adult erythrocytes is the band 3 glycoprotein (Childs et al., 1979), which also carries ABH blood group antigen activity. Other substances on mature erythrocytes, notably band 4.5 glycoproteins and some glycolipids, also carry I and ABH activities, but Fukuda et al. (1979) showed that the antigenic shift from i to I expression was at least partly due to changes in the carbohydrate structure carried by a single type of polypeptide, the band 3 protein. These authors compared the carbohydrate structures of the band 3 glycoprotein from cord and adult blood and concluded that the I-positive adult band 3 contained branched polylactosamine structures, whereas the cord blood band 3 contained the linear structures associated with i activity. Thus the band 3 protein (which has an AMW of about 90K, and 5–8% carbohydrate) resembles the high-molecular-weight proteins of lymphocytes in bearing increasingly branched oligosaccharide chains on more mature cell types.

A comparison of the results with those discussed in Sections III and IV suggests some general conclusions:

- It is commonly observed that a *particular protein may be differently glycosylated* at various stages in the differentiation of the cells producing it. This is clearly the case for the Thy-1 antigen, very probably true for lymphocyte high-molecular-weight (L-CA) glycoproteins, and likely for the LSGP family.

- This observation strengthens the idea that *different carbohydrate chains have different, specific functions* and argues against suggestions that the only role for carbohydrate is a general one such as stabilizing protein structure, protecting polypeptide chains from proteolysis, or allowing transport of membrane proteins to the cell surface (although the presence of oligosaccharides may in specific cases be necessary for a particular protein to be stable, indigestible, or transportable; see the case of Thy-1, page 93). However, the idea that changes in carbohydrate structure are accompanied by changes in function is so far supported by experimental evidence only in the case of the proposed correlation between total sialic acid content and ability of lymphoid cells to circulate.

- There is a tendency, at least in cells of the hemopoietic system, toward *increased carbohydrate chain complexity with increasing cellular differentiation*. This is seen in the increased branching of carbohydrate structures on adult as opposed to fetal red blood cells, and in the addition of sialic acid to many proteins of mature T cells. It is a likely cause for the changes in lectin and antibody binding of L-CA molecules on mature peripheral lymphocytes as opposed to thymocytes, as well as for the suggested changes in oligosaccharide structure of LSGP that accompany the differentiation of resting T cells into cytotoxic T cells.

- Changes in carbohydrate structure are probably due to *activation of specific glycosylating enzymes* (note the good correlation between sialic acid content and sialyl transferase activity in thymocytes and peripheral T cells) and not simply to changes in glycoprotein catabolic rates or in rates of membrane protein turnover. The glycosylating enzymes may affect many glycoproteins (e.g., sialyl transferase) or be more specific (e.g., the enzyme(s) postulated to act on LSGP during cytotoxic T-cell differentiation).

- Finally, it is noteworthy that the three major thymocyte surface proteins described in Section III each have *different carbohydrate structures*. These proteins are relatively well characterized; only the glycoproteins of erythrocytes have been studied to the same degree. The relationships between glycoprotein structure and cellular function are still mysterious, and here the lymphocyte is the obvious candidate for study, since its behavior is undeniably more fascinating than that of an erythrocyte.

ACKNOWLEDGMENTS

I am very grateful to R. Hooghe for providing Fig. 2c; to A. Williams for providing unpublished data; to W. R. A. Brown, D. Hoessli, J. Kaufman, and A.

Williams for stimulating discussion; and to W. Breisinger and M. Bühler for help in preparing the manuscript. The Basel Institute for Immunology was founded and is supported by F. Hoffmann-La Roche Ltd., Basel, Switzerland.

VI. REFERENCES

Ades, A. W., Zwerner, R. K, Acton, R. T., and Balch, C. M., 1980, *J. Exp. Med.* **151**:400–406.

Allan, D., and Crumpton, M. J., 1970, *Biochem. J.* **120**:133–143.

Altevogt, P., Kurnick, J. T., Kimura, A. K., Bosslet, K., and Schirrmacher, V., 1982, *Eur. J. Immunol.* **12**:300–307.

Andersson, L. C., Gahmberg, C. G., Kimura, A. K., and Wigzell, H., 1978, *Proc. Natl. Acad. Sci. U.S.A.* **75**:3455–3458.

Atkinson, P. H., and Hakimi, J., 1980, in: *The Biochemistry of Glycoproteins and Proteoglycans* (W. J. Lennarz, ed.), pp. 191–239, Plenum Press, New York.

Auchincloss, H., Ozato, K., and Sachs, D. H., 1982, *J. Immunol.* **128**:1584–1589.

Axelsson, B., Kimura, A., Hammarström, S., Wigzell, H., Nilsson, K., and Mellstedt, H., 1978, *Eur. J. Immunol.* **8**:757–764.

Bach, F. H., Alter, G. J., Widmer, M. B., Segal, M., and Dunlap, B., 1981, *Immunol. Rev.* **54**:5–26.

Barclay, A. N., Letarte-Muirhead, M., Williams, A. F., and Faulkes, R. A., 1976, *Nature (London)* **263**:563–567.

Bron, C., Schmid, M., Corradin, G., Glasebrook, A. L., Engers, H. D., Horwath, C., Cerottini, J. C., and MacDonald, H. R., 1981, in: *Mechanisms of Lymphocyte Activation* (K. Resch and H. Kirchner, eds.), pp. 198–201, Elsevier/North-Holland, Amsterdam.

Brown, W. R. A., and Williams, A. F., 1982, *Immunology* **46**:713–726.

Brown, W. R. A., Barclay, A. N., Sunderland, C. A., and Williams, A. F., 1981, *Nature (London)* **289**:456–460.

Campbell, D. G., Gagnon, J., Reid, K. B. M., and Williams, A. F., 1981, *Biochem. J.* **195**:15–30.

Carlsson, S., and Stigbrand, T., 1982, *Eur. J. Biochem.* **123**:1–7.

Carter, P. B., and Sunderland, C. A., 1980, *Immunogenetics* **10**:583–593.

Childs, R. A., and Feizi, T., 1981, *Biochem. Biophys. Res. Commun.* **102**:1158–1164.

Childs, R. A., Feizi, T., and Tonegawa, Y., 1979, *Biochem. J.* **181**:533–538.

Coffman, R. L., and Weissman, I. L., 1981, *J. Exp. Med.* **153**:269–279.

Coffman, R. L., and Weissman, I. L., 1981, *Nature (London)* **289**:681–683.

Cohen, F. E., Novotny, J., Sternberg, M. J. E., Campbell, D. G., and Williams, A. F., 1981, *Biochem. J.* **195**:31–40.

Conzelmann, A., Pink, J. R., Acuto, D., Mach, J. P., Dolivo, S., and Nabholz, M., 1980, *Eur. J. Immunol.* **10**:860–868.

Cotmore, S. F., Crowhurst, S. A., and Waterfield, M. D., 1981, *Eur. J. Immunol.* **11**:597–603.

Crumpton, M. J., and Snary, D., 1974, in: *Contemporary Topics in Molecular Immunology,* Volume 3 (G. L. Ada, ed.), pp. 27–56, Plenum Press, New York.

Cullen, S. E., Kindle, C. S., Shreffler, D. C., and Cowing, C., 1981, *J. Immunol.* **127**:1478–1484.

Dalchau, R., and Fabre, J. W., 1979, *J. Exp. Med.* **149**:576–591.

Dalchau, R., and Fabre, J. W., 1981, *J. Exp. Med.* **153**:753–765.

Dalchau, R., Kirkely, J., and Fabre, J. W., 1980, *Eur. J. Immunol.* **10**:737–744; 745–749.

de Sousa, M., 1981, *Lymphocyte Circulation: Experimental and Clinical Aspects*, Wiley, New York, p. 81.

Despont, J.-P., Abel, C. A., and Grey, H. M., 1975, *Cell. Immunol.* **17**:487–494.

Dunlap, B., Bach, F. H., and Bach, M. L., 1978, *Nature (London)* **271**:253–255.

Dunlap, B., Mixter, P. F., Koller, B., Watson, A., Widmer, B., and Bach, F. H., 1980, *J. Immunol.* **125**:1829–1831.

Fukuda, M., and Fukuda, M. N., 1981, *J. Supramol. Struc.* **17**:313–324.

Fukuda, M., Fukuda, M. N., and Hakomori, S., 1979, *J. Biol. Chem.* **254**:3700–3703.

Gahmberg, C. G., 1981, in: *New Comprehensive Biochemistry*, Volume 1: *Membrane Structure* (J. B. Finean and R. M. Michell, eds.), pp. 127–160, Elsevier/North-Holland, Amsterdam.

Gahmberg, C. G., and Andersson, L. C., 1977, *J. Biol. Chem.* **252**:5888–5894.

Gahmberg, C. G., and Andersson, L. C., 1982, *Eur. J. Biochem.* **122**:581–586.

Gahmberg, C. G., Häyry, P., and Andersson, L. C., 1976, *J. Cell. Biol.* **68**:642–653.

Glasebrook, A. L., Sarmiento, M., Loken, M. R., Dialynas, D. P., Quintans, J., Eisenberg, L., Lutz, C. T., Wilde, D., and Fitch, F. W., 1981, *Immunol. Rev.* **54**:225–266.

Goldstein, I. J., and Hayes, C. E., 1978, *Adv. Carbohydr. Chem. Biochem.* **35**:127–340.

Hammarström, S., 1972, in: *Methods in Enzymology*, Volume 28B (V. Ginsburg, ed.), pp. 368–383, Academic Press, New York.

Hayman, M. J., and Crumpton, M. J., 1972, *Biochem. Biophys. Res. Commun.* **47**:923–930.

Hellström, V., Dillner, M.-L., Hammarström, S., and Perlmann, P., 1976, *Scand. J. Immunol.* **5**:45–54.

Hoessli, D., and Vassalli, P., 1980, *J. Immunol.* **125**:1758–1763.

Hoessli, D., Vassalli, P., and Pink, J. R. L., 1980a, *Eur. J. Immunol.* **10**:814–821.

Hoessli, D., Bron, C., and Pink, J. R. L., 1980b, *Nature (London)* **283**:576–578.

Hoessli, D., Pink, J. R. L., Hooghe, R., Schreier, M., and Vassalli, P., 1982, in: *Protides of the Biological Fluids*, Volume 29 (H. Peeters, ed.), pp. 71–74, Pergamon Press, Oxford.

Hooghe-Peters, E., and Hooghe, R. J., 1982, *J. Neuroimmunol.* **2**:191–200.

Hubbard, S. C., and Ivatt, R. J., 1981, *Annu. Rev. Biochem.* **50**:555–583.

Irlé, C., Piguet, P.-F., and Vassalli, P., 1978, *J. Exp. Med.* **148**:32–45.

Judd, W., Poodry, C. A., Broder, S., Friedman, S. M., Chess, L., and Strominger, J. L., 1980, *Proc. Natl. Acad. Sci. U.S.A.* **77**:6805–6809.

Kaladas, P. M., Kabat, E. A., Kimura, A., and Ersson, B., 1981, *Mol. Immunol.* **18**:969–977.

Kamarck, M. E., and Gottlieb, P. D., 1980, *Mol. Immunol.* **17**:1117–1127.

Kaufmann, Y., and Berke, G., 1981, *J. Immunol.* **126**:1443–1446.

Kimura, A. K., and Wigzell, H., 1978, *J. Exp. Med.* **147**:1418–1434.

Kincade, P. W., Lee, G., Watanabe, T., Sun, L., and Scheid, M. P., 1981, *J. Immunol.* **27**:2262–2268.

Kornfeld, R., and Kornfeld, S., 1980, in: *The Biochemistry of Glycoproteins and Proteoglycans* (W. J. Lennarz, ed.), pp. 1–34, Plenum Press, New York.

Ledbetter, J. A., and Herzenberg, L. A., 1979, *Immunol. Rev.* **47**:63–90.

Letarte, M., and Meghji, G., 1978, *J. Immunol.* **121**:1718–1725.

Lotan, R., and Nicolson, G. L., 1979, *Biochim. Biophys. Acta* **559**:329–376.

MacDonald, H. R., Mach, J. P., Schreyer, M., Zaech, P., and Cerottini, J. C., 1981, *J. Immunol.* **126**:883–886.

Michaelson, J., Scheid, M., and Boyse, E. A., 1979, *Immunogenetics* **9**:193–197.

Morishima, Y., Ogata, S., Collins, N. H., Dupont, B., and Lloyd, K. O., 1982, *Immunogenetics* **15**:529–535.

Morrison, M., and Schonbaum, G. R., 1976, *Annu. Rev. Biochem.* **45**:861–888.

Neufeld, E. F., and Ashwell, G., 1980, in: *The Biochemistry of Glycoproteins and Proteoglycans* (W. J. Lennarz, ed.), pp. 241–265, Plenum Press, New York.

Nilsson, S. F., and Waxdal, M. J., 1976, *Biochemistry* **15**:2698–2705.

Omary, M. B., and Trowbridge, I. S., 1980, *J. Biol. Chem.* **255**:1662–1669.

Omary, M. B., Trowbridge, I. S., and Battifora, I., 1980a, *J. Exp. Med.* **152**:842–852.

Omary, M. B., Trowbridge, I. S., and Scheid, M. P., 1980b, *J. Exp. Med.* **151**:1311–1316.

Pink, J. R. L., Fedecka-Bruner, B., Coltey, M., Peault, B. M., and Le Douarin, N. M., 1981, *Eur. J. Immunol.* **11**:517–520.

Pink, J. R. L., Hoessli, D., Tartakoff, A., and Hooghe, R., 1983, *Mol. Immunol.* (in press).

Rose, M. L., 1982 *Immunology Today* **3**:6–8.

Rose, M. L., and Malchiodi, F., 1981, *Immunology* **42**:583–591.

Saito, M., and Osawa, T., 1980, *Carbohydr. Res.* **78**:341–348.

Saito, M., Toyoshima, S., and Osawa, T., 1978, *Biochem. J.* **175**:823–831.

Sarmiento, M., Glasebrook, A. L., and Fitch, F. W., 1980, *Proc. Natl. Acad. Sci. U.S.A.* 77:1111–1115.
Sarmiento, M., Loken, M. R., and Fitch, F. W., 1981, *Hybridoma* 1:13–26.
Sarmiento, M., Loken, M. R., Trowbridge, I. S., Coffman, R. L., and Fitch, F. W., 1982, *J. Immunol.* 128:1676–1684.
Schmidt-Ullrich, R., Mikkelsen, R. B., and Wallach, D. F. H., 1978, *J. Biol. Chem.* 253:6973–6978.
Schreier, M. H., Iscove, N. N., Tees, R., Aarden, L., and von Boehmer, H., 1980, *Immunol. Rev.* 51:315–336.
Sharon, N., 1980, in: *Progress in Immunology IV* (M. Fougereau and J. Dausset, eds.), pp. 254–278, Academic Press, New York.
Sharon, N., 1983, *Adv. Immunol.* (in press).
Siadak, A. W., and Nowinski, R. C., 1980, *J. Immunol.* 125:1400–1401.
Sidman, C. L., Forni, L., Köhler, G., Langhorne, J., and Fischer Lindahl, K., 1980, in: *Basel Institute for Immunology Annual Report*, pp. 61–62, Hoffmann–La Roche, Basel.
Standring, R., and Williams, A. F., 1978, *Biochim. Biophys. Acta* 508:85–96.
Standring, R., McMaster, W. R., Sunderland, C. A., and Williams, A. F., 1978, *Eur. J. Immunol.* 8:832–839.
Stutman, O., 1978, *Immunol. Rev.* 42:138–184.
Sunderland, C. A., McMaster, W. R., and Williams, A. F., 1979, *Eur. J. Immunol.* 9:155–159.
Thomas, D. G., Calderon, R. A., and Blaxland, L. J., 1978, *Nature (London)* 275:711–715.
Trowbridge, I. S., 1978, *J. Exp. Med.* 148:313–328.
Trowbridge, I. S., Weissman, I. L, and Bevan, M. J., 1975, *Nature (London)* 256:652–654.
Trowbridge, I. S., Nilsen-Hamilton, M., Hamilton, R. T., and Bevan, M. J., 1977, *Biochem. J.* 163:211–217.
Trowbridge, I. S., Hyman, R., and Mazauskas, C., 1978, *Cell* 14:21–32.
von Boehmer, H., and Haas, W., 1981, *Immunol. Rev.* 54:27–56.
Watson, A., Dunlap, B., and Bach, F. H., 1981, *J. Immunol.* 127:38–42.
Williams, A. F., 1982, *Biosci. Rep.* 2:277–287.
Williams, A. F., and Gagnon, J., 1982. *Science* 216:696–703.
Yogeeswaram, G., and Salk, P. L., 1981, *Science* 212:1514–1516.

The Receptor on Mast Cells and Related Cells with High Affinity for IgE

Henry Metzger

Section on Chemical Immunology
Arthritis and Rheumatism Branch
National Institute of Arthritis, Diabetes, Digestive and Kidney Diseases
National Institutes of Health
Bethesda, Maryland 20205

I. INTRODUCTION

Mast cells, basophils, and related tumor lines have a glycoprotein on their surface membrane that binds monomeric immunoglobulin E (IgE) with exceptionally high affinity. When the cell-bound IgE reacts with a multivalent antigen the cells rapidly degranulate—a reaction that has been shown to be mediated by the membrane glycoprotein.

This review describes what is known about the nature and mode of action of this component. I shall refer to it as "the" receptor for IgE, recognizing that there are in fact many receptors capable of binding at least aggregated IgE. These others are likely to play significant roles in regulating the biosynthesis and functioning of IgE, but, in terms of the properties listed above, the receptor that serves as the focus of this review is unique.

Many of the detailed studies of this receptor have utilized a neoplastic line of rat cells—the rat basophilic leukemia (RBL) originally discovered by Eccleston *et al.* (1973). However, the available evidence indicates that, as far as the structure and basic functioning of the receptor are concerned, the facts we have learned also apply to the receptor on normal cells. Detailed study of the receptor

Abbreviations used in this chapter: IgE, immunoglobulin E; PAGE, polyacrylamide gel electrophoresis; RBL, rat basophilic leukemia; SDS, sodium dodecylsulfate.

has been pursued by several groups for about ten years and several reviews of the subject have appeared. In this summary I shall emphasize the newer data, many of them unpublished at the time this chapter was completed.

II. BINDING OF IgE

A. Methods

Binding studies in this system can be performed with excellent precision and reasonable accuracy. Purified IgE is radiolabeled and the specific activity determined on the basis of some estimate of protein concentration. If one wishes to express the specific activity in molar terms the molecular weight of the IgE must be incorporated into the calculation. The IgE is mixed with cells or some alternative preparation of receptors (Metzger *et al.*, 1976; Rossi *et al.*, 1977), and the IgE bound to receptors is separated from unbound ligand. Nonspecific binding is estimated by performing a control experiment in the presence of a large excess of unlabeled IgE. For certain studies it is important to determine the fraction of ligand that is bindable, since some of the IgE may be inactive either prior to or after radiolabeling. This fraction can be determined by exposing the IgE to a large excess of receptors. With care, preparations of IgE that are ≥90% active can be obtained.

When such well-characterized IgE is exposed to a preparation of receptors, a finite amount becomes bound and adding additional IgE or allowing the reaction to proceed for longer times reveals no further binding. The saturation value obtained in this way defines the concentration of binding sites.

B. Mechanism of Binding

Early studies (Kulczycki and Metzger, 1974) demonstrated that the binding of IgE to the receptors on cells was consistent with a simple bimolecular reaction:

$$L + R \rightleftharpoons LR \qquad (1)$$

That is, the initial rate of binding was linearly proportional to the initial concentration of IgE (L) and the concentration of cells [and therefore by implication the initial concentration of binding sites (R)]. Similarly the rate of dissociation appeared to be proportional to the concentration of bound IgE, although only a small fraction of the reaction could be studied at that time. No unusual effects were observed when small variations in temperature, pH, or several constituents of the medium were imposed.

However, the interaction of a ligand with receptors on a cell may be more complicated than it at first appears, since the binding sites are not distributed homogeneously throughout the solution. A useful discussion of how this aspect of the reaction can be incorporated into kinetic studies has been given by DeLisi (1981). The reaction is dissected into two stages:

$$L + R \underset{k_-}{\overset{k_+}{\rightleftharpoons}} L \ldots R \underset{k_{-1}}{\overset{k_1}{\rightleftharpoons}} LR \qquad (2)$$

The concentrations of the "encounter complex," $L \ldots R$, and the bonded state, LR, are determined by the interplay of the concentrations of the free ligand and receptor, the "diffusive rate constants," k_+ and k_-, and the "reaction rate constants," k_1 and k_{-1}. If the rate-limiting step in the forward reaction is the formation of the encounter complex, i.e., $k_+ \ll k_1$, then it can be shown that the rate of formation of the bonded state LR may be relatively insensitive to the number of unoccupied receptors *per cell* until that value falls to a relatively small fraction of the total. Contrariwise, if the reaction is diffusion-limited, the dissociation from the bounded state to free reactants can be shown to be directly related to the number of unoccupied binding sites.

We have recently reexamined the reaction of IgE with cell-bound receptors in order to determine whether or not the reaction was diffusion-controlled (Wank *et al.*, 1983). The rate of binding of labeled IgE was determined using cells whose number of binding sites was systematically varied by preincubating the cells with unlabeled IgE. The effect of receptor occupancy on the rate of dissociation was studied by comparing the dissociation of labeled IgE in the presence and absence of unlabeled IgE. Figure 1 shows that the initial rate of binding is proportional to the number of receptors per cell and Fig. 2 shows that the rate of dissociation is independent of the number of unoccupied receptors. These results demonstrate that the reaction is *not* diffusion-controlled and that it is not significantly affected by the inhomogeneous distribution of receptors in the suspension of cells.

This finding permits one to compare the rate constants for the reaction of IgE with cell-bound receptors to the values obtained with receptors solubilized by treating the cells with nonionic detergents (Table I). Whereas the rates of dissociation are similar, the forward rate constant for the reaction with the cell-bound receptors is substantially smaller than that for the reaction of IgE with soluble receptors. The explanation for this apparent discrepancy is uncertain. Since it is the forward rather than the reverse rate constant that is affected it appears unlikely that changes in the conformation of the receptor induced by solubilization with detergent account for the difference. Rather we have postulated that a "gating effect" of other membrane components on the intact cell may be responsible (Wank *et al.*, 1983). If so, then one predicts that the rate of binding of IgE to cells treated with proteases or glycosidases to which the recep-

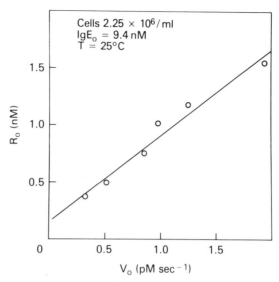

Figure 1. Effect of varying the number of unoccupied receptors *per cell* on the initial rate of binding (V_0). R_0, concentration of unoccupied receptors at the start of the experiment; IgE_0, concentration of labeled IgE at the start of the experiment. From Wank *et al.* (1983).

tor is resistant, or to liposomes into which purified receptors have been incorporated, should be enhanced. It is interesting that Pecoud *et al.* (1981) observed an apparent 2-fold increase in the initial binding velocity, and a parallel 1.6-fold increase in the apparent K_A, after treatment of cells with neuraminidase. Qualitatively this is what one would predict from such a gating effect. However, studies on the soluble receptor would need to be performed in order to rule out an effect on the receptor itself.

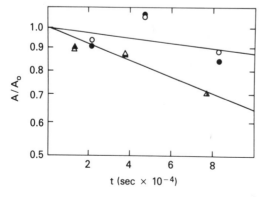

Figure 2. Rates of dissociation of [^{125}I]-IgE from cells in the presence and absence of unlabeled IgE. Circles, 24°C; triangles, 37°C. Open symbols, no IgE; filled symbols, with unlabeled IgE. The ordinate is a log scale that shows the bound [^{125}I]-IgE as a fraction of the amount bound at time = 0. From Wank *et al.* (1983).

Table I. Rate Constants for Binding of IgE to
Receptors on Cells or in Detergent Extracts
at $20°C^a$

	k_f $(M^{-1} sec^{-1} \times 10^{-5})$	k_r $(sec^{-1} \times 10^6)$
Cells	1.2	1.3
Extract	37	0.64^b

[a]From Wank et al. (1983).
[b]From Rossi et al. (1977).

C. Binding Parameters; Valence

Typical rate constants for the reaction of IgE with the cell-bound or soluble receptor have already been noted (Table I) and the subject has been reviewed previously (Metzger and Bach, 1978; Froese, 1980). In view of the critical role of aggregation in the functioning of this system (Section VI.A.1) the valence of the receptor is of particular interest. A variety of studies from our own group have demonstrated that the receptor can bind only one molecule at a time regardless of whether the valence is assessed on intact cells (Mendoza and Metzger, 1976; Schlessinger et al., 1976) or in detergent extracts (Rossi et al., 1977; Newman et al., 1977; Kanellopoulos et al., 1980). Claims to the contrary (Ishizaka and Ishizaka, 1975; Kulczycki et al., 1979), we feel, have experimental complexities associated with them, as discussed elsewhere (Mendoza and Metzger, 1976; Kanellopoulos et al., 1979).

D. Specificity of Binding

The receptor that binds monomeric IgE with high affinity is highly specific with respect to the native conformation of IgE, the species of IgE, and the isotype of the immunoglobulin. There have been reports that suggest there may be different isotypes (or allelic variants) of human and rat IgE that bind with different avidity (Conroy et al., 1979; Lehrer, 1981), but more direct analyses are needed before the bases for the observations are clarified. A recent report by Sterk and Ishizaka (1982) is interesting in that it suggests that normal mouse mast cells have two high-affinity receptors for IgE. One of these cannot distinguish between mouse and rat IgE, binding both with an apparent affinity of $\sim1.6 \times 10^9$ (BALB/c) to 3×10^9 (CBA/J). The other binds mouse IgE as tightly but binds rat IgE very weakly. This clearly implies a heterogeneity of the receptor population. Whether it involves small differences of otherwise similar receptors or two basic types of receptors will need to be explored by other than binding studies.

E. Sequelae of Binding

There is no evidence that the binding of monomeric IgE to the receptor on cells in and of itself induces significant changes in the cell. The bound IgE persists on the cell surface for long periods of time as assessed by radioautography of tumor cells reacted with radiolabeled IgE (Isersky *et al.*, 1979)—a finding consistent with a variety of much earlier observations on the persistence of passive sensitization *in vivo*. Studies with the cultured tumor cells also showed that occupancy of the receptors with IgE affected neither the overall growth properties of the cells nor the number of unoccupied receptors (Isersky *et al.*, 1979).

It is worth noting that recent data on the Fc receptor for immunoglobulin on macrophages suggest a different set of events (Segal *et al.*, 1983a,b). Those receptors appear to undergo a continuous cycle of internalization and the degree to which the immunoglobulin is internalized is related to its ability to bind to the receptors (see also Section VI.B.4).

III. BINDING SITES ON IgE

It has been possible to prepare a variety of proteolytic digestion products from human IgE and to test their activity or structure after treatment under conditions known to affect the binding of the intact IgE. In brief, all of the studies are consistent with the principal site of binding on IgE being related to the $C_\epsilon 3$ or $C_\epsilon 4$ domains or both, although this is largely based on indirect data (Dorrington and Bennich, 1978). In a detailed study Bennich *et al.* (1977) were unable to substantiate the observation that a pentapeptide from the $C_\epsilon 2$ region had binding activity (Hamburger, 1975). Despite a single report that indicated otherwise (Fritsche and Spiegelberg, 1978), it so far has not been possible to develop a method for preparing Fc fragments from rodent IgE reproducibly. The fragment corresponding to $F(ab')_2$—which contains the $C_\epsilon 2$ domains—does not bind to the receptor (Ellerson *et al.*, 1978; Perez-Montfort and Metzger, 1982).

Two studies have demonstrated that rat IgE becomes relatively resistant to proteolytic attack when it is bound to mast cells (Ellerson *et al.*, 1978) or a tumor analog (Isersky *et al.*, 1979). Such studies are difficult to compare with the digestion of unbound IgE because the conditions are perforce quite different. For example, in the study by Ellerson *et al.*, cells that carried a maximum of 0.4 μg of IgE per ml were reacted with 250 μg/ml enzyme whereas 2000–5000 μg/ml of unbound IgE were reacted with 20–50 μg/ml enzyme—a 400- to 1000-fold difference in the product of the concentrations of the reactants!

We recently explored a different approach. IgE–α-chain complexes (Section IV.B) were purified from cells that had been loaded with radiolabeled rat or mouse IgE prior to solubilization with nonionic detergent. We compared the rate

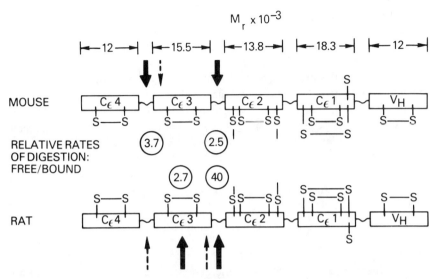

Figure 3. Diagram of approximate locations of trypsin cleavage sites on mouse and rat ε chains. Homology of both chains with human ε chain has been assumed for the location, type, and number of disulfide bonds. The unbonded sulfhydryl groups on the $C_\epsilon 1$ domains represent the sites of the heavy-chain/light-chain disulfides; those on the $C_\epsilon 2$ domains, heavy-chain/heavy-chain disulfides. A molecular scale shows the molecular weight of the domains, including the carbohydrate side chains, for human ε chain. The bold arrows show the principal cleavage sites. The dashed arrows show sites of cleavage that generate fragments whose buildup and decay could not be measured accurately. The numbers in the circles are the ratios of the rate constants for digestion of unbound IgE (free) and IgE–receptor complexes (bound) by trypsin at the site shown by the respective bold arrow. From Perez-Montfort and Metzger (1982).

of proteolysis of the bound IgE by trypsin with the rate for unbound IgE under exactly the same conditions. The results are summarized in Fig. 3. The figure shows the principal sites of cleavage and relative rates of digestion for free versus bound IgE. It appeared that cleavage between both the $C_\epsilon 3$ and $C_\epsilon 4$ and $C_\epsilon 2$ and $C_\epsilon 3$ domains is markedly retarded for mouse IgE bound to receptor. A somewhat analogous situation prevailed with respect to rat IgE although here the inhibition of cleavage at the $C_\epsilon 2:C_\epsilon 3$ junction was more complete. These results suggest that the receptor is interacting with the IgE well up along the Fc region. It is particularly interesting that the inhibition of cleavage by the receptor affects both ε chains. Since, except at the points of contact, all sites on the chains are rotated 180° with respect to each other, it suggests that there is a measure of bilateral symmetry to the receptor (Section IV.B.3).

The sequence analysis of rat IgE is being pursued (H. Bennich, personal communication) and when it becomes practical to identify specific regions, for example from peptide "fingerprints," it may be of interest to perform double-labeling studies with free and receptor-bound IgE in order to identify the sites of interaction more precisely.

Kulczycki and Vallina (1981) prepared IgE that was deficient in carbohydrate by culturing the rat tumor IR162, which produces a monoclonal IgE (Bazin et al., 1974), in the presence of tunicamycin. They observed that both pauci- and nonglycosylated IgE could bind specifically to the receptor, although the affinity of these preparations relative to native IgE was not assessed. Since the affinity of the native IgE is so high, a substantial reduction in activity (several orders of magnitude) might be missed unless explicitly tested for.

IV. STRUCTURE OF THE RECEPTOR

A. General Comments

Although considerable information has been obtained about the receptor some of the inherent weaknesses in the analyses must be appreciated. Almost all of the analyses involve labeling of the receptor and such studies obviously can only detect those polypeptides that became labeled with a given technique. With one exception (Fewtrell et al., 1981) (Section IV.B.5.c), all the studies have involved solubilization, and this assumes that there are no polypeptides lost when the membrane is disrupted (Section IV.C.5). If denaturants are subsequently used during the purification (Kulczycki et al., 1979) the potential problem is aggravated. While cross-linking reagents may prevent such losses (Holowka et al., 1980; Holowka and Metzger, 1982) they obviously can only do so if there are suitable residues sufficiently close to be bonded by the particular reagent employed.

B. The α Chain

Much of the older data have been reviewed previously—most recently by Froese (1980) and Metzger et al. (1982)—and these will be dealt with only briefly; some newer results will be dealt with in more detail. The α chain has been isolated by three principal methods: (1) by immunoprecipitation from detergent extracts of cells using either IgE plus anti-IgE (Conrad et al., 1976; Kulczycki et al., 1976) or antireceptor antibodies (Isersky et al., 1978; Froese et al., 1982b); (2) by elution with denaturants from columns to which IgE has been covalently bound and which had been loaded with detergent extracts of cells (Kulczycki et al., 1976; Rossi et al., 1977; Conrad and Froese, 1978a; Kulczycki and Parker, 1979; Froese et al., 1982a); or (3) by using haptenated IgE and eluting the IgE–receptor complexes from a column conjugated with antihapten antibodies with hapten (Conrad and Froese, 1978b; Kanellopoulos *et al.*, 1979), or using an IgE with antihapten activity which, after being bound to receptors, is adsorbed on a column conjugated with hapten and eluted with hapten after washing (Holowka and Metzger, 1982).

1. Molecular Weight

In all instances, if the material is *thoroughly* washed only an $M_r \simeq 50,000$ component is observed regardless of whether the receptor is labeled *in situ* by surface-labeling the cells, by allowing the cells to incorporate radioactive amino acids or monosaccharides, or by labeling after purification.[*] Similarly, staining gels on which the receptor was electrophoresed in sodium dodecylsulfate (SDS) with Coomassie Blue reveals only this single component (Kanellopoulos *et al.*, 1979). Much higher molecular weights are estimated from the position at which the receptor or receptor-IgE complexes are eluted from a gel filtration column run with nonionic detergents (Conrad *et al.*, 1976; Rossi *et al.*, 1977; Kulczycki and Parker, 1979). As noted (Rossi *et al.*, 1977; Newman *et al.*, 1977) such estimates are not meaningful because they fail to account for any bound detergent, or for hydrodynamic "shapes" that deviate substantially from spherical symmetry.

We recently reexamined the molecular weight of the α chain by gel permeation chromatography in 6 M guanidine HCl (Kumar and Metzger, 1982). This procedure appears to give more accurate estimates for glycoproteins than most other methods because both the unknowns and standards are likely to form random coils with a constant ratio of mass to Stokes radius (Leach *et al.*, 1980). In our experiments the α chains eluted in a peak that was as narrow as those obtained with the protein standards used to calibrate the column. This was surprising since on gel electrophoresis in SDS the band given by the α chain is extraordinarily broad. The latter finding plus the observation that different sections of such broad bands gave narrower, appropriately shifted bands when reelectrophoresed (Holowka *et al.*, 1980; Goetze *et al.*, 1981) suggested considerable heterogeneity. The data from the chromatography in 6 M guanidine indicate that this heterogeneity may not be due simply to variations in mass.

The molecular weight determined by Kumar and Metzger (1982) is less than the previous "best" estimates (Kanellopoulos *et al.*, 1980) (Table II). However, even chromatography in 6 M guanidine has given inaccurate molecular weights; in particular the aberrant estimates all appear to be 13 ± 1% too low (Leach *et al.*, 1980). If this were true of the α chain, then the "correct" molecular weight would be 44,000—close to the extrapolated molecular weight from

---

[*]The one exception to this statement is the so-called "H-component," which is observed when columns conjugated with IgE are loaded with crude detergent extracts, washed, and subsequently eluted with denaturant. The nature of this component has been reviewed by Froese (1980).

Table II. Comparison of Molecular Weights Obtained for the
α Chain and Its Fragments by Different Methods[a]

Enzyme treatment	Method of analysis		
	Composition[b]	SDS–PAGE[c]	Guanidine HCl column
None	50 ± 3	47, 54	38.5 ± 1.6 (4)[d]
Endoglycosidase	(35 ± 3)[e]	35	27.3 ± 0.3 (3)
Papain	–	30 and 34	21.5 ± 1.0 (2)
Bromelain			
Limited	–	30 and 34	21.5 ± 1.6 (2)
Extensive	–	24	13.3 ± 1.5 (2)
	–	16	5.2 ± 0.8 (2)

[a]Values are molecular weights $\times$ 10^{-3}.
[b]Data from Kanellopoulos et al. (1980).
[c]The lower value for the untreated α chain is based on an extrapolation (Kanellopoulos et al., 1980). All other values are from Goetze et al. (1981).
[d]Values shown are the means and standard deviations for the number of analyses shown in parentheses.
[e]The value shown is the estimate for the α subunit free of carbohydrate.

Table III. Composition of the α Chain of the Receptor for IgE[a]

Amino acid	Residues/mole	Amino acid	Residues/mole	Monosaccharide	Residues/mole
Lysine	30.8	Cysteic acid	7.27	Fucose	6.9 ± 1.0
Histidine	6.04	Valine	24.4	Mannose	27 ± 3.0
Arginine	8.37	Methionine	2.80	Galactose	40 ± 2.0
Aspartic acid	40.2	Isoleucine	21.9	Glucosamine	27
Threonine	17.3	Leucine	23.9	Sialic acid	?
Serine	32.2	Tyrosine	13.5	ΣM_r	15,000
Glutamic acid	23.6	Phenylalanine	12.6		
Proline	8.99	Tryptophan	2.5		
Glycine	19.4	ΣM_r	35,000		
Alanine	14.6				

[a]Data from Kanellopoulos et al. (1980).

analyses on SDS gels and from compositional data (Table III) (see also Section IV.B.5.c).

2. Carbohydrate

That radioactive precursors of oligosaccharides became incorporated into α chains (Kulczycki et al., 1976) and that receptors bound to various lectins (Helm et al., 1979; Helm and Froese, 1981a) first provided direct and indirect evidence that this subunit is a glycopeptide. Compositional analysis first indicated that approximately one-third of the mass of the α chain was contributed by carbohydrate (Kanellopoulos et al., 1980) (Table III). Subsequently, characterization of the product obtained by digestion with an endoglycosidase (Goetze et al., 1981) and from cells grown in the presence of tunicamycin (Hempstead et al., 1981a) gave similar estimates. An apparent discrepancy in these results considering the specificity of the oligosaccharidase used and the effects of tunicamycin has been discussed (Kumar and Metzger, 1982).

There is also some uncertainty about the presence of sialic acid. We failed to get unequivocal evidence for sialic acid residues in our compositional analyses (Kanellopoulos et al., 1980). Nevertheless, prior treatment with neuraminidase increases the susceptibility of the α chains to oligosaccharidases (Goetze et al., 1981) and to tritiation by galactose oxidase and [^{3}H]-NaBH$_4$ (Pecoud et al., 1981). It is possible that sialic acid residues were lost during the preparative steps for the compositional analyses. The estimates of molecular weight of the receptor have varied somewhat when different sublines of the RBL lines of cells were tested (reviewed in Froese, 1980). Nevertheless, the tryptic maps of surface-labeled α chains from various preparations appeared similar (Pecoud and Conrad, 1981); likewise the heterogeneity observed on SDS gels (see Section IV.B.1) appears reduced when oligosaccharidase-treated α chains or chains from cells treated with tunicamycin are examined (Goetze et al., 1981; Hempstead et al., 1981a). Both these observations are consistent with the apparent heterogeneity being related to the carbohydrate moiety.

The α chain synthesized by cells treated with tunicamycin appears to retain substantial binding activity for IgE (Hempstead et al., 1981a) although, as with the analogous study on IgE, a significant decrease in affinity cannot be ruled out on the basis of the studies performed. As already noted (Section II.B) the increase in the apparent forward rate constant for the binding of IgE to cells that have been treated with neuraminidase might be related to effects on surrounding structures rather than on the α chain itself, but this possibility needs to be tested explicitly.

3. Substructures

When isolated α chains are reacted in SDS with a variety of proteases a uniform pattern emerges. Regardless of whether the chains have been labeled intrinsically or extrinsically, a single digestion product can be obtained that contains virtually all of the label (Goetze et al., 1981). Recent analyses by chromatography in guanidine HCl (Kumar and Metzger, 1982) have confirmed that the molecular weight of the digested material is almost precisely one-half that of the intact chain (Table II). A variety of experimental approaches were unsuccessful in separating the two halves; however, some results suggested to us differences in their properties. Thus it appeared that one of them (α2) moved slightly more rapidly on gel electrophoresis in SDS, was preferentially modified by surface-labeling, had less abundant carbohydrate, and was preferentially cleaved to a smaller fragment by bromelain, compared to the other portion (α1) (Goetze *et al.*, 1981). Nevertheless, until these fragments have been separated and characterized more fully, their significance is uncertain.

We have not been able to renature the products (or the intact α chain) from SDS so that reactivity with either IgE or antireceptor antibodies is restored. Attempts to use an alternative strategy, namely to produce "active" fragments by digesting the native uncomplexed receptor in crude extracts or purified IgE-receptor complexes, have not been successful either (Section IV.B.5.a).

As noted in Section III, the digestion of *both* ϵ chains of IgE is retarded when the IgE is bound to α chains. As we have noted elsewhere (Goetze *et al.*, 1981; Perez-Montfort and Metzger, 1982; Kumar and Metzger, 1982) it is interesting to speculate that the bilateral symmetry of the receptor suggested by that result might be accounted for by the bilateral symmetry of the α chain that the experiments on the fragmentation of the α chains suggest.

4. Composition and Peptide Analyses

Analyses of the amino acids of the α chain shows that there should be $\simeq$40 sites cleavable by trypsin per 35,000 daltons of peptide (Table III). In one study employing tryptic cleavage of α chains labeled by the lactoperoxidase method, 18 peptides were observed (Pecoud and Conrad, 1981). The method of labeling will certainly modify tyrosines and potentially phenylalanines and histidines. There are a total of $\simeq$30 such residues per α chain (Table III)—more than enough to account for the number of peptides seen. However, it seems likely that the number of discrete peptide sequences is overestimated by this technique because of the heterogeneity of the α chain when examined by either gel electrophoresis in SDS (Sections IV.B.1, 2) or isoelectric focusing (Hempstead *et al.*, 1981a). It is also possible that variations in the amount of mono- versus diiodotyrosine could affect the results. Incomplete digestion can produce artifactual heterogeneity, but since the authors found no variation in the patterns with time of digestion, it is likely that all cleavable bonds were broken. Receptors from several RBL lines showed indistinguishable patterns. As noted by the authors, this finding is consistent with differences in glycosylation accounting for the heterogeneity of this polypeptide.

Hempstead *et al.* (1981a) examined the tryptic peptides prepared from α chains obtained from cells that had incorporated [³H] leucine by reverse-phase high-pressure liquid chromatography using water/acetonitrile gradients. They observed four major peaks, at least one of which is likely to represent three closely eluting peptides, and one minor component. This is a much smaller number than that described by Pecoud and Conrad, although the method of labeling should, if anything, have led to a contrary result. The α chains from tunicamycin-treated cells showed about ten discernable components—eight of which differed from those obtained from α chains derived from untreated cells.

5. Other Properties

Some additional properties of the α chains are worth recording for the sake of completeness, although the findings cannot yet be incorporated into the model of the receptor.

a. Susceptibility to Proteases. We previously observed that when unoccupied receptors in crude extracts were warmed to 25° or 37°C, rapid loss of binding activity was observed as assayed by the soluble receptor assay (Rossi *et al.*, 1977). If the receptors had been preloaded with IgE no such loss was evident. We postulated that proteolytic enzymes in the crude extract might be cleaving the unoccupied receptors more rapidly than those to which IgE was bound. We have since tested to see if we could cleave α chains in nonionic detergent extracts and obtain fragments similar to those we have prepared by digestion of α chains in SDS (Section IV.B.3). We have confirmed that indeed the α chains are more resistant to proteolytic attack in the presence of bound IgE, but have found that even the unoccupied chains are relatively resistant. Furthermore, definable fragments have not so far resulted. We have reconfirmed the loss of activity [as measured by the $(NH_4)_2SO_4$ assay] when crude extracts are warmed to 37°C, but when such material is precipitated with IgE and anti-IgE, no bands other than the usual band of α chains are observed on gel electrophoresis. Roth and Froese (1982) have reported similar results.

b. Binding of Detergent. The receptor for IgE can be solubilized from cells by a variety of detergents. Initial studies employed Nonidet P40 or the related Triton X-100 (Conrad *et al.*, 1976; Kulczycki *et al.*, 1976; Rossi *et al.*, 1977). We have recently shown that the detergents octylglucoside and sodium cholate and the zwitterionic detergent 3-[(3-cholamidopropyl)dimethylamonio]-1-propane-sulfate (Hjelmeland, 1980) were equally effective (Rivnay and Metzger, 1982). In contrast to other surface-labeled proteins, which are only partially recovered in the detergent extract (Isersky *et al.*, 1982a; Rivnay and Metzger, 1982), receptor-IgE complexes are solubilized fully.

When IgE–α-chain complexes are purified they appear to be soluble and unaggregated even after rigorous removal of detergent (S. Wank, B. Rivnay, and H. Metzger, unpublished observations). Nevertheless when such purified IgE–α-chain complexes are chromatographed on columns of agarose in the presence of nonionic detergent they elute at a volume much different than that for free IgE, suggesting that the Stokes radius has increased substantially owing to the binding of detergent. Conrad *et al.* (1976) removed Nonidet P40 from crude extracts of cells with beads of polystyrene–divinylbenzene. Nevertheless virtually all of the IgE–receptor complexes remained soluble. We have observed the same result using nonionic detergents that have a higher critical micelle concentration than Nonidet P40 and which can therefore be more efficiently removed by dialysis. It seems likely that under such conditions the complexes interact with lipids in the crude extract (Rivnay and Metzger, 1982). We have not so far had success using "charge shift electrophoresis" to analyze the binding of detergent to the receptor (R. Perez-Montfort and H. Metzger, unpublished observations). The compositional analyses of α chains showed a "hydrophobicity index" (as determined by the method of Barrantes, 1975) that was intermediate between the average for peripheral versus integral membrane proteins (Kanellopoulos et al., 1980).

   c. *Inactivation by Radiation.* There are few methods available by which the potential interaction of the receptor with other cellular components can be analyzed. If such interactions are weak or transient or require special conditions, they may be undetectable when one solubilizes the cell, owing to the consequent dilutional and other disruptive effects. The use of cross-linking reagents provides one approach, but there are many reasons why such experiments may have so far failed to demonstrate reactions of the receptor with other cellular components. An alternative approach is target analysis using high-energy radiation (Kempner and Schlegel, 1979). With this method it is potentially possible to demonstrate interactions of a macromolecule in unfractionated biological material (even whole cells) provided that a discrete functional assay is available. We recently examined the receptor for IgE using this technique. The function we monitored was the capacity of the irradiated material to bind IgE. If only the intact α chain was required, then one would predict that a "target size" equivalent to at least the mass of the α chain should have been found. If the conformation of the α chain was affected by the β subunit (Section IV.C) or by some still unidentified other component, a larger "target" might have been detected. Surprisingly the target size was *smaller* than our best estimates for the mass of the α chain (Fewtrell et al., 1981). Several explanations for these unexpected results are possible. One is that they are simply due to experimental error. If the results of chromatography in guanidine HCl are correct as they stand (Section IV.B.1) then the average value obtained—38,500—is close to the value obtained for the IgE-binding activity on intact cells by target analysis—37,300. One would then have to assume that previous estimates of the molecular weight, e.g., by gel electrophoresis in SDS, were substantially too high and similarly that the target size determined for the solubilized receptor—28,000—was substantially too low. Since in the radiation inactivation experiments calibration markers were used that gave the expected molecular weights, this is hard to explain. An alternative possibility, viz. that the method of radiation inactivation is detecting functional domains in the α chains, is a more attractive explanation, but one that is difficult to validate. It is notable that IgE—which, like others immunoglobulins, is known to have discrete, relatively independent domains—also gave a target size substantially smaller than the whole molecule when its capacity to bind to receptors was assessed (Fewtrell et al., 1981).

C. The β Chain

1. Detection

When the molecular weight of the component that binds IgE in a detergent extract was assessed from sedimentation and diffusion data using an assay for soluble receptors, a molecular weight of 77,000 was estimated for the receptor free of detergent (Newman et al., 1977). Although we could not exclude experimental error, this seemed like a substantial discrepancy with the molecular weight determined for the α chain (Section IV.B.1). We decided to use cross-linking reagents to test whether the native receptor might consist of a dimer of α chains or α chains associated with a previously undetected second chain. Initial results showed that after cross-linking the labeled α chains had shifted to a higher molecular weight when tested by gel electrophoresis (cited in Metzger, 1978). Further analysis showed that a second component of molecular weight 30,000–35,000 had become cross-linked to the α chain, yielding a complex of ≃90,000 (Holowka et al., 1980). This result and the fact that it could be observed on intact cells as well as in extracts of the cells was for us the critical finding; it demonstrated that at least some of the small amounts of a 30,000-molecular-weight component(s), which can sometimes be seen in preparations that appear otherwise relatively pure (Kulczycki and Parker, 1979; Helm and Froese, 1981b), was not simply a co-purifying contaminant (see also Section IV.D).

2. Molecular Weight; Fragments

So far only gel electrophoresis in SDS has been used to determine the molecular weight of the isolated β chain. The value obtained—30,000–35,000—is approximately the same as that calculated for the difference between the molecular weight of the principal cross-linked product and that of the α chain. We were initially puzzled to find that the cross-linked receptors on partially purified membrane particles were considerably smaller (Holowka and Metzger, 1982). We ultimately surmised that proteolytic splitting of the β component was occurring since addition of two protease inhibitors, leupeptin, and pepstatin, largely prevented formation of the smaller component (Holowka and Metzger, 1982). Our provisional estimates were that the larger fragment, β1, had a molecular weight of 20,000 and that the smaller region, β2, had a molecular weight of ≃15,000.

3. Composition

The 35,000-dalton component that can be cross-linked to α becomes labeled with ^3H when cells are grown in a mixture of $[^3H]$-amino acids but not when they are grown in radioactive glucosamine or mannose (Holowka and Metzger, 1982).

The component referred to by Hempstead et al. (1981a) as "receptor-associated protein" has a similar molecular weight (which does not change when observed in extracts from cells treated with tunicamycin). It was also shown to be labeled when extracts from cells grown in [^{3}H]leucine and [^{35}S]methionine were examined but not when the cells were grown in [^{14}C]glucosamine or [^{14}C]mannose. The tryptic peptides of the "receptor-associated protein" appear to be quite different from those of α chains (Hempstead *et al.*, 1981a).

When RBL cells are incubated with ^{32}P and the receptor is isolated by several different methods, the principal phosphorylated component that is regularly observed is a component whose mobility on gel electrophoresis before and after cross-linking is precisely like that of the β chain (Fewtrell *et al.*, 1982). By electrophoretic analysis of the acid hydrolysate, the incorporated ^{32}P had the same mobility as O-phosphoserine. The only other component observed that does not appear in control precipitates is an $M_r \simeq 14,000$ component that by a variety of criteria is consistent with the postulated smaller cleavage product of β, β2. We observed no significant phosphorylation of the α chain. Hempstead *et al.* (1981b) using normal mast cells reported that small amounts of ^{32}P were incorporated into α chains, although they were minimal compared to the amount incorporated into these chains after reacting the cells with the ionophore A23187. They failed to observe labeling of a component in the 30,000–35,000 range before or after reaction with A23187. However, under the conditions they employed for purifying the receptor, it is virtually certain that the β chains would have been lost.

The incorporation of ^{32}P into β is likely not to be related simply to the biosynthesis of β (Fewtrell *et al.*, 1982). The reasoning behind this statement is as follows: At least when filled with monomeric IgE, the receptor (as defined by the bound IgE) persists on the cell surface (Isersky *et al.*, 1979). Since β appears to be firmly bound to α in crude cell extracts (Holowka and Metzger, 1982; S. A. Wank and H. Metzger, unpublished observations) it is reasonable to suppose that they are firmly associated in the plasma membrane. Therefore, any ^{32}P incorporated into β chains after saturation of the receptors with IgE should have been incorporated into receptors previously inserted into the surface membrane. That the specific activity of ^{32}P-labeled β chains relative to the recovered bound IgE is quantitatively unchanged regardless of whether incorporation is performed before or after the addition of IgE completes the argument.

It should be mentioned that labeling with neither iodonaphthylazide (Section IV.C.4) nor ^{32}P has so far been sufficiently intense to make it a practical way of following β in experiments designed to investigate its interaction with α (Section IV.C.2.d).

4. Extrinsic Labeling Properties

When chemically cross-linked receptors are isolated from cells whose membrane proteins have been modified by surface-labeling techniques, the α chain of the $\alpha:\beta$ complex but not the β chain is labeled (Holowka *et al.*, 1980). On the other hand, when cells or membranes are reacted with the hydrophobic probe iodonaphthylazide (Bercovici and Gitler, 1978) only the β and not the α is found to be labeled (Holowka *et al.*, 1981). In preparations where the protease activity was not inhibited with leupepsin and pepstatin much or virtually all of the label may appear in an $M_r = 20,000$ fraction (Holowka *et al.*, 1981). RBL cells and normal rat peritoneal cells gave similar results. It is this same component, $\beta1$ (Section IV.C.2) that becomes cross-linked to the α chain.

5. Association with α Chain

The most practical method we have so far found to explore how α and β are associated is to use cross-linking reagents: α chains are radioiodinated by surface-labeling cells with the lactoperoxidase method, the cells are reacted with amidi-nated IgE, and they are then solubilized with detergent. After processing of the extract by different procedures, the extent to which β remains associated with α is assessed by cross-linking of the specimen with dimethylsuberimidate. The bound IgE is precipitated with anti-IgE, and the SDS extract of the precipitate is analyzed by gel electrophoresis. A shift in the apparent molecular weight of the α chains from 50,000 to 85,000–90,000 indicates the presence of the β chain. This assay is clearly cumbersome and progress has been slow. Recent experiments (Rivnay *et al.*, 1982) have employed a mouse IgE hybridoma with antidinitro-phenyl activity (Liu *et al.*, 1980) by which the complexes are adsorbed to trini-trophenyl-lysyl-Sepharose beads (Holowka and Metzger, 1982). After washing with the desired solvents, the complexes are released with dinitrophenyl hapten and the eluate is cross-linked and then analyzed. The loss of β seen by washing with detergent alone can be largely prevented by washing with (unlabeled) deter-gent extracts of tumor cells, dialyzed extracts, and mixtures of detergent with lipids isolated from the tumor. The β chains in such partially purified $\alpha:\beta$ com-plexes can then be labeled extrinsically, so that we now have a simpler assay for exploring conditions required for $\alpha:\beta$ association.

Once the best conditions by which the $\alpha:\beta$ complex can be purified without loss of β are found, the native stoichiometry of $\alpha:\beta$ can be determined more rigorously. However, it is almost certain that one and only one β chain is asso-ciated with each α chain. This conclusion is derived largely from the results of the cross-linking studies. In some experiments essentially all of the α becomes cross-linked. Nevertheless only two types of cross-linked product are observed (under conditions where no cleavage of β occurs). One is the 90,000-dalton species already referred to; the other is material that fails to penetrate the gel. Significantly no components are observed at molecular weights $\simeq 120,000$, 130,000, 150,000, . . . such as would be expected for $\alpha_1\beta_2$, $\alpha_2\beta_1$, $\alpha_1\beta_3$, and so forth. When the entire preparation is reduced in order to break the cross-links formed by the dimethyl dithiobispropionimidate, only α and β chains are observed. These results are most consistent with the fundamental structural unit for the receptor being $\alpha_1\beta_1$. The failure of some of the cross-linked species to penetrate into the gel seems most likely to result from inadequate penetration of SDS into the cross-linked species.

The molecular weight analyses of Newman et al. (1977) suggested a value of 80,000 for the native receptor in crude extracts. This is gratifying close to the expected weight for the $\alpha_1\beta_1$ complexes. Nevertheless, it may be worthwhile to reexamine the native receptor once the conditions for stabilizing its polypeptide chain structure have been defined.

D. Other Chains

Helm and Froese (1981b) have drawn attention to a $\simeq 70,000$-dalton component that they observed in immunoprecipitates from extracts of labeled cells (see also Froese, 1980). The nature of this material has not been characterized further.

It has already been mentioned that even in the absence of cross-linking reagents, a component having a molecular weight similar to that of β can be variably detected. It is not, however, the only component observed (e.g., Fig. 5 in Kulczycki and Parker, 1979; Holowka et al., 1980; Holowka and Metzger, 1982). Thus at least two additional components—$M_r \simeq 40,000$–45,000—appear to travel with the receptor for IgE particularly under conditions where the association of α and β is preserved (Rivnay et al., 1982). It is not possible at this stage to state whether these components are specifically associated with the receptor for IgE. That the β can be cross-linked to α and is associated with α in a fixed stoichiometry is about as firm evidence as one can hope to get that the association between the chains is physiological. We are convinced that applying such rigorous criteria before accepting that a component forms part of the receptor is essential. Whether one terms such components "subunits" or not is largely a question of semantics at present. That the translational diffusion constant of the receptors in the plane of the membrane is well below that expected for freely mobile components could be due to interactions of the receptor with other cellular constituents (Schlessinger et al., 1976).

V. ARRANGEMENT OF THE RECEPTOR IN MEMBRANES

The arrangement of the receptor for IgE in the plasma membrane has been partially clarified. Early studies using IgE conjugated with ferritin demonstrated that the binding sites appeared to be diffusely distributed over the surface of the cell (Sullivan *et al.*, 1971; Becker *et al.*, 1973; Lawson *et al.*, 1975). That IgEs that bore distinguishable fluorescent labels were independently mobile (Mendoza and Metzger, 1976; Schlessinger *et al.*, 1976) provided further evidence that the receptors are not normally clustered. As the structure of the receptor has become better understood it has been possible to ask more specific topographical questions.

A. Methods of Study

Modification of the receptor with reagents whose distribution can be surmised has been the most common strategy tried. Cells or membranes are reacted with either labeling reagents or degradative enzymes and the receptor is then isolated and examined. The results are compared to some standard preparation. For example, if the isolated receptor is sensitive to a particular degradative enzyme when isolated in its soluble form but not *in situ*, then the site of enzymatic attack is said to be "unexposed" in the latter situation. One can begin to "map" various discrete regions of the receptor using such criteria. Note, however, that if the fully solubilized receptor is *not* modified by the method used the experiment is uninformative.

All of the receptors under consideration are exposed on the surface of the cell when the number of binding sites on intact cells is compared to the number in detergent extracts (Rossi *et al.*, 1977). Thus we need not concern ourselves with a substantial fraction of receptors whose distribution (and hence exposure) might be quite different than that of those disposed on the cell surface.

B. Disposition of the α Chain

Since α chains that have been freed of all other polypeptides bind IgE (Kanellopoulos *et al.*, 1979, 1980; Kulczycki and Parker, 1979; Holowka *et al.*, 1980), the binding site on the receptor for IgE must be on the α chain. Because these sites are on the surface, the α chain must be exposed on the surface. Other, circumstantial, evidence for this is that surface iodination of cells by the lactoperoxidase method leads to labeling of the α chain (Conrad and Froese, 1976; Kulczycki *et al.*, 1976); iodogen (Markwell and Fox, 1978) gives similar results (N. Kumar and H. Metzger, unpublished observations), as does labeling with galactose oxidase and $NaBH_4$ (Pecoud and Conrad, 1981). Since both of the postulated domains of the α chain are likely to contain carbohydrate and possibly both contain some of the surface label it is likely that both α1 and α2 are exposed (Goetze *et al.*, 1981).

The α chain *in situ* appears to be resistant to proteolytic attack (Metzger *et al.*, 1976; Isersky *et al.*, 1979, 1982b); since the α chains in the solubilized receptor are also relatively resistant (N. Kumar and H. Metzger, unpublished observations) the experiments are not informative. Surface-labeling of the α chains is blocked when IgE is bound (Conrad and Froese, 1976). When the receptor is then solubilized and labeling of it attempted again, no modification, at least by lactoperoxidase, is observed (Pecoud and Conrad, 1981). Thus the failure of chains complexed with IgE to become labeled on various preparations of membranes (Pecoud and Conrad, 1981; Isersky et al., 1982a) is uninterpretable.

It is not clear whether the α chain interacts with the lipid bilayer. As already noted (Section IV.B.5.b) the amino acid composition data yield a hydrophobicity index that is borderline, but about the same as that of glycophorin. The latter is thought to interact with the bilayer through a short helical segment (Marchesi et al., 1976). If binding of detergent is used as a criterion, the results are mixed (Section IV.B.5.b). That the α chain is *not* labeled with the hydrophobic probe iodonaphthylazide is not very informative—there are too many explanations for such negative results.

C. Disposition of the β Chain

The β chain is modified by the hydrophobic probe iodonaphthylazide exclusively in that region of the chain dubbed β1 (Section IV.C.2). It does not incorporate oligosaccharide precursors and is not observed in extracts of cells reacted with lactoperoxidase under conditions where β was proven to be present (Holowka et al., 1980, 1981; Holowka and Metzger, 1982). These latter results are all consistent with—but by no means prove—the supposition that the β chain is not exposed on the surface of the cell. On the other hand, β is cleaved *in situ* in the absence of the protease inhibitors leupepsin and pepstatin and the smaller fragment that appears to have been cleaved off intact, β2, is phosphorylated (Section IV.C.3). These findings have been tentatively interpreted as indicating that β2 penetrates the cytoplasmic surface of the bilayer. Attempts to label extrinsically this portion on membrane fragments have so far not been successful (Isersky et al., 1982a).

D. Model of Receptor

On the basis of the data that have been reviewed in the previous sections we prepared a schematic drawing of how the two components of the receptor, α and β, might be incorporated into the plasma membrane (Fig. 4) (Goetze et al., 1981; Fewtrell et al., 1982). It must be emphasized, as we did in the original work, that the chief usefulness of the model is to assist us in articulating specific questions that can be explored experimentally. While we are confident that over the five-year period since we drew our first model (Metzger, 1978) some progress has

Figure 4. Schematic representation of the receptor for IgE. This figure, a modified version of the preferred model (A) shown in Fig. 9 of Goetze *et al.* (1981), shows the presumptive location of the O-phosphoserine residue(s). As in the original figure, the horizontal line represents the surface of the outer leaflet of the plasma membrane bilayer, the hatched areas represent carbohydrate, the black areas represent sites of high susceptibility to proteolysis, the single asterisk represents the principal site of surface-labeling, the double asterisk represents the site of labeling by iodonaphthylazide, and the circles represent spheres whose volumes are proportional to their masses. The figure is drawn to scale using the best information available in 1982. From Fewtrell *et al.* (1982).

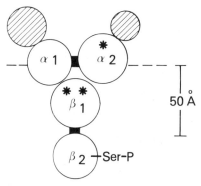

been made, it is likely that results over the next five-years will require major revisions in the current schema.

VI. MECHANISM OF RECEPTOR ACTION

A. Molecular Requirements for Triggering of Secretion

1. Importance of Aggregation

Although some controversy had (has?) persisted, it has been long recognized that aggregation of the IgE bound to the surface of mast cells and basophils by antigen—or in the laboratory by some other means—is a critical step. Only the elucidation of the biochemical details will provide proof, but the current consensus (Metzger and Ishizaka, 1982) is that what aggregation of IgE accomplishes is to bring about close association between previously separated receptors for IgE.

Three principal observations form the foundation for this formulation:

1. The receptors *in situ* are univalent (Mendoza and Metzger, 1976; Schlessinger *et al.*, 1976).
2. The receptors are mobile (Sullivan *et al.*, 1971; Becker *et al.*, 1973; Carson and Metzger, 1974; Lawson *et al.*, 1975).
3. Multivalent antibodies to the receptor for IgE, can by themselves trigger cells (T. Ishizaka *et al.*, 1977; Isersky *et al.*, 1978).

Observation (1) indicates that the primary process is *inter*molecular rather than *intra*molecular; observation (2), that the molecules that mediate the reaction need not be closely adjacent prior to triggering; and observation (3), that the important molecules are the receptors and not the IgE.

A quantitative analysis of how multivalent binding of a ligand either directly (e.g., with antireceptor antibodies) or indirectly (e.g., by binding of multivalent antigen to IgE bound to receptors) increases the temporal stability of receptor clusters has been presented (DeLisi, 1980). It is still not understood, however, what is meant by, or rather what is required of, the "association." That is, it is not known how "close" the receptors have to get together. It is possible that the receptors must make van der Waals contact, e.g., in order to form an active site, or to produce a mutual conformational change or the like (intrinsic mechanism). It is also possible that simply having receptors at a sufficiently high local concentration will permit some other—presumably multivalent—molecule to interact with them (extrinsic mechanism). The alternative mechanisms have also been referred to as "direct" or "linkage" models (Metzger, 1977). We have made an attempt to investigate this question by using cross-linking reagents. We triggered cells with preaggregated IgE and reacted the cells with cross-linking reagents to see if multimers of receptors were formed. Although we saw no evidence for such covalently linked receptors (Holowka et al., 1980) the negative results are not really definitive.

The group headed by McConnell has been exploring the usefulness of using monofunctional ligands incorporated into liposomes or planar membranes as a tool for studying triggering of mast cells coated with specific IgE. They observed that even highly mobile hapten ligands could stimulate release apparently because of clustering of the IgEs induced by the antibody–antigen reaction at the sites of cell–lipid monolayer contact (Weis et al., 1982). Those observations indicate that the receptors need only be very indirectly linked in order to promote a response. The results are consistent with either an "intrinsic" or an "extrinsic" mechanism.

2. Extent of Clustering Required

The question of how much clustering of the receptors is required for triggering is usefully divided into two questions, the answers to which, though related, have quite different implications.

a. Size of Clusters. A variety of experimental approaches suggested that, whereas aggregation of IgE was necessary, the degree of aggregation did not have to be extensive (K. Ishizaka and Ishizaka, 1968; Becker et al., 1973; Siraganian et al., 1975; Lawson et al., 1975). Some of the data suggested that dimers might be sufficient (K. Ishizaka and Ishizaka, 1968; Siraganian et al., 1975), but the possibility that tiny amounts of larger aggregates might be the active species could not be excluded.

Quantitative studies using preformed, defined aggregates of IgE eliminated this possibility and demonstrated unequivocally that dimers of IgE (and therefore of receptors) were adequate to induce release (Segal et al., 1977; Fewtrell and Metzger, 1980; Kagey-Sobotka et al., 1981). It is interesting, however, that the efficacy of larger oligomers appears to be greater at least when tested in some systems. With respect to human basophils, it could not be ruled out that oligomers larger than dimers are simply increasing the probability of generating dimers of the receptor (Kagey-Sobotka et al., 1981). With the rat tumor cells, the differences between the dimers and trimmers or higher oligomers did not seem explicable on such grounds alone (Fewtrell and Metzger, 1980).

The minimal cluster size presumably is directly related to the mechanism by which receptors trigger the initial biochemical event. It is for this reason that we referred to the minimal cluster size as the "unit signal" (Segal et al., 1977).

b. Number of Clusters. The number of unit signals required to trigger release is a different aspect of the role of aggregation of receptors and is likely to be related to many more cellular events than the initial perturbation. Several factors appear to be involved. Normal cells (and to a much more limited extent the tumor cells so far reported on) (Fewtrell et al., 1979), have a mechanism by which the signal generated can be rendered ineffective. The process is termed "desensitization" (Lichtenstein, 1971). It refers to the finding that cells whose receptors are putatively triggered will not degranulate under conditions such as deprivation of Ca^{2+} or low temperature even when the permissive conditions are subsequently restored (Lichtenstein and Osler, 1964; Osler et al., 1968). The system can be manipulated in such a way that the desensitization is "receptor-specific" (Sobotka et al., 1979; Siraganian and Kimberly, 1979; MacGlashan and Lichtenstein, 1981). That is, if other receptors on the same cells are then stimulated, perfectly normal release ensues. The mechanism of desensitization appears to have similar requirements with respect to clustering of receptors as the stimulatory reaction (Kagey-Sobotka et al., 1981). Thus it appears that the amount of secretion is determined by the balance between stimulation and inactivation (Dembo et al., 1979). The desensitization mechanism is kinetically saturable so that the rate of generation of signals appears to be critical. This can explain the observation that, at least with normal mast cells, the secretory response to increasing doses of preformed aggregates of IgE continues to increase over a range well beyond the cells' capacity to bind IgE (Fewtrell and Metzger, 1980). This must mean that the *rate* of formation of clusters rather than only the total *number* of clusters is significant. Related observations are that if the stimulus is topographically localized local degranulation is observed (Lawson et al., 1978). One explanation of this phenomenon is that the "signal" becomes inactivated rather than simply diluted or prevented from reaching other "compartments." Likewise the number of clusters required to induce the initial quanta of release is proportionately much smaller than that required for further degranulation, i.e., the dose–response curve is much too flat (Fewtrell and Metzger, 1980).

It follows that secretion is a poor (albeit experimentally simple and physiologically relevant) measure of activation of receptors. What one can conclude is that, using efficient preparations of preaggregated IgE or efficient cross-linking ligands and active cells the number of clusters required for substantial release can be quite small—on the order of hundreds or less per cell (Fewtrell and Metzger, 1980).

B. Consequences of the Association of Receptors

1. General Comments

Very little is known about the biochemical changes that ensue following the clustering of receptors and one can only recount largely negative (and largely unpublished) results that have limited value even to exclude certain mechanisms. Nevertheless, it is worthwhile to review the approaches that are available for study. The problem simply stated is this: The evidence is good that association of receptors is the initial critical event but the immediate consequences are unknown. How then does one design practical experiments, i.e., experiments whose complexity bears some reasonable relationship to the usefulness of what is likely to be learned? Two major strategies can be delineated. The first is a direct approach; one seeks changes in the receptor or in its associations with other cellular components. The second is an indirect approach; one searches for perturbations in general and hopes to relate these to the action of the receptors.

2. Changes in the Structure of the Receptor

Changes in the structure of the receptor imply an intrinsic mechanism. So far only limited experiments have been performed or at least published. The simplest approach is to look for changes in either of the polypeptide chains of the receptor, in their size or modification (e.g., phosphorylation, methylation). It can be argued that even this approach may be more difficult than anticipated because we know that only a small fraction of the receptors *need* to be clustered in order to get substantial stimulation (Section VI.A.2.b). We do not know what happens if a large number of receptors is clustered. Do all of them generate the initial signal or is there something that limits the initial perturbation? If the latter, the putative changes might be restricted to a tiny proportion of the molecules. The experiments that demonstrate "receptor-specific" desensitization (Section VI.A.2.b) give one hope that this is not the case. Those experiments show that even after a substantial number of receptors have been clustered (under desensitizing conditions) the remaining ones remain capable of generating a normal response. An optimistic interpretation is that one can anticipate a stoichiometric relationship between the number of receptors clustered and the extent of the initial biochemical perturbation.

So far we have observed no changes in either the size or the phosphorylation of the α or β chains or—by using cross-linking reagents—in their interaction with each other or with other cellular components (J. D. Taurog and H. Metzger, unpublished observations; Holowka *et al.*, 1980; Fewtrell *et al.*, 1981). However, those initial experiments need to be extended if one wishes to exclude such changes more definitively.

One further cautionary note is necessary. Changes should ideally be sought under conditions where the cell is minimally perturbed. Otherwise changes may be induced (or observed) as a *consequence* of the perturbation and will not reflect the initiating signal. A case in point is the observation by Hempstead *et al.* (1981b) that the α chain of the receptor becomes phosphorylated when cells are stimulated to secrete. In this instance stimulation was induced with the ionophore A23187, which is unlikely to involve the receptors for IgE in its mechanism of release. Therefore, whatever may be the significance of the phosphorylation (the authors propose that it may be related to a feedback mechanism) it is unlikely to be related to the event *initiated* by the receptor. Had similar findings been observed with receptor-induced release the results could easily have been misinterpreted. Thus blocking the pathway at a point as proximal to the initiation event as possible may be important in order to obviate such confusion.

3. Functional Changes

It is possible that the unclustered receptor is a zymogen that when aggregated becomes an active enzyme; alternatively it may become an ion channel. In either case the isolated receptor would exhibit an intrinsic function. It should be possible to explore several such possibilities directly by preparing liposomes containing purified receptors or IgE–receptor complexes. Our group has begun exploring this approach using, as a first criterion for successful reconstitution of the receptor, its ability to be reincorporated into liposomes after being solubilized from cells. Initial studies revealed that several factors are important: the nature of the lipid, of the detergent, and of the detergent/lipid ratio (Rivnay and Metzger, 1982). A substantial proportion of such reincorporated receptor–IgE complexes appear to be oriented in such a way that the IgE can be stripped off under conditions (Kulczycki and Metzger, 1974) where specific binding activity of the receptors is maintained (Rivnay and Metzger, 1982). Reconstituted receptors are likely to provide powerful tools for studying the structure of the receptor. Their usefulness for functional studies will importantly depend upon whether the action of the receptor has an "intrinsic" aspect or occurs entirely via an "extrinsic" mechanism (see Section VI.B.4).

4. Changes in the Interaction of the Receptor with Other Cellular Components

One change in the receptor that occurs as a consequence of clustering has been identified: the receptors are internalized (Isersky *et al.*, 1982b). The observations (so far made only on RBL cells) are that monomeric IgE persists for long times on the surface of the cell; it slowly dissociates but is not appreciably internalized (Isersky *et al.*, 1979). However, when preaggregated dimers or trimers of IgE are reacted with cells, the IgE and, as far as one can tell, the receptors to which they are bound disappear from the surface of the cell (Isersky *et al.*, 1982b). The phenomenon is distinctly different from that recently proposed for the Fc$_\gamma$ receptor on macrophages (Segal *et al.*, 1983a,b). In the latter instance there appears to be a regular cyclical traffic of receptors between the plasma membrane and the cytoplasm; aggregates of IgG are thought to internalize in preference to monomers because they bind more firmly, *not* because they signal a change in cycling of receptors. This is clearly a different situation than in the case of the high-affinity receptor for IgE where clustering *induces* the internalization.

The phenomena of internalization and stimulation of the cell have not been compared; the available data at first glance suggest that the phenomena are independent sequelae of receptor clustering. Thus, the dramatic difference between dimers and trimers in their capacity to induce secretion from RBL cells (Fewtrell and Metzger, 1980) is not mirrored in the speed or extent to which they are internalized (Isersky *et al.*, 1982b). But one must be cautious. In the studies on internalization the entire population of bound oligomers was monitored; in the studies of secretion a minor subpopulation could have been sufficient to trigger the release observed (Section VI.A.2.b).

It has not so far been possible to manipulate this system in such a way that the cells can complete the process of degranulation in the absence of the continued clustering of receptors. Using hapten-specific IgE and a hapten conjugate to generate clustering, it is observed that addition of monovalent hapten causes an immediate cessation of release of mediators (Kagey-Sobotka *et al.*, 1982). In these experiments, performed on human basophils, it is difficult to distinguish whether the added hapten is preventing the clustering of additional receptors or is causing the deaggregation of existing clusters or both. With RBL cells, which desensitize more slowly, clustering of receptors can be induced under conditions nonpermissive for secretion, the cells washed, permissive conditions reintroduced, and release then monitored. The results suggest that disrupting preformed aggregates prevents further release (C. Fewtrell and H. Metzger, unpublished observations). Thus there is no evidence for an intermediate that is sufficiently long-lived that, when the clusters which engendered it are disrupted, it can continue to function. Incidentally these results also suggest that internalized clustered receptors also do not form a stable intermediate of secretion. Concanavalin A stimulates cells by aggregating IgE via the carbohydrate on the immunoglobulin (Keller, 1973; Magro, 1974; Fewtrell *et al.*, 1979). That concanavalin A bound to beads stimulates localized degranulation (Lawson *et al.*, 1978) also suggests that the signal is generated by receptors at the surface of the cell and that internalization is not a necessary step.

Internalization is an example of a mechanism that might be purely "extrinsic."

The clustering that is induced by the ligand may simply hold the receptors in a configuration such that some other element (e.g., a cytoskeletal component) could form stable bonds with the receptors. The receptor would simply serve as a passive link between the stimulating ligand and the hypothetical element; the receptor thus would subserve a role entirely analogous to that currently postulated for IgE. Such a mechanism has recently been modeled mathematically for receptors in general by Brandts and Jacobson (1983).

5. Other Changes

The search for early changes in cellular elements other than the receptor that result from receptor clustering has followed three approaches: (1) looking for measurable changes in some biochemical parameter, (2) blocking pathways with inhibitors, and, more recently, (3) selection of cell variants deficient in certain pathways, coupled with complementation studies. The articles by T. Ishizaka (1982), Winslow and Austen (1982), and Siraganian et al. (1982) that appeared in a recent symposium proceedings, give an excellent overview of the status of this area.

I shall limit my own very brief discussion strictly to what such studies have so far contributed and can be expected to achieve with respect to understanding the mechanism of action of the receptor per se. Clearly the entire biochemical pathway of exocytosis is a complex phenomenon of which the receptor forms only a small part.

In previous sections the need for a suitable assay for the initiation of the biochemical pathway induced by clustering of receptors was stressed. No study has yet appeared in which the stoichiometric relationship between clustering of receptors and the changes, studied by the first approach referred to above, have been correlated. (The other approaches do not lend themselves to this type of analysis.) Whether the perturbation measured—such as fluxes of Ca^{2+} (Foreman et al., 1977; T. Ishizaka et al., 1979), methylation of lipids (Hirata et al., 1979; T. Ishizaka et al., 1980), or changes in levels of cyclic adenosine monophosphate (Holgate et al., 1980) or a protein kinase (Winslow et al., 1981)—is an immediate or somewhat more distal consequence of receptor clustering is not as critical as determining that it is quantitatively and temporally appropriately coupled.

Once such a perturbation has been identified it may be possible to determine which cellular component(s) is responsible. If it is the receptor itself, then the approach referred to earlier, of preparing liposomes into which purified receptors have been incorporated, should be highly useful. If the immediate consequence involves a mixed mechanism, i.e., one in which the receptor interacts with a second component but in more than a passive way, the problem becomes much more complex. Molecular complementation and in situ radiation inactivation have been profitably employed for the study of receptors for hormones. Cross-linking reagents have received less attention than they probably deserve, perhaps because the number of reagents that are readily available is still limited.

VII. SUMMARY

Study of the cell-surface receptor for IgE has provided a rough outline of its structure. The protein contains an α subunit that is a glycopeptide exposed on the external surface of the plasma membrane. This chain binds monomeric IgE on a mole/mole basis with high affinity and specificity. *In situ* it interacts with a second subunit, β, which is more deeply imbedded in the membrane. Clustering of the receptor into dimers and higher oligomers stimulates exocytosis of those cells on which the receptor resides. The most pressing stuctural–functional problem is defining how association of receptors with each other initiates the biochemical events leading to degranulation. An essential step will be to identify biochemical phenomena that are stoichiometrically linked to the clustering of the receptors.

ACKNOWLEDGMENTS

I should like to acknowledge the many individuals with whom I have worked in my own laboratory and to note that it is unlikely that there are any ideas expressed in this review that have not been engendered by active discussions with them. I should like to express special thanks to my most recent younger collaborators, Drs. Fewtrell, Finbloom, Goetze, Holowka, Kanellopoulos, Kumar, Perez-Montfort, Rivnay, and Wank, as well as to Dr. Isersky, who has been with my group from the outset of our detailed exploration of this area.

VIII. REFERENCES

Barrantes, F. J., 1975, *Biochem. Biophys. Res. Commun.* **62**:407–414.
Bazin, H., Querijean, P., Beckers, A., Heremans, J. F., and Dessy, F., 1974, *Immunology* **26**: 713–723.
Becker, K. E., Ishizaka, T., Metzger, H., Ishizaka, K., and Grimley, P., 1973, *J. Exp. Med.* **108**:394–409.
Beenich, H., Ragnarsson, U., Johansson, S. G. O., Ishizaka, K., Ishizaka, T., Levy, D. A., and Lichtenstein, L. M., 1977, *Inst. Arch. Allergy Appl. Immunol.* **53**:459–468.
Bercovici, T., and Gitler, C., 1978, *Biochemistry* **17**:1484–1489.
Brandts, J. F., and Jacobson, B. S., 1983, *Surv. Synth. Pathol. Res.* (in press).
Carson, D. A., and Metzger, H., 1974, *J. Immunol.* **113**:1271–1277.
Conrad, D. H., and Froese, A., 1976, *J. Immunol.* **116**:319–326.
Conrad, D. H., and Froese, A., 1978a, *J. Immunol.* **120**:429–437.
Conrad, D. H., and Froese, A., 1978b, *Immunochemistry* **15**:283–288.
Conrad, D. H., Berczi, I., and Froese, A., 1976, *Immunochemistry* **13**:329–332.

Conroy, N. C., Adkinson, N. F., and Lichtenstein, L. M., 1979, *Int. Arch. Allergy Appl. Immunol.* **60**:106–109.

DeLisi, C., 1980, *Q. Rev. Biophys.* **13**:201–231.

DeLisi, C., 1981, *Mol. Immunol.* **18**:507–511.

Dembo, M., Goldstein, B., Sobotka, A. K., and Lichtenstein, L. M., 1979, *J. Immunol.* **123**: 1864–1872.

Dorrington, K. J., and Bennich, H., 1978, *Immunol. Rev.* **41**:3–25.

Eccleston, E., Leonard, B. J., Lowe, J. S., and Welford, H. J., 1973, *Nature (London) New Biol.* **244**:73–76.

Ellerson, J. R., Karlson, T., and Bennich, H., 1978, in: *Protides of the Biological Fluids*, Volume 25 (H. Peeters, ed.), pp. 739–742, Pergamon Press, New York.

Fewtrell, C., and Metzger, H., 1980, *J. Immunol.* **125**:701–710.

Fewtrell, C., Kessler, A., and Metzger, H., 1979, *Adv. Inflamm. Res.* **1**:205–221.

Fewtrell, C., Kempner, E., Poy, G., and Metzger, H., 1981, *Biochemistry* **20**:6589–6594.

Fewtrell, C., Goetze, A., and Metzger, H., 1982, *Biochemistry* **21**:2004–2010.

Foreman, J. C., Hallet, M. B., and Mongar, J. L., 1977, *J. Physiol.* **271**:193–214.

Fritsche, R., and Spiegelberg, H. L., 1978, *J. Immunol.* **121**:471–478.

Froese, A., 1980, *Crit. Rev. Immunol.* **1**:79–132.

Froese, A., Helm, R. M., Conrad, D. H., Isersky, C., Ishizaka, T., and Kulczycki, A., Jr., 1982a, *Immunology* **45**:107–116.

Froese, A., Helm, R. M., Conrad, D. H., Isersky, C., and Ishizaka, T., 1982b, *Immunology* **45**:117–123.

Goetze, A., Kanellopoulos, J., Rice, D., and Metzger, H., 1981, *Biochemistry* **20**:6341–6349.

Hamburger, R. N., 1975, *Science* **189**:389–390.

Helm, R. M., and Froese, A., 1981a, *Int. Arch. Allergy Appl. Immunol.* **65**:81–84.

Helm, R. M., and Froese, A., 1981b, *Immunology* **42**:629–636.

Helm, R. M., Conrad, D. H., and Froese, A., 1979, *Int. Arch. Allergy Appl. Immunol.* **58**: 90–98.

Hempstead, B. L., Parker, C. W., and Kulczycki, A., Jr., 1981a, *J. Biol. Chem.* **256**:10717–10723.

Hempstead, B. L., Kulczycki, A., Jr., and Parker, C. W., 1981b, *Biochem. Biophys. Res. Commun.* **98**:815–822.

Hirata, F., Axelrod, J., and Crews, F. T., 1979, *Proc. Natl. Acad. Sci. U.S.A.* **76**:4813–4816.

Hjelmeland, L. M., 1980, *Proc. Natl. Acad. Sci. U.S.A.* **77**:6368–6370.

Holgate, S. T., Lewis, R. A., and Austen, K. F., 1980, in: *Progress in Immunology*, Volume IV (M. Fougereau and J. Dausset, eds.), pp. 847–859, Academic Press, New York.

Holowka, D., and Metzger, H., 1982, *Mol. Immunol.* **19**:219–222.

Holowka, D., Hartman, H., Kanellopoulos, J., and Metzger, H., 1980, *J. Receptor Res* **1**: 41–68.

Holowka, D., Gitler, C., Bercovici, T., and Metzger, H., 1981, *Nature (London)* **289**:806–808.

Isersky, C., Taurog, J. D., Poy, G., and Metzger, H., 1978, *J. Immunol.* **121**:549–558.

Isersky, C., Rivera, J., Mims, S., and Triche, T., 1979, *J. Immunol.* **122**:1926–1936.

Isersky, C., Rivera, J., Triche, T. J., and Metzger, H., 1982a, *Mol. Immunol.* **19**:925–941.

Isersky, C., Rivera, J., Mims, S., Segal, D. M., and Triche, T., 1982b, *Fed. Proc.* **41**:824 (abstr. 3240).

Ishizaka, K., and Ishizaka, T., 1968, *J. Immunol.* **101**:68–78.

Ishizaka, T., 1982, *Fed. Proc.* **41**:17–21.

Ishizaka, T., and Ishizaka, K., 1975, *Ann. N.Y. Acad. Sci.* **254**:462–475.

Ishizaka, T., Chang, T. H., Taggart, M., and Ishizaka, K., 1977, *J. Immunol.* **119**:1589–1596.

Ishizaka, T., Foreman, J. C., Sterk, A. R., and Ishizaka, K., 1979, *Proc. Natl. Acad. Sci. U.S.A.* **76**:5858–5862.

Ishizaka, T., Hirata, F., Ishizaka, K., and Axelrod, J., 1980, *Proc. Natl. Acad. Sci. U.S.A.* **77**:1903-1906.

Kagey-Sobotka, A., Dembo, M., Goldstein, B., Metzger, H., and Lichtenstein, L. M., 1981, *J. Immunol.* **127**:2285-2291.

Kagey-Sobotka, A., MacGlashan, D. W., and Lichtenstein, L. M., 1982, *Fed. Proc.* **41**: 12-16.

Kanellopoulos, J., Rossi, G., and Metzger, H., 1979, *J. Biol. Chem.* **254**:7691-7697.

Kanellopoulos, J. M., Liu, T. Y., Poy, G., and Metzger, H., 1980, *J. Biol. Chem.* **255**: 9060-9066.

Keller, R., 1973, *Clin. Exp. Immunol.* **13**:139-147.

Kempner, E. S., and Schlegel, W., 1979, *Anal. Biochem.* **92**:2-10.

Kulczycki, A., Jr., and Metzger, H., 1974, *J. Exp. Med.* **140**:1676-1695.

Kulczycki, A., Jr., and Parker, C. W., 1979, *J. Biol. Chem.* **254**:3187-3193.

Kulczycki, A., Jr., and Vallina, V. L., 1981, *Mol. Immunol.* **18**:723-731.

Kulczycki, A., Jr., McNearney, T. A., and Parker, C. W., 1976, *J. Immunol.* **117**:661-665.

Kulczycki, A., Jr., Hempstead, B. L., Hofmann, S. L., Wood, E. W., and Parker, C. W., 1979, *J. Biol. Chem.* **254**:3194-3200.

Kumar, N., and Metzger, H., 1982, *Mol. Immunol.* **19**:1561-1567.

Lawson, D., Fewtrell, C., Gomperts, B., and Raff, M. C., 1975, *J. Exp. Med.* **142**:391-402.

Lawson, D., Fewtrell, C., and Raff, M. C., 1978, *J. Cell Biol.* **79**:394-400.

Leach, B. S., Collawn, J. F., Jr., and Fish, W. W., 1980, *Biochemistry* **19**:5741-5747.

Lehrer, S. B., McCants, M. L., Farris, P. N., and Bazin, H., 1981, *Immunology* **44**:711-716.

Lichtenstein, L. M., 1971, *J. Immunol.* **107**:1122-1129.

Lichtenstein, L. M., and Osler, A. G., 1964, *J. Exp. Med.* **120**:507-530.

Liu, F. T., Bohn, J. W., Ferry, E. L., Yamamoto, H., Molinaro, C. A., Sherman, L. A., Klinman, N. R., and Katz, D. H., 1980, *J. Immunol.* **124**:2728-2736.

MacGlashan, D. W., Jr., and Lichtenstein, L. M., 1981, *J. Immunol.* **127**:2410-2414.

Magro, A. M., 1974, *Nature (London)* **249**:572-573.

Marchesi, V. T., Furthmayr, J. H., and Tomita, M., 1976, *Annu. Rev. Biochem.* **45**:667-698.

Markwell, M. A. K., and Fox, C. F., 1978, *Biochemistry* **17**:4807-4817.

Mendoza, G. R., and Metzger, H., 1976, *Nature (London)* **264**:548-550.

Metzger, H., 1977, in: *Receptors and Recognition*, Volume 4 (P. Cuatrecasas and M. F. Greaves, eds.), pp. 73-102, Chapman and Hall, London.

Metzger, H., 1978, *Immunol. Rev.* **41**:186-199.

Metzger, H., and Bach, M., 1978, in: *Immediate Hypersensitivity* (M. Bach, ed.), pp. 561-588, Marcel Dekker, New York.

Metzger, H., and Ishizaka, T., (Chrmn.), 1982, *Fed. Proc.* **41**:7-34.

Metzger, H., Budman, D., and Lucky, P., 1976, *Immunochemistry* **13**:417-423.

Metzger, H., Goetze, A., Kanellopoulos, J., Holowka, D., and Fewtrell, C., 1982, *Fed. Proc.* **41**:8-11.

Newman, S. A., Rossi, G., and Metzger, H., 1977, *Proc. Natl. Acad. Sci. U.S.A.* **74**:869-872.

Osler, A. G., Lichtenstein, L. M., and Levy, D. A., 1968, *Adv. Immunol.* **8**:183-231.

Pecoud, A., and Conrad, D., 1981, *J. Immunol.* **127**:2208-2214.

Pecoud, A. R., Ruddy, S., and Conrad, D. H., 1981, *J. Immunol.* **126**:1624-1629.

Perez-Montfort, R., and Metzger, H., 1982, *Mol. Immunol.* **19**:1113-1125.

Rivnay, B., and Metzger, H., 1982, *J. Biol. Chem.* **257**:12800-12808.

Rivnay, B., Wank, S. A., Poy, G., and Metzger, H., 1982, *Biochemistry* **21**:6922-6927.

Rossi, G., Newman, S. A., and Metzger, H., 1977, *J. Biol. Chem.* **252**:704-711.

Roth, P. A., and Froese, A., 1982, *Immunol. Lett.* **4**:159-165.

Schlessinger, J., Webb, W. W., Elson, E. L., and Metzger, H., 1976, *Nature (London)* **264**: 550-552.

Segal, D. M., Taurog, J. D., and Metzger, H., 1977, *Proc. Natl. Acad. Sci. U.S.A.* **74**:2993–2997.

Segal, D. M., Dower, S. K., and Titus, J. A., 1983a, *J. Immunol.* **130**:130–137.

Segal, D. M., Titus, J. A., and Dower, S. K., 1983b, *J. Immunol.* **130**:138–144.

Siraganian, R. P., and Kimberley, A. H., 1979, *J. Immunol.* **122**:1719–1725.

Siraganian, R. P., Hook, W. A., and Levine, B. B., 1975, *Immunochemistry* **12**:149–157.

Siraganian, R. P., McGivney, A., Barsumian, E. L., Crews, F. T., Hirata, F., and Axelrod, J., 1982, *Fed. Proc.* **41**:30–34.

Sobotka, A. K., Dembo, M., Goldstein, B., and Lichtenstein, L. M., 1979, *J. Immunol.* **122**:511–517.

Sterk, A. R., and Ishizaka, T., 1982, *J. Immunol.* **128**:838–843.

Sullivan, A. L., Grimley, P. M., and Metzger, H., 1971, *J. Exp. Med.* **134**:1403–1416.

Wank, S. A., DeLisi, C., and Metzger, H., 1983, *Biochemistry* **22**:954–959.

Weis, R. M., Balakarishnan, K., Smith, B. A., and McConnell, H. M., 1982, *J. Biol. Chem.* **257**:6440–6445.

Winslow, C. M., and Austen, K. F., 1982, *Fed. Proc.* **41**:22–29.

Winslow, C. M., Lewis, R. A., and Austen, K. F., 1981, *J. Exp. Med.* **154**:1125–1133.

Human Immunoregulatory Molecules: Interleukin 1, Interleukin 2, and B-Cell Growth Factor

Lawrence B. Lachman

Immunex Corporation
Seattle, Washington 98101

and

Abby L. Maizel

Department of Pathology
Division of Pathobiology
M. D. Anderson Hospital and Tumor Institute
Houston, Texas 77030

I. INTRODUCTION

Intensive investigations over the past several years have clearly indicated that a significant degree of immune regulation is accomplished by soluble mediators. Among the host of potential immune regulators that have been described to date, the interleukins have been the most fully characterized. Yet many aspects of both the biochemistry and the cell biology of these factors remain to be determined. In an attempt to place some of the areas of current investigational interest into perspective, a brief historical overview of each factor will be undertaken. This historical overview will detail our knowledge of the biochemical properties attributed to each factor when first described. This latter point will be of significance in our subsequent attempts to unravel the biological properties of each factor and how it mediates those effects that lead to a competent immune response.

II. HISTORY

A. Lymphocyte-Activating Factor or Interleukin 1

Lymphocyte-activating factor, currently known as interleukin 1 (IL-1), was first described following a series of experiments in which it was observed that macrophages released a soluble mediator (IL-1), which was mitogenic for mouse thymocytes (Gery and Waksman, 1972). The macrophages seemed to require "activation" in order to release this mitogenic molecule(s) and lipopolysaccharide was demonstrated to be a most efficacious stimulant. Among the biological properties of IL-1 that were initially defined was the fact that, although this monokine was mildly mitogenic for quiescent murine thymocytes, IL-1 was much more active in the presence of a comitogen such as phytohemagglutinin (PHA) or concanavalin A (Gery et al., 1972). Specifically, culturing mouse thymocytes with both IL-1 and PHA led to a synergistic proliferative response that was greater than the mitogenesis seen with either agent alone. Thus, firmly established by the initial investigators in this area were the findings that IL-1 was a macrophage product, that macrophages required activation for release of the monokine, and that this factor(s) was mitogenic for unstimulated as well as lectin-stimulated murine thymocytes.

A subsequent finding of significance was the demonstration that not only was IL-1 produced by those normal murine monocytes recently isolated from the peritoneum, but that several murine monocytic cell lines also retained the capability of producing IL-1 upon exogenous stimulation (Lachman et al., 1977). The proliferactive properties of the IL-1 derived from the monocytic cell lines remained constant in that it was weakly mitogenic for unstimulated mouse thymocytes and highly mitogenic for those cells that had been lectin-stimulated. This observation was also of significance since it demonstrated that IL-1 production by macrophages was relatively stable phenotypically since it was not invariably lost by those cells established in continuous culture. Macrophage cell lines proved to be invaluable as a reproducible source of large quantities of IL-1 and remain today the standard source for murine IL-1. Human IL-1 has also been produced from several sources. Until the recent past, IL-1 has mainly been derived from stimulated monocytes placed in short-term culture. These monocytes have been prepared from peripheral venous blood of either normal donors, patients with acute monocytic leukemia (AMOL), or patients with acute myelomonocytic leukemia (AMML) (Lachman et al., 1978). The monocytes from the leukemic peripheral blood may be isolated in high yields and have provided a needed resource for the generation of large quantities of human IL-1. The monocytic cells from the leukemic sources, as of this date, have only been used in short-term primary culture and have not been adapted successfully to continuous culture. A recent finding that should be of significant importance for the future generation of large quantities of human IL-1 is that the U937 cell line will produce substantial quantities of the monokine upon exogenous stimulation (Palacios et al., 1982). This continuous monocytic line was originally derived from a patient with a histiocytic lymphoma and may prove to be an important resource in future studies on the molecular characterization of human IL-1.

B. T-Cell Growth Factor or Interleukin 2

The aforementioned observation that the mitogenic effects of IL-1 plus PHA were synergistic rather than additive became the focus of considerable experimental interest. Among the host of possible explanations for this synergistic effect was the speculation that the mitogenicity mediated by a lectin, in the presence of a monokine, may be modulated through another signal. After years of intensive investigation by several laboratories it became evident that this speculation was, in fact, a possibility. A sequential series of events that has gained wide acceptance encompasses the observations that a subset of thymus-derived lymphocytes, following activation by lectins, becomes sensitive to the effects of the monokine IL-1, with the resultant production of a second lymphokine, termed interleukin 2 (IL-2) (Smith et al., 1980; Larsson et al., 1980; Gillis and Mizel, 1981; Maizel et al., 1981a). It is this second mediator, IL-2, that actually stimulates a subset of lectin-activated T lymphocytes into the S phase of the cell cycle (Smith et al., 1980). Therefore, the lymphokine IL-2 is thought to represent the proximate mitogenic stimulus while the monokine IL-1 acts as an amplification factor in the production of IL-2.

The multitudinous studies that reinforced the concept that IL-2 was the mitogenic stimulus for T lymphocytes began with the observation that normal human T lymphocytes could be grown in continuous culture dependent upon a factor(s) present in the culture supernatant from lectin-stimulated mononuclear cells (conditioned medium) (Morgan et al., 1976; Ruscetti et al., 1977). The successful long-term growth of cultured T cells required an initial lectin- and/or antigen-dependent activation step. Following this activation signal it was shown that cell growth was thereafter dependent only upon continuous replenishment of the conditioned medium, which contained factor(s) supportive of T-cell growth (for review see Ruscetti and Gallo, 1981). At this juncture, the factor responsible for this cellular proliferation was termed T-cell growth factor (TCGF). Recently the nomenclature was revised such that the factor responsible for the long-term growth of cultured T cells was renamed IL-2 (Aarden et al., 1979).

Since the initial description of T-cell growth factor a plethora of studies directed at the elucidation of the cell biological processes associated with the growth factor and at the biochemical characterization of the factor have appeared (for review see Gillis *et al.*, 1982). IL-2 (TCGF) was shown not only to support the growth of polyclonally activated T-cell populations but also to support the growth of functionally distinct subpopulations. Specifically, "educated" cytotoxic T cells, antigen-specific helper T cells, and natural killer cells could be shown to grow in culture dependent upon IL-2. In addition, the phenotypic expression of membrane antigens on the continuously cultured T cells faithfully correlated with their functional capabilities.

Subsequent to the demonstrations that IL-2 could effectively support normal T-cell proliferation (both human and murine), many laboratories began to explore the interrelationships between the interleukins. Central to the hypotheses that were subsequently formulated were three essential observations. The first was that adherent accessory cells (i.e., cells of the monocyte–macrophage series) were apparently required for optimal T-cell mitogenesis in response to either lectin or antigen stimulation (Rosenstreich *et al.*, 1976; Lipsky *et al.*, 1976; Maizel *et al.*, 1979). The second observation was that cells of the monocytic series were capable of producing IL-1 and that this monokine was capable of promoting mitogenesis in lectin-stimulated cells of the T lineage. Third, only IL-2 was capable of sustaining the long-term proliferation of cultured T cells. From these observations the previously mentioned theoretical construct was proposed that IL-1 functioned to modulate the production of IL-2 and that IL-2 actually stimulated S-phase entry of the activated T cells. For the experimental verification of this scheme it was necessary to demonstrate that the role of the monocyte in T-cell mitogenesis could at least partially be substituted by the monokine IL-1 and that IL-1 could modulate the T-cell dependent production of IL-2. Both of these requirements were, in fact, confirmed experimentally. It was demonstrated that IL-1 could partially substitute for the intact monocyte in lectin-stimulated human T-cell mitogenesis (Maizel *et al.*, 1981b), and it was shown that IL-1 could effectively substitute for the monocyte in antigen-stimulated systems, given a limiting number of accessory cells putatively required for antigen presentation (Mizel and Ben-Zvi, 1980). It was also confirmed that the production of IL-2 by a population of activated T lymphocytes was modulated in part by the availability of the monokine IL-1 (Smith *et al.*, 1980; Larsson *et al.*, 1980). A significant relationship existed between IL-2 production and IL-1 availability when a fixed number of activated T cells were titrated with increasing amounts of IL-1. Therefore, a relatively coherent picture of T-cell mitogenesis had been formulated and experimentally confirmed. The lectin (and/or antigen) functioned to activate a subset of T cells to become responsive thereafter to IL-1 stimulation for IL-2 production. The lectin also functioned to induce receptors on lymphocytes that were requied for IL-2 absorption (Bonnard *et al.*, 1979; Larsson, 1981; Robb *et al.*, 1981). IL-1 functioned as a differentiation-amplification signal in the production of IL-2, and IL-2 actually served as the mitogenic stimulus necessary for T-cell S-phase entry.

C. B-Cell Growth Factor

With the clear demonstration of the existence of a T-cell-specific growth factor and the demonstration of the bimodal amplification network involving IL-1 and IL-2, attention turned to the definition of those requirements essential for B-cell proliferation. Initial experimentation on the role of soluble factors in B-cell proliferation revealed that conditioned media derived from either lectin-stimulated normal human peripheral blood lymphocytes or murine antigen-specific helper T cells (grown in the presence of irradiated accessory cells) were capable of promoting S-phase entry in a subpopulation of B lymphocytes (Ford *et al.*, 1981; Andersson and Melchers, 1981; Sredni *et al.*, 1981). Similar B-cell growth factor(s) (BCGF) were also observed in conditioned media from two cell lines of at least a putative neoplastic origin. These murine lines were phorbol-ester-stimulated EL-4 thymoma cells and lectin-stimulated T hybridoma cells (FS6 14.13) (Howard *et al.*, 1981, 1982). Yet conditioned media sources such as those mentioned above contain multiple functional biological activities. Therefore, the question that readily became apparent was whether one of the known biological activities present in the various conditioned media sources [e.g., IL-1, IL-2, or T-cell replacing factor (TRF)] was responsible for B-cell mitogenesis or whether B-cell S-phase entry was under the control of a specific unique cytokine. Several laboratories subsequently performed a series of biological experiments that indicated that the latter possibility was, in fact, the strongest alternative.

The most convincing experiments ruling out the role of IL-2 in B-cell proliferation relied upon the fact that activated T lymphocytes can effectively adsorb IL-2 from conditioned media preparation. Work in both human and murine systems revealed that, when activated B cells were exposed to conditioned media containing B-cell mitogenic activity from which IL-2 had been adsorbed by prior exposure to T-cell blasts, the B-cell mitogenic activity will still present and in several instances was even enhanced (Andersson and Melchers, 1981; Maizel *et al.*, 1982a; Duncan *et al.*, 1982). The possibility that B-cell proliferation was being stimulated by a factor or group of factors operationally similar to the lymphokine(s), termed TRF, was also ruled out by several biological experiments. Data derived from human and murine B-cell lines maintained in suspension culture revealed that, although addition of TRF-containing supernatants to growing B cells could be demonstrated to induce immunoglobulin secretion, growth could effectively be maintained independently of both the differentiative signal and the differentiative response (Sredni *et al.*, 1981; Howard *et al.*, 1981). The possible role of IL-1 as a B-cell-growth-promoting agent has been somewhat more difficult to resolve than the roles of the abovementioned cytokines. The ability of clonally derived T-cell populations to produce B-cell mitogenic factors would seem to argue against IL-1, a known macrophage product, being the sole factor involved in the observed stimulation of growth. Furthermore, the ability of supernatants from T-cell hybidomas (i.e., conditioned media known to be devoid of IL-1 activity) to support the clonal expansion of B lymphocytes, grown in limiting dilution cultures, would also militate against IL-1 being the only factor responsible for B-cell proliferation (Wetzel *et al.*, 1982). These experimental observations are somewhat in contradiction to initial work in the murine system that has indicated that, once B-cell proliferation has been established, conditioned media known to contain IL-1 could putatively support continued cellular expansion (Howard *et al.*, 1981). What ultimate role IL-1 plays in these systems remains to be determined fully. Definitive confirmation of the existence of a unique BCGF, suggested by the above phenomenological data, will be seen in subsequent sections, in which the biochemical separation of such a specific factor will be described.

III. PURIFICATION AND CHEMICAL CHARACTERIZATION OF IL-1, IL-2, AND BCGF

The biochemical separation of the previously described cytokines and the subsequent utilization of these moieties in discriminating biological assays has added more than suggestive evidence for the definitive existence of specific factors regulating both T-cell and B-cell proliferation. The availability of purified material should greatly aid in future studies concerned with the molecular characterization of each specific factor. Future determination of amino acid sequence, development of nucleotide probes, synthesis of peptide fragments, and eventual utilization of all these modalities should greatly expand our understanding of cellular immunological function and the basic cell biology of mammalian cell proliferation. The following section will not exhaustively review the area of cytokine purification, but it will summarize the biochemical properties of IL-1, IL-2, and BCGF and emphasize those areas in need of future exploration.

A. Biochemical Characteristics of Human IL-1

Human IL-1 has been produced and purified from those monocytes found in normal venous peripheral blood and from those monocytes found in peripheral blood of patients with AMOL or AMML. The specific activity of the IL-1 that is produced by the malignant cells is no greater than that produced by the normal population when calculated on a per-cell basis. Yet, considering the markedly increased numbers of monocytes in the leukemic stages of the abovementioned diseases, a significantly greater amount of IL-1 may be isolated from a single donor with either AMOL or AMML.

Recently, human IL-1 produced by these leukemic monocytes was purified to apparent homogeneity (Lachman, 1983). The procedure involved multiple steps, including molecular weight fractionation, isoelectric focusing, and sodium dodecylsulfate–polyacrylamide gel electrophoresis (SDS–PAGE) (Fig. 1). The utilization of gel electrophoresis took advantage of the relatively low molecular weight of human IL-1 (11,000) in order to separate the monokine from the residual proteins remaining after isolectric focusing. The incorporation of a denaturing gel system was chosen because of the observation that, if purification was attempted using electrophoresis under nondenaturing conditions (tris–glycine buffer), IL-1 could be isolated in high yield, yet the preparation was not homogeneous. SDS–PAGE allowed for the isolation of an apparently homogeneous protein. The significant disadvantage of the denaturing procedure lay in the fact that the monokine, as isolated from the SDS gels, retained only a fraction of that activity originally applied to the system. Interestingly, this sensitivity to SDS appeared to be unique to human IL-1 in that previous reports did not indicate the same finding for murine IL-1. Therefore, although human IL-1 seemingly was purified to homogeneity, the pure material was suitable for chemical but not biological experiments. For most biological experiments, human IL-1 was purified by nondenaturing gel electrophoreses and most recently by high-pressure liquid chromatography. The molecular weight, isoelectric point, and sensitivities to degradative enzymes, heat, and pH extremes were determined for highly purified IL-1 derived from the leukemic source and are summarized in Table I.

B. Biochemical Characteristics of Human IL-2

Human IL-2 has been produced and purified from two major sources. The first and most common is lectin-stimulated normal peripheral blood mononuclear cells. The second source is from a cell line designated Jurkat-FHCRC (Gillis and Watson, 1980). The Jurkat cell line derives from a patient with a T-cell lymphoma. The suffix of the cell line is of significance since there are many substrains of the Jurkat line currently available that have been shown to be poor producers of IL-2, while the population indicated above routinely produces large quantities of the lymphokine. The most efficacious stimulant for IL-2 release by the Jurkat cell line is a combination of the lectin PHA and the phorbol ester, phorbol myristic acetate (PMA). Although lectin stimulation alone results in significant release of IL-2 from the cell line, the combined use of PHA and PMA results in substantially greater production.

Human IL-2 produced from the Jurkat line has been purified by multiple steps, including sequential gel filtration, ion-exchange chromatography, preparative isoelectric focusing, and SDS–PAGE (Gillis et al., 1982). Electroelution of that material stainable on the polyacrylamide gels reveals that a single protein

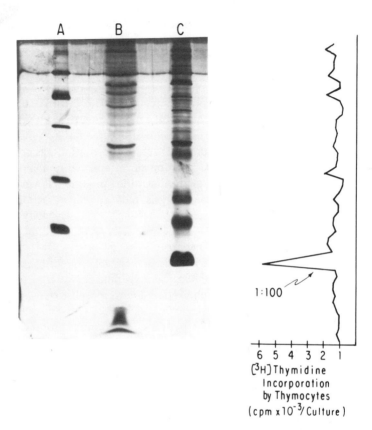

Figure 1. Analytical and preparative SDS–PAGE of human IL-1. Human IL-1, derived from AMOL cells, was purified through diafiltration and isoelectric focusing. Control medium, with no cells, was processed in the same fashion. Fractions of pH 6.8–7.2, from the isoelectric focusing columns, were lyophilized and applied to an analytical slab gel and a preparative tube gel. Lanes A, B, and C refer to the analytical slab gel. Lane A contains molecular weight markers of 94K, 67K, 43K, 30K, 20.1K, and 14.4K. Lane B contains control medium processed by diafiltration and isoelectric focusing. Lane C contains medium conditioned by AMOL cells (i.e., contains IL-1) and processed by diafiltration and isoelectric focusing. Proteins were visualized by silver staining. The thymidine incorporation profile was derived from elution and subsequent assay of samples from the preparative tube gels, which contained AMOL-derived IL-1. Examination of lanes B and C of the slab gel reveals the presence in lane C (experimental lane) of a darkly staining protein of approximately 11,000 daltons, which is absent from lane B (control lane). The 11,000-dalton material contained the majority of IL-1 activity as determined by elution of unstained material from the preparative gels. Repeat SDS–PAGE of the active material eluted from the preparative gels demonstrated that the protein was homogeneous.

Table I. Chemical and Physical Characteristics
of Human IL-1

Molecular weight	11,000[a]
Isoelectric point	7.0[b]
Protease sensitivity	Trypsin
	Chymotrypsin
Chemical sensitivity	Sodium dodecylsulfate
Chemical insenstivity	2-Mercaptoethanol
	Neuraminidase
	Sodium periodate
	Iodoacetamide
Temperature stability	56°C, 60 min: stable
	100°C, 2 min: unstable
pH stability	pH 3–10: stable

[a] The molecular weight was that derived from SDS–PAGE of
IL-1 that had been purified by molecular weight diafiltration, isoelectric focusing, and SDS–PAGE. The initial conditioned medium, for the IL-1 purification, was derived from
monocytes of a patient with AMOL. This source of IL-1 was
used for the majority of the values reported in this table.
[b] The isoelectric point noted in the table represents the major
species found in those IL-1 preparations recovered from the
purification scheme described in footnote a. Minor species
amounting to only a fraction of the total activity have not
been included.

band, migrating with an apparent molecular weight of 13,500, contains the
majority of activity. It should be emphasized that IL-2 produced by lectin-
activated normal mononuclear cells is characterized by greater molecular heterogeneity than the IL-2 produced by the Jurkat line (Robb and Smith, 1981). This
finding is of importance in the purification mentioned above when considerations
of true homogeneity are made.

In addition to the Jurkat line being a valuable source of large quantities of
active lymphokine that are suitable for purification, the line has also been
extremely useful as a source of radiolabeled factor. Specifically, IL-2 has been
prepared from Jurkat cells grown in the presence of either [^{35}S] methionine or
mixtures of radiolabeled amino acids (Gillis et al., 1982; Robb et al., 1981).
Utilization of the labeled factor has facilitated the acquisition of important information concerning the molecular composition of the growth-promoting agent.
Furthermore, radiolabeled IL-2 has been utilized in the development of an assay
for the study of the specific IL-2 cell-surface receptor.

The purification of human IL-2 from peripheral blood mononuclear cells has
been somewhat more difficult than its purification from the Jurkat line consider-

ing the evidence, mentioned previously, that normal mononuclear-cell-derived IL-2 possesses greater molecular heterogeneity. Some of this heterogeneity has been shown to be attributable to the method of production of the factor (Welte *et al.*, 1982). Yet several laboratories have successfully purified human mono-nuclear-cell-derived IL-2 to an extent approaching homogeneity. One purification scheme possessing considerable efficacy utilizes lectin-stimulated peripheral-blood-lymphocyte-conditioned media that are produced in serum-free conditions (Mier and Gallo, 1982). The isolation procedure involves multiple steps, including ion-exchange chromatography on DEAE–Sepharose, repeated gel filtration through Ultrogel AcA54, and preparative SDS–PAGE. The active fractions iso-lated from the SDS gels have a molecular weight of 13,000 and this material, extracted from the gels, migrates as a predominant single band when rerun on analytical SDS gels.

Another purification scheme for human IL-2 also utilized serum-free condi-tions but incorporated multiple initial stimulation steps for the induction of high levels of IL-2 (Welte *et al.*, 1982). Pooled mononuclear cells from multiple donors were stimulated first by Sendai virus for 12 hr and thereafter by lectin for 48 more hr. An additional increase in IL-2 production was achieved by costimula-tion with Daudi cells. The IL-2 present in the conditioned medium was subse-quently purified to high specific activity and relatively high yield by ion-exchange chromatography on DEAE–cellulose, gel filtration through Ultrogel AcA44, and sequential chromatography on blue agarose and procion-red agarose. The IL-2 produced in the absence of Daudi costimulation possessed a molecular weight of 16,000 and 17,000 on SDS–PAGE. The IL-2 produced in the presence of costimulation possessed a molecular weight of 14,000 on denaturing gel electrophoresis.

Table II summarizes the chemical and physical characteristics of human IL-2 as prepared by the methods described above. Every effort has been made to distinguish those characteristics that are unique to the Jurkat-derived IL-2 or have not been determined for both sources of the factor.

C. Biochemical Characteristics of Human BCGF

Of the three cytokines being evaluated in this review, human BCGF is the one most recently defined biologically and biochemically. The body of literature currently available on human BCGF is relatively small, yet this area of investiga-tion is being pursued intensively. The information in this section should therefore be considered as the result of only the initial attempts at understanding the biochemistry of this unique factor. The separation scheme to be described does not represent a complete purification protocol. It is directed at the analytical demonstration that BCGF is a unique lymphokine.

Table II. Chemical and Physical Characteristics of Human IL-2

Molecular weight	13,000–16,000[a]
Isoelectric point	6.5–6.8[b]
	7.8–8.1
Protease sensitivity	Trypsin
	Chymotrypsin
Chemical sensitivity	Sodium dodecylsulfate[c]
Chemical insensitivity	2-Mercaptoethanol
	Urea (2–4 M)
	Neuraminidase
Temperature sensitivity	56°C, 60 min: stable
	70°C, 30 min: unstable
pH stability	pH 3–10: stable

[a] The molecular weight range given in the table was derived from those values seen on SDS–PAGE from IL-2 produced from several sources. Human IL-2 produced from lectin-stimulated peripheral blood lymphocytes has been shown to possess molecular weights, under denaturing conditions, ranging experimentally from 13,000 to 16,000. The incorporation of stimulating factors, other than lectins, during the IL-2 production phase has been reported to alter the predominant molecular weight species, although values still fall essentially within the range (Welte *et al.*, 1982).

[b] The isoelectric points have been presented as two sets of ranges. The pI 6.5–6.8 range refers to the predominant species experimentally found with IL-2 prepared from mononuclear cells of peripheral venous blood. The 7.8–8.1 range incorporates those values predominantly seen with IL-2 prepared from the Jurkat line and those values found with IL-2 prepared from normal mononuclear cells after neuraminidase treatment. Minor species have not been included in the table.

[c] The effect of sodium dodceylsulfate on the biological activity of IL-2 has been reported to be somewhat variable. The sensitivity to SDS reported in the table refers to 0.1% SDS, at 70°C, for longer than 15 min (Gillis *et al.*, 1982).

Human peripheral blood mononuclear cells provided the source for generation of the B-cell mitogenic factor. Lectin-stimulated mononuclear cells from multiple donors were pooled and cultured for 72 hr in serum-free conditions (Maizel *et al.*, 1982a,b). The conditioned medium was subsequently fractionated by ammonium sulfate precipitation (50–80% saturation), DEAE–Sephadex chromatography, and sequential gel filtration on columns packed with Bio-Gel P30 and Bio-Gel P100. During the fractionation procedures all samples were assayed routinely for multiple biological activities, including the ability to in-

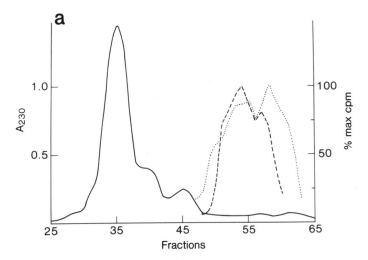

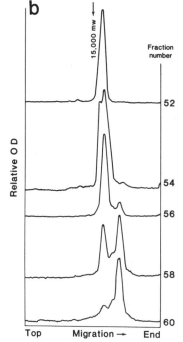

Figure 2. (a) Bio-Gel P100 gel filtration of human TCGF and BCGF. Conditioned medium, derived from 72-hr lectin-stimulated peripheral blood lymphocytes, was fractionated by ammonium sulfate precipitation, DEAE–Sephadex chromatography, and Bio-Gel P30 filtration. The fractions from the P30 column containing TCGF and BCGF activity were concentrated and applied to a Bio-Gel P100 gel filtration column. Fractions were collected and subsequently tested for the ability to promote the long-term growth of cultured T cells (IL-2) and the ability to promote B-cell S-phase entry (BCGF) using a thymidine incorporation assay (Maizel *et al.*, 1982a). The optical density at 230 nm (A_{230}) was also included. The results are presented as percentage maximal cpm in order to assess factor separation more effectively. The maximal activity in the presence of growth factor measured on T cells in long-term culture was 40,000–45,000 cpm per 2×10^5 cells when labeled with 1 μCi [^{3}H]-Tdr (6 Ci/mmole) for the last 16 hr of assay. The maximal activity measured on quiescent T cells activated with lectin and growth factor was 18,000–20,000 cpm per 2×10^5 cells. The maximal activity measured on B cells stimulated with growth factor in the presence of 0.01% sheep erythrocytes was 14,000–17,000 cpm per 2×10^5 cells. The maximal activity as measured on B cells with growth factor in the presence of 3 μg insolubilized anti-IgM was 30,000–35,000 cpm. (——) O.D. at 230 nm; (----) T-cell activity; (· · · ·) B-cell activity.

(b) SDS–PAGE of Bio-Gel P100 gel filtration fractions. P100 gel filtrations were labeled *in vitro* by reductive methylation in the presence of [^{3}H]formaldehyde. The labeled fractions were electrophoresed on a 15% polyacrylamide gel under denaturing conditions. The gel was autoradiographed and subsequently scanned. The figure represents the scan of the autoradiograph in the regions of the peak of TCGF activity and the peak of BCGF activity. The fraction numbers listed refer to the same fraction numbers as in Fig. 2a.

duce the T-cell-dependent production of IL-2, the ability to maintain the long-term growth of cultured T cells, and the ability to induce S-phase entry in purified human B lymphocytes exposed to sheep red blood cells and/or anti-IgM. Those activities associated with the long-term growth of cultured T cells (IL-2), the amplification of IL-2 production (IL-1), and the stimulation of B-cell S-phase entry (BCGF) were seen to copurify during ammonium sulfate precipitation and DEAE–Sephadex chromatography. The subsequent gel filtration procedure on the low-molecular-weight exclusion column provided separation of the IL-1 activity from the activities associated with IL-2 and BCGF. The IL-1 appeared at a greater elution volume on the Bio-Gel P30 column, corresponding to a lower apparent molecular weight. Documentation that this lower-molecular-weight material was IL-1 was supported by the data that this material could augment the T-cell-dependent production of IL-2 in the presence of lectin, yet was without detectable activity in those assays measuring the long-term growth of cultured T cells.

Those fractions exhibiting maximal BCGF and IL-2 activity were next applied to a column packed with a higher-molecular-weight exclusion gel (Bio-Gel P100). Isolation and assay of the chromatographic samples from this column revealed a separation between the T-cell-active fractions and the B-cell-active fractions. Although the peaks overlapped, there were several fractions that consistently stimulated significant B-cell proliferative activity while lacking demonstrable T-cell activity (Fig. 2a). The molecular weight of those proteins that eluted in the fractions enriched for B-cell activity and those that eluted in the fractions enriched for T-cell activity was determined by PAGE. The collected fractions from the Bio-Gel P100 column were radiolabeled *in vitro* by reductive methylation. The labeled fractions were electrophoresed under denaturing conditions and the gel was autoradiographed. A scan of the autoradiograph revealed a predominant protein species of 14,000–15,000 daltons in those fractions enriched for T-cell growth and a predominant moiety of 12,000–13,000 daltons in those fractions possessing B-cell stimulatory activity in the absence of IL-2 activity (Fig. 2b).

Further documentation that the activity present in the fractions enriched for B-cell proliferation was being modulated by a protein distinct from that factor stimulating T-cell proliferation was provided by biological adsorption of the partially purified samples. As mentioned in previous sections, activated T lymphocytes were capable of specifically adsorbing IL-2 from growth factor preparations. When the P100 chromatographic samples, enriched for B-cell activity, were subjected to adsorption by T blasts, the activity associated with B-cell proliferation remained intact. Futhermore, adsorption of the fractions enriched for B-cell activity with activated B cells led to a diminution of the B-cell proliferative activity, indicating that activated cells of the B lineage may specifically adsorb BCGF from growth factor preparations. Verification of the existence of a specific factor stimulating B-cell proliferation was also achieved biochemically.

For this demonstration, those P100 gel filtration fractions enriched for B-cell stimulatory activity were pooled from multiple column chromatographic separations. The fractions were concentrated and rechromatographed on a lower-molecular-weight exclusion gel. Collection and reassay of the material eluting from the column revealed again that the B-cell-proliferation-stimulating activity could be demonstrated in the absence of T-cell-proliferation-stimulating activity.

Therefore, through a combination of biochemical and biological techniques, the existence of a specific factor responsible for the stimulation of B-cell proliferation has been demonstrated. A summary of the chemical and physical characteristics of human BCGF that have been demonstrated thus far is presented in Table III. It should again be emphasized that a significant degree of investigation

Table III. Chemical and Physical Characteristics of Human BCGF

Molecular weight	12,000–13,000[a]
Isoelectric point	6.3–6.6
Protease sensitivity	Trypsin
Chemical sensitivity	–[b]
Chemical insensitivity	2-Mercaptoethanol
Temperature stability	56°C, 10 min: stable[c]
	56°C, 60 min: unstable
	100°C, 5 min: unstable
pH stability	pH 3–8: stable

[a] The molecular weight given in the table refers to values found on SDS–PAGE of those purification fractions possessing B-cell proliferative activity in the absence of detectable T-cell activity (see text). Conditioned medium prepared from lectin-stimulated peripheral blood lymphocytes was fractionated by ammonium sulfate precipitation, DEAE–Sephadex chromatography, and sequential gel filtration. The fractions possessing activity specifically for B cells, derived from the final gel filtration, were utilized for the assessment of molecular weight by SDS–PAGE.

[b] Not done. As was discussed in the text, BCGF has been described only in the recent past. The values presented in the table represent the initial data on characteriziation; new data are presently being accumulated.

[c] BCGF, prepared as described in footnote a, appeared to possess more heat sensitivity than either IL-1 or IL-2. The actual data revealed that heating a preparation of BCGF, stabilized with 0.1% polyethyleneglycol (6000 MW), for 15 min at 56°C resulted in a 22% loss of activity. Heating for 30 min at 56°C resulted in a 45% loss of activity, and heating at 56°C for 60 min resulted in greater than 70% loss of activity.

remains to be done in the area of the biochemical characterization and purification of human BCGF. This field is still in its infancy and the prospects for future understanding are exciting.

IV. BIOLOGICAL PROPERTIES OF IL-1, IL-2, AND BCGF

As mentioned in the introduction, this article will not exhaustively review the literature concerning the biological properties of IL-1, IL-2, and BCGF. It is hoped that this section will highlight the most interesting new findings concerning the properties of IL-1, IL-2, and BCGF.

A. Biological Properties of IL-1

The number of biological activities attributed to IL-1 has been rapidly increasing and has firmly established the central role of IL-1 in immunomodulation (for review see Mizel, 1982; Lachman, 1983; Oppenheim et al., 1982). Some of the most interesting recent experiments have involved in vivo testing. Human IL-1 that has been partially purified by diafiltration and isoelectric focusing has been injected intravenously into several different species of experimental animals (Lachman, 1983). First and foremost it should be emphasized that human IL-1 prepared as described above is free of detectable concentrations of endotoxin. This has been confirmed both by in vivo determinations and by the in vitro Limulus amebocyte assay. Injection of endotoxin-free IL-1 into rabbits resulted in the generation of a monophasic fever. The kinetics of this temperature elevation were distinctly different from those due to endotoxin. This observation was further confirmed by experiments using endotoxin-tolerant rabbits, in which IL-1 could also induce a characteristic fever response. The ability of endotoxin-free IL-1 to induce a characteristic fever in an experimental animal has led to the widely held belief that interleukin 1 and endogenous pyrogen are probably the same factors (Rossenwasser and Dinarello, 1981; Murphy et al., 1980).

The intravenous administration of IL-1 into rats also modulated the numbers of specific cells in the peripheral circulation. Injection of IL-1, prepared through isoelectric focusing, resulted in a relatively rapid increase in the concentration of peripheral blood polymorphonuclear leukocytes within 90 min of exposure. The absolute increase in cells was 8000 granulocytes/mm^3. Again it should be emphasized that the ability to elevate the number of plasma granulocytes was unique to the soluble mediator and was not shared by endotoxin. Twenty-four hours subsequent to IL-1 injection, the experimental animals also experienced significant increases in the plasma levels of fibrinogen and acute phase reactant proteins. These two effects were ascribed to a soluble factor termed leukocyte endogenous mediator (Kampschmidt *et al.*, 1980), which is now thought to be identical to IL-1.

The *in vitro* properties of IL-1 have also been receiving significant attention. In addition to the immunomodulating effects mentioned in the previous sections, recent work has suggested that a macrophage-derived product, presumably IL-1, could also function as a growth factor for human fibroblasts (Schmidt *et al.*, 1982). The histological demonstration that macrophages occur at the site of wound healing provides further suggestive evidence for this contention (Leibovich and Ross, 1975). More definitive support for the identity between that macrophage product stimulating fibroblast proliferation and IL-1 has been accumulated in a study documenting the copurification of these two activities. Experiments have documented that the activity ascribed to IL-1 and the activity associated with fibroblast proliferation copurify through isoelectric focusing followed by sequential high-pressure liquid chromatography columns (Postlethwaite *et al.*, 1983).

B. Biological Properties of IL-2

The biological role of IL-2 as an immunostimulant intimately involved in the control of T-cell proliferation has been firmly established by numerous investigations. The *in vitro* functions mediated by this factor have been well delineated and have been the subject of several comprehensive reviews (Gillis *et al.*, 1982; Farrar *et al.*, 1982; Ruscetti and Gallo, 1981). Some of the most interesting recent experimental observations have been in the area of *in vivo* testing, in experimental animals, of the immunomodulating agent. One series of experiments has focused on whether the documented *in vitro* requirement for IL-2 in the generation of alloreactive cytotoxic lymphocytes could also be demonstrated *in vivo* subsequent to the administration of purified IL-2 (Gillis *et al.*, 1982). The purified lymphokine was inoculated into a series of experimental animals that had been immunized with allogeneic tumor cells. It was demonstrated that intraperitoneal administration of IL-2 in alloimmunized mice resulted in an approximately twofold augmentation of effector cell lytic activity, which was mediated by cells of T lineage.

Experiments were also undertaken to demonstrate the efficacy of *in vivo* IL-2 administration on natural killer (NK) cell cytoxicity (Gillis *et al.*, 1982). Mice were inejcted intraperitoneally with purified IL-2. Forty-eight hours later spleen cells were removed and NK activity determined. *In vivo* administration of IL-2 resulted in a marked augmentation of splenic cytotoxic cell activity. Furthermore, the cytotoxicity was specific for NK-susceptible cells, with NK-tolerant cells being resistant to the effect. Therefore, IL-2 administration, intraperitoneally, effectively augmented both alloimmune cytotoxic lymphocyte responses and NK-cell activity.

Another interesting series of experiments examined the role of the intravenous administration of IL-2 on the generation of immunocompetent T cells in *nu/nu* mice. Mice carrying this mutation do not usually contain detectable levels of immunocompetent T cells. Experimental *nu/nu* animals treated with heterologous erythrocytes and a partially purified preparation of IL-2 were subsequently shown to be capable of generating helper T cells (Stotter *et al.*, 1980). It should be emphasized that in this system the generation of specific helper T-cell populations required the simultaneous administration of antigen and the lymphokine. Alloreactive cytotoxic lymphocytes also were generated in the nude mouse by a protocol in which IL-2 was injected with allogeneic stimulator cells (Wagner *et al.*, 1980).

The ability to demonstrate an effect when IL-2 is administered intravenously depends upon multiple parameters. One parameter of importance is potential serum inhibitors. In this regard, it has been demonstrated the normal mice contain high levels of an IL-2 inhibitor whereas sera of athymic *nu/nu* mice do not (Hardt *et al.*, 1981). The absence of the inhibitor in the nude mouse may partially explain the efficacy of IL-2 administration in this experimental animal. Yet more significant is the fact that the presence of inhibitors to IL-2 in normal experimental populations may indicate a significant biological control mechanism. Because of the nonspecific nature of the IL-2 signal, the presence of inhibitors could be presumed to function by limiting the scope of action of the lymphokine.

C. Biological Properties of Human BCGF

The investigation into the mode of action of human BCGF is presently in its early stages of development. Several interesting and substantial observations have already been compiled that reveal intriguing aspects of the cell biology of the human B lymphocyte (for review see Maizel *et al.*, 1983). Following an activation event(s) (Zubler and Kanagawa, 1982) a subpopulation of human B lymphocytes has been shown to acquire sensitivity to the subsequent effects of growth factors, resulting in a proportion of the population going through the S phase of the cell cycle. As previously demonstrated, one factor responsible for this growth is specific for B lymphocytes and is different from the cytokines discussed in this review. A question of importance that has recently been investigated concerns the cellular sources responsible for the B-cell-specific factor.

Recent investigations revealed that the T lymphocyte plays a central role in the production of this factor. Initial work in the murine system demonstrated that factors capable of stimulating B-cell proliferation could be derived from putatively neoplastic thymoma cells and/or T hybridoma cells (Howard *et al.*, 1981). Evidence that a normal thymus-derived cell also produced BCGF recently was found from experiments utilizing normal human peripheral blood mononuclear cells (Maizel *et al.*, 1983). For these studies human T cells, B cells, and monocytes were purified from peripheral venous blood. The cell populations were lectin-stimulated, either alone or in combination, for a period of 72 hr. At this time, the conditioned media were clarified and purified through DEAE–Sephadex chromatography. The amount of activity promoting B-cell mitogenesis was determined in comparison to a known standard, and units of activity were calculated. It was demonstrated that lectin-stimulated T cells, by themselves, were poor producers of human BCGF. Addition of monocytes to the T-cell cultures resulted in a substantial augmentation of factor production. Lectin-stimulated T lymphocytes, in the presence of 10% added monocytes, produced at least fivefold more factor than those lectin-activated T lymphocytes cultured alone. In another series of experiments, those lectin-activated T cells, cultured with monocytes, were further cocultured with syngeneic B cells. Of interest was the observation that this cultivation led to a further substantial increase in factor production, which was approximately double that seen with lectin-activated T cells and monocytes. Culture of lectin-stimulated monocytes or B lymphocytes alone or in combination without the presence of T cells failed to result in substantial factor generation.

Experiments were next conducted to verify further the role of the T cell in the production of B-cell stimulatory factors. Lectin-exposed T cells, monocytes, and B lymphocytes were cultured together for 24 hr. Following this preincubation period, the cells were repurified and placed alone in culture for an additional 72 hr. The conditioned media from this secondary 72-hr cultivation period were fractionated through DEAE–Sephadex and the units of BCGF activity were determined. From these experiments it could again be seen that the T lymphocyte was focal for factor production. During the secondary culture period, the activated T lymphocytes that initially had been placed together with monocytes, either alone or in combination with B cells, continued to produce B-cell-stimulatory factors, while the non-T cells failed to produce significant amounts of these factors. Therefore, these experiments reinforced the concept that the T lymphocyte plays a central role in the production of a B-cell mitogenic factor. The T-cell-dependent production of the factor(s) was markedly augmented by the presence of both a monocyte and a B lymphocyte. The mechanisms by which the cell types interacted to augment factor production are currently under investigation.

Another interesting question that has received considerable attention concerns the biological role of soluble factors in the induction of a B-cell differentiative response. An aspect of this question that is particularly relevant to the present discussion concerns the role of BCGF in this differentiative response.

One would presume that the *in vivo* biological response to an antigenic challenge would involve the clonal expansion of a specific B-cell population in association with the secretion of specific immunoglobulin. Understanding the mechanistic events in a differentiative response, however, requires dissection of the proliferative and differentiative events at the molecular level. The demonstration that B-cell proliferation can occur in the absence of significant immunoglobulin secretion, and, conversely, that a differentiative response can be induced in the absence of cell growth, would suggest that these events are in fact controlled separately. Both of these biological situations recently have been demonstrated to occur under the appropriate *in vitro* circumstances. Stimulation of human B lymphocytes in the presence of sheep erythrocytes and purified human BCGF induces S-phase entry in a proportion of the cells. Simultaneous determination of the degree of immunoglobulin secretion has been consistently negative (Maizel *et al.*, 1982a). Therefore, utilizing relatively purified growth factors, one may induce proliferation without differentiation.

The converse experimental situation has also been demonstrated *in vitro*. Antigen-stimulated populations of human B cells, cultured with a small number of adherent accessory cells and irradiated T cells, may be induced to secrete IgM in the presence of soluble factor preparations, lacking BCGF, that have been derived from peripheral blood mononuclear cells. Simultaneous measurement of S-phase entry among these cells has revealed that the IgM secretory response may occur in the essential absence of S-phase entry. Therefore, it would appear that these two events may be separated biologically. Furthermore, these experimental situations underscore the specificity of the BCGF entity. This factor appears to possess both target cell and functional specificity.

V. CONCLUSIONS AND PERSPECTIVES

From the information presented in the previous sections it is hoped that a relatively clear picture has emerged concerning the role of soluble factors in B- and T-cell proliferation as it is currently understood. It has been shown that the ability to mount a proliferative response is dependent upon a complex series of cellular interactions, which are partially mediated through low-molecular-weight proteins. These proteins appear to function in much the same manner as hormonal agents. The growth factors have been shown to be effective at concentrations of 10^{-10}-10^{-12} M and to require cellular receptors for the transmission of their effects. These factors also possess target cell and functional specificity in much the same fashion as hormonal agents. The interleukins, including BCGF, also possess many similarities to the other mammalian growth factors that previously have been described. The factors share similarities in molecular weight, cell cycle specificity, and mechanism of action.

Future studies on the molecular biology of the interleukins and BCGF should greatly expand our understanding of both the cell biology of lymphoid cells and the mechanisms underlying mammalian cell proliferation in general. In addition, the potential use of these agents for *in vivo* immunomodulation is exciting from a clinical perspective. This area of investigation is still in its infancy, yet, given the nature of the studies that have already been completed, it should yield important information that may be of significant utility.

ACKNOWLEDGMENTS

This work was supported in part by NIH grant CA21927, an institutional grant from the Interferon Research Fund, and a grant from the Faisal Foundation. We would like to acknowledge the excellent secretarial assistance of Linda Kimbrough in the preparation of this chapter.

VI. REFERENCES

Aarden, L. A., *et al.*, 1979, *J. Immunol.* **123**:2928.

Andersson, J., and Melchers, F., 1981, *Proc. Natl. Acad. Sci. U.S.A.* **78**:2497.

Bonnard, G. D., Yasaka, D., and Jacobson, D., 1979, *J. Immunol.* **123**:2704.

Duncan, M. R., George, F. W., and Hadden, J. W., 1982, *J. Immunol.* **129**:56.

Farrar, J. J., Benjamin, W. R., Hilfiker, M. D., Howard, M., Farrar, W. L., and Farrar, J.-F., 1982, *Immunol. Rev.* **63**:129.

Ford, R. J., Mehta, S. R., Franzini, D., Montagna, R., Lachman, L., and Maizel, A. L., 1981, *Nature (London)* **294**:261.

Gery, I., and Waksman, B. H., 1972, *J. Exp. Med.* **136**:143.

Gery, I., Gershon, R. K., and Waksman, B. H., 1972, *J. Exp. Med.* **136**:128.

Gillis, S., and Mizel, S. B., 1981, *Proc. Natl. Acad. Sci. U.S.A.* **78**:1133.

Gillis, S., and Watson, J., 1980, *J. Exp. Med.* **152**:1709.

Gillis, S., Mochizuki, D. Y., Conlon, P. J., Hefeneider, S. H., Ramthun, C. A., Gillis, A. E., Frank, M. B., Henney, C. S., and Watson, J. D., 1982, *Immunol. Rev.* **63**:167.

Hardt, C., Rollinghoff, M., Pfizenmaier, K., Mosmann, H., and Wagner, H., 1981, *J. Exp. Med.* **154**:262.

Howard, M., Kellser, S., Chused, T., and Paul, W. E., 1981, *Proc. Natl. Acad. Sci. U.S.A.* **78**:5788.

Howard, M., Farrar, J., Hilfiker, M., Johnson, B., Takatsu, K., Hamaoka, T., and Paul, W. E., 1982, *J. Exp. Med.* **155**:914.

Kampschmidt, R. F., Pullian, L. A., and Upchurch, H. F., 1980, *J. Lab. Clin. Med.* **95**:616.

Lachman, L. B., 1983, *Fed. Proc.* (in press).

Lachman, L. B., Hacker, M. P., Blyden, G. T., and Andschumacher, R. E., 1977, *Cell. Immunol.* **34**:416.

Lachman, L. B., Moore, J. O., and Metzger, R. S., 1978, *Cell. Immunol.* **41**:199.

Larsson, E. L., 1981, *J. Immunol.* **126**:1323.

Larsson, E. L., Iscove, N. N., and Coutinho, A., 1980, *Nature (London)* **283**:664.

Leibovich, S. J., and Ross, R., 1975, *Am. J. Pathol.* **78**:71.

Lipsky, P. E., Ellner, J. J., and Rosenthal, A. S., 1976, *J. Immunol.* **116**:868.

Maizel, A. L., Mehta, S. R., and Ford, R. J., 1979, *Cell Immunol.* **48**:383.

Maizel, A. I., Mehta, S. R., Hauft, S., Franzini, D., Lachman, L. B., and Ford, R. J., 1981a, *J. Immunol.* **127**:1058.

Maizel, A. L., Mehta, S. R., Ford, R. J., and Lachman, L. B., 1981b, *J. Exp. Med.* **153**:470.

Maizel, A. L., Sahasrabuddhe, C., Mehta, S., Morgan, J., Lachman, L., and Ford, R. J., 1982a, *Proc. Natl. Acad. Sci. U.S.A.* **79**:5998.

Maizel, A. L., Sahasrabuddhe, C., Mehta, S., Morgan, J., Lachman, L., and Ford, R. J., 1982b, *UCLA Symp. Mol. Cell. Biol.* **24**:197.

Maizel, A. L., Mehta, S., Kouttab, N., Morgan, J., Ford, R., and Sahasrabuddhe, C., 1983, *Fed. Proc.* (in press).

Mier, J. W., and Gallo, R. C., 1982, *J. Immunol.* **128**:1122.

Mizel, S. B., 1982, *Immunol. Rev.* **63**:51.

Mizel, S. B., and Ben-Zvi, A., 1980, *Cell Immunol.* **54**:382.

Morgan, D. A., Ruscetti, F. W., and Gallo, R. C., 1976, *Science* **193**:1007.

Murphy, P. A., Simon, P. L., and Willoughby, W. F., 1980, *J. Immunol.* **124**:2498.

Oppenheim, J. J., Stadler, B. M., Siraganian, R. P., Mage, M., and Matheson, B., 1982, *Fed. Proc.* **41**:257.

Palacios, R., Ivhed, I., Sideras, P., Nelsson, K., Sugawara, I., and Fernandez, C., 1982, *Eur. J. Immunol.* **12**:895.

Postlethwaite, A. E., Lachman, L. B., Mainardi, C. L., and Kang, A. H., 1983, *J. Exp. Med.* **157**:801.

Robb, R. J., and Smith, K. A., 1981, *Mol. Immunol.* **18**:1087.

Robb, R. J., Munck, A., and Smith, K. A., 1981, *J. Exp. Med.* **154**:1455.

Rosenstreich, D. L., Farrar, J. J., and Dougherty, S., 1976, *J. Immunol.* **116**:131.

Rossenwasser, L. J., and Dinarello, C. A., 1981, *Cell Immunol.* **63**:134.

Ruscetti, F. W., and Gallo, R. C., 1981, *Blood* **57**:359.

Ruscetti, F. W., Morgan, D. A., and Gallo, R. C., 1977, *J. Immunol.* **119**:131.

Schmidt, J. A., Mizel, S. B., Cohen, D., and Green, I., 1982, *J. Immunol.* **128**:2177.

Smith, K. A., Lachman, L. B., Oppenheim, J. J., and Favata, M. D., 1980, *J. Exp. Med.* **151**:1551.

Sredni, B., Sieckmann, D. G., Kumagar, S., House, S., Green, I., Paul, W. E., 1981, *J. Exp. Med.* **154**:1500.

Stotter, H., Rude, E., and Wagner, H., 1980, *Eur. J. Immunol.* **10**:719.

Wagner, H., Hardt, C., Heeg, K., Rollinghoff, M., and Pfizenmaier, K., 1980, *Nature (London)* **284**:278.

Welte, K., Wang, C. Y., Mertelsmann, R., Venuta, S., Feldmann, S. P., and Moore, M. A. S., 1982, *J. Exp. Med.* **156**:454.

Wetzel, G. D., Swain, S. L., and Dutoon, R. W., 1982, *J. Exp. Med.* **156**:306.

Zubler, R. H., and Kanagawa, O., 1982, *J. Exp. Med.* **156**:415.

Immunoglobulin Structure–Function Correlates: Antigen Binding and Idiotypes

Stuart Rudikoff

Laboratory of Genetics
National Cancer Institute
National Institutes of Health
Bethesda, Maryland 20205

I. INTRODUCTION

During the past few years our understanding of the mechanisms involved in the generation of antibody diversity has greatly increased from studies of monoclonal antibodies (hybridomas) and the use of recombinant DNA technology. While much attention has appropriately been focused on these developments, it is nonetheless surprising how little we actually know about the function of these molecules at the molecular level. Since we assume that the primary role of antibodies is to bind antigens, it is obvious that a detailed analysis of this process is essential to an understanding of the mechanisms by which antibodies carry out their biological functions.

Abbreviations used in this chapter: V_L, variable segment of the immunoglobulin light chain or the corresponding gene encoding this region; J_L, joining segment of the immunoglobulin light chain or the corresponding gene encoding this region; C_L, constant region of the immunoglobulin light chain or the corresponding gene encoding this region; V_H, variable segment of the immunoglobulin heavy chain or the corresponding gene encoding this region; J_H, joining segment of the immunoglobulin heavy chain or the corresponding gene encoding this region; C_H, constant region of the immunoglobulin heavy chain or the corresponding gene encoding this region; D_H, "diversity" segment of the immunoglobulin heavy chain or the corresponding gene encoding this region (the D segment varies in size from probably one to a few amino acids and is included in the third complementarity-determining region); Ars, arsonate; CRI, cross-reactive idiotype; DNP, dinitrophenyl; IdI, individual idiotype; IdX, cross-reactive idiotype; NIP, nitroiodophenylacetate; NP, nitrophenylacetyl; PC, phosphocholine; SRBC, sheep red blood cells.

Many of the early studies addressing the problem of structure–function relationships employed homogeneous immunoglobulins produced by human myelomas (reviewed by Potter, 1973; Seligmann and Brouet, 1973) or mouse plasmacytomas (Potter, 1975; Potter *et al.*, 1975) as sources of material to avoid the problem of antibody heterogeneity. In addition, several immunization protocols were developed that produced essentially homogeneous antibodies (Krause, 1970, 1971; Haber, 1971; Eichmann, 1972; Braun and Jaton, 1974). The contribution to this field of the mouse plasmacytoma system developed by Michael Potter and Melvin Cohn cannot be overemphasized. The homogeneous immunoglobulins produced by mouse plasma cell tumors have provided the initial materials, as well as model systems, employed in many of the studies addressing antibody structure–function relationships. The identification of mouse myeloma proteins that bound chemically defined haptenic determinants (Cohn, 1967; Eisen *et al.*, 1968; Potter and Leon, 1968; Potter, 1970; Vicari *et al.*, 1970; Sher and Tarikas, 1971) provided immunochemists with many of the tools necessary to examine these problems. The introduction of the hybridoma technology by Kohler and Milstein (1975, 1976) has made the variety of materials available essentially unlimited.

Initial approaches to characterize the antibody combining site of heterogeneous antibody populations involved studies to determine the size of the area complementary to haptenic determinants as well as attempts to define regions of the site involved in antigen binding by the use of affinity labeling reagents. Kabat (1956, 1957, 1960), in a series of experiments employing anticarbohydrate antibodies, used oligosaccharides of increasing length to define the optimal size of carbohydrate determinants complementary to the binding site. Experiments designed to characterize the antibody combining site chemically were subsequently performed by the use of affinity labeling reagents that were irreversibly bound to the antibody molecule (Metzger *et al.*, 1963, 1964; Good *et al.*, 1967; Wofsy and Parker, 1967; Singer and Thorpe, 1968). Affinity labeling of heterogeneous populations created considerable difficulty in characterizing various parameters of the reaction and precise location of the label. This technique met with more success when applied to homogeneous immunoglobulins with defined hapten-binding specificities (Metzger and Potter, 1968; Goetzle and Metzger, 1970; Haimovich *et al.*, 1970; Metzger *et al.*, 1971; Givol *et al.*, 1971; Chesebro and Metzger, 1972). In these instances, peptides to which labeling reagents attached could then be isolated and characterized. One of the limitations of this technique derives from the uncertainty of whether the labeling group is attached to areas of the hapten intimately involved in antibody contact or is located distal to regions of interaction. Second, most affinity labeling reagents react specifically with one, or at most a few, amino acid side chains (i.e., tyrosine and lysine), limiting their effectiveness to the presence of reactive amino acids.

Until 1974 one of the significant problems encountered in attempts to address the questions of antibody structure–function was the lack of X-ray crystallographic data defining the antibody molecule three-dimensionally. In 1974 two Fab' structures were reported (Poljak *et al.*, 1974; Segal *et al.*, 1974), thus filling in a large gap in our knowledge of the antibody molecule. Unfortunately, no new detailed structures of known antigen-binding proteins have been described since then, although an Fab structure has been reported for the human myeloma protein, Kol (Marquardt *et al.*, 1980). Thus, many of the questions raised by these models remain to be answered. With the availability of the three-dimensional structures and a continuing accumulation of a variety of additional biochemical data, many facets of the antibody structure–function problem can now be more adequately analyzed. In the present review I will address two major problems in this area: (1) the correlations between antibody structure and antigen binding for which significant data are now available and (2) the structure of variable region antigenic determinants (idiotypes), which have become a source of increased interest in immunology as a result of their postulated role in immune networks and immune regulation (Jerne, 1974).

II. GENERAL STRUCTURE

Previously, it has been possible to represent the generalized structure of an immunoglobulin molecule in a rather simplistic schematic form. However, with the recent contributions of X-ray analysis, additional protein sequence data, and molecular biology, the perception of the immunoglobulin molecule has changed drastically. In terms of a generalized structure the polypeptides comprising the immunoglobulin molecule remain a ~23,000-dalton light chain and a ~50,000-dalton heavy chain, which are usually found in a basic subunit consisting of two light and two heavy chains. Each of these chains is composed of an NH_2-terminal variable region (~100 amino acids) and a carboxy-terminal constant region (~100 amino acids in light chains and 300–400 amino acids in heavy chains, depending on the particular class). It is the variable regions of the light and heavy chains that are involved in the formation of the antigen-binding site and that will be of particular importance to the concepts of structure–function relations addressed herein.

To review briefly some general features of immunoglobulin variable regions, it should be recalled that variable regions of light and heavy chains each contain three areas identified by Kabat and co-workers (T. T. Wu and Kabat, 1970; Kabat and Wu, 1971) as exhibiting a much higher degree of amino acid sequence variation than the remainder of the variable regions. These segments were termed *hypervariable* or *complementarity-determining* and were predicted to be brought into close proximity in three-dimensional folding of the immunoglobulin molecule to form the antigen-binding surface. X-ray crystallographic analyses (Poljak et al., 1974; Segal et al., 1974) have directly confirmed this prediction in that the immunoglobulin variable and constant regions are folded into compact domains (Fig. 1) and that the six complementarity-determining regions of the light and heavy chains are brought into close proximity at the "tip" of the molecule to form the antigen-binding surface. Recent studies at both the protein and nucleic acid levels have revealed additional complexities in that both light and heavy chain variable regions are assembled as the products of multiple gene elements.

For the purpose of the following discussion I will use murine κ light chains and heavy chains as models since considerable data are available in these systems. The principles derived from these experimental models appear to be applicable to all other immunoglobulin systems currently under investigation. Immuno-globulin light chains are generated from three gene segments (Brack et al., 1978; Weigert et al., 1978; Max et al., 1979; Sakano et al., 1979), designated variable (V_L), joining (J_L), and constant (C_L). The κ-chain V_L segment encodes amino acids 1-95 of the variable region; J_L, amino acids 96-113; and C_L, the entire constant region. Position 96, encoded by the J_L segment, is the last residue in the third light chain complementarity-determining region, thus potentially en-abling substitutions at this position to introduce diversity into the antigen-binding site. Heavy chains are similarly encoded by variable (V_H) (Early et al., 1980; Sakano et al., 1980), joining (J_H) (Rao et al., 1979; Bernard and Gough, 1980; Early et al., 1980; Schilling et al., 1980; Sakano et al., 1980), and constant (C_H) (Honjo and Kataoka, 1978; Yaoita and Honjo, 1980; Rabbitts et al., 1980; Shimazu et al., 1981) gene segments and in addition employ a third variable region segment, "D" (D_H) (Early et al., 1980; Sakano et al., 1980, 1981; Kuro-sawa and Tonegawa, 1982). The V_H gene encodes amino acids 1-~95; D_H, a por-tion of the third complementarity region; J_H, amino acids 100b-113[*], and C_H, the entire constant region. For variable regions, BALB/c mice appear to possess >100 germline V_L and >100 germline V_H genes (Hood et al., 1976; Potter, 1977; Seidman et al., 1978; Lenhard-Schuller et al., 1978; Cory and Adams, 1980; Davis et al., 1980; Cory et al., 1981), four functional J_L genes (Max et al., 1979; Sakano et al., 1979), four J_H genes (Sakano et al., 1980), and an undeter-mined but probably large (>20) number of D genes (Early et al., 1980; Sakano et al., 1980, 1981; Kurosawa and Tonegawa, 1982).

Before attempting to consider structure–function relations, we will first address possible mechanisms and the extent of structural diversity generated by these mechanisms within the system. Immunoglobulin structural diversity can be generated in a variety of ways:

1. Significant diversity exists as a result of the large germline repertoire of V genes. This diversity may be further amplified by the potential random association of light and heavy chains.

[*]Numbering used throughout is according to Kabat et al. (1979).

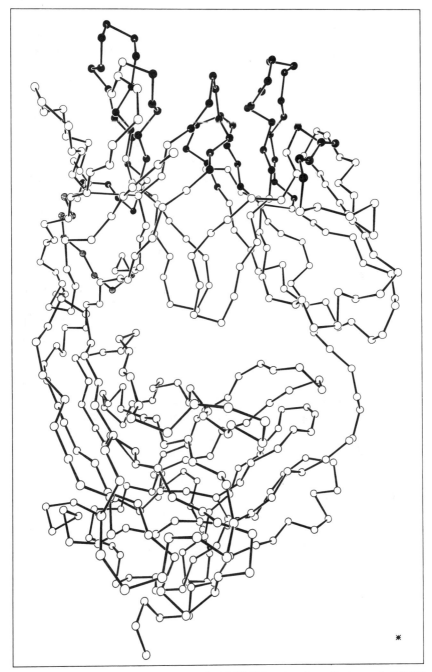

Figure 1. Three-dimensional structure of the M603 Fab, taken from Davies *et al.* (1975b). Complementarity-determining regions are indicated by solid circles.

2. An extremely large degree of diversity is generated by the association of various gene segments. For example, the pairing of a single V_L gene with four different J_L genes (Weigert *et al.*, 1978; Rudikoff *et al.*, 1980) can produce four structurally different light chains. Assuming 100 different V_L genes and four J_L genes, 400 light chains can be assembled. The diversity inherent in heavy chains is even greater in that two recombinations, V_H-D_H and D_H-J_H, occur between three genetic elements (Early *et al.*, 1980; Sakano *et al.*, 1980).

3. Alterations in the sites of recombination between the various gene segments create amino acid sequence differences at V_L-J_L (Weigert *et al.*, 1978, 1980; Max *et al.*, 1979; Sakano *et al.*, 1979; Rudikoff *et al.*, 1980) and V_H-D_H-J_H (Rao *et al.*, 1979; Early *et al.*, 1980; Sakano *et al.*, 1980, 1981; Schilling *et al.*, 1980; Gough and Bernard, 1981; Kurosawa and Tonegawa, 1982) boundaries.

4. Somatic point mutations occur throughout immunoglobulin V genes (Weigert *et al.*, 1970, 1978; Cesari and Weigert, 1973; Bernard *et al.*, 1978; Gearhart *et al.*, 1981; Bothwell *et al.*, 1981; Crews *et al.*, 1981; Selsing and Storb, 1981; Cook *et al.*, 1982; Rudikoff *et al.*, 1982).

5. Gene conversion may occur between related members of immunoglobulin families (Clarke *et al.*, 1982).

It is thus clear that a variety of mechanisms operate to generate a vast amount of structural diversity within immunoglobulins. A major point that must be stressed is that *structural* diversity does not equal *functional* diversity in that all amino acid substitutions will not produce alterations in antigen-binding specificity. Therefore, one of the most important immunochemical questions remaining to be answered is that of the relationship between amino acid substitutions produced by these various genetic mechanisms and functional diversity at the phenotypic level as exemplified by changes in antigen binding.

III. STRUCTURAL CORRELATES OF ANTIGEN BINDING

This section will present data relating to the structure of the antibody combining site and the apparent function of segments of the antibody variable region in antigen binding. Systems selected are those for which sufficient structural and functional analyses are available to be deemed appropriate in the above context. As will be seen, many of the models described in Section IV also present data pertinent to the topic of structure–function. Inclusion in the idiotype section is merely for convenience and is not intended to indicate a lesser contribution to the first topic.

The first system to generate significant structure–function correlates was the study of myeloma proteins binding the haptenic determinant dinitrophenyl (DNP). Several myeloma proteins binding DNP with high affinities have been described (Eisen *et al.*, 1968; Jaffe *et al.*, 1971) and analyzed to varying degrees. This system has been reviewed extensively (see Potter, 1977) and will therefore not be presented in detail. The most widely studied of the DNP binding myeloma proteins, M315, has been characterized as to the binding of hapten by equilibrium dialysis (Eisen *et al.*, 1968; Pecht *et al.*, 1972), fluorescence quenching (Eisen *et al.*, 1968, Eisen, 1971; Michaelides and Eisen, 1974), and temperature jump relaxation spectrometry (Pecht *et al.*, 1972; Haselkorn *et al.*, 1974). Additional analyses using affinity labeling reagents (Metzger and Potter, 1968; Goetzl and Metzger, 1970; Haimovich *et al.*, 1970, 1972; Givol *et al.*, 1971) and nuclear magnetic resonance employing hapten spin-labeled probes (Dwek *et al.*, 1975, 1977; Sutton *et al.*, 1977; Wain-Hobson *et al.*, 1977; Dower *et al.*, 1977) have produced an informative body of data on the binding of hapten by this protein. Subsequent to the availability of three-dimensional structures, hypothetical models have been constructed of M315 and, using additional physical-chemical data, detailed models of the DNP binding site have been generated (Padlan *et al.*, 1976b; Dwek *et al.*, 1977; Dower *et al.*, 1977). The accumulated data on this system have permitted a detailed assessment of the likely molecular interactions between DNP and antibody.

A. Phosphocholine

Much of the informative data currently available on the structure–function question are derived from the widely studied murine phosphocholine (PC) system. This system originated with the description of a series of mouse plasmacytomas reacting with various bacterial polysaccharides (Cohn, 1967; Potter and Lieberman, 1970; Potter, 1977). It was later shown that the haptenic moiety with which these proteins reacted was, in fact, PC (Leon and Young, 1971). Recent studies have demonstrated the biological importance of these proteins in that immunoglobulins expressing these variable regions are protective against *Streptococcus pneumoniae* infections (Briles *et al.*, 1981a, b). Subsequent to the initial observations, a number of primary amino acid sequences, a three-dimensional structure, and a gene family analysis have been determined for PC-binding antibodies.

PC-binding antibodies in all inbred strains of mice tested (Claflin, 1976; Claflin and Rudikoff, 1976) employ essentially three light chains, as represented by the BALB/c myeloma proteins T15, M603, and M167. These three light chains differ considerably in amino acid sequence and are members of different V_K subgroups. The heavy chains from these proteins are similar in sequence and are all members of the same subgroup (Potter, 1977). The Fab' fragment from one of these, M603, has been crystallized and a three-dimensional structure determined

to 3.1-Å resolution (Segal et al., 1974). An analysis of the M603 structure de-
lineates many of the principles of immunoglobulin structure–function relations
inherent to the antibody molecule itself. First, from Fig. 1 it can be seen that
the Fab' is a compact domain structure with the six hypervariable regions
clustered at the "tip" to form the antigen-binding surface. The antigen-binding
surface of M603 is a large wedge-shaped cavity approximately 12 Å deep, 15 Å
wide, and 20 Å long (Fig. 1). One of the most dramatic observations inherent
in the structure is the degree to which the lengths of the hypervariable regions
determine the shape of the binding surface and consequently the nature of the
antigen with which it can interact. The M603 light chain has an unusually long
first hypervariable region (L1)[*] containing an insertion of six amino acids. The
large loop containing L1 not only gives considerable depth to the cavity but also
effectively shields L2 from the antigen-binding cavity. Thus, in the M603 structure the antigen-binding surface is actually composed of only five of the hypervariable regions. In the heavy chain the H2 region has a two-amino-acid insertion
and H3 is also quite long. The net effect of these long hypervariable regions is
the creation of the cavity seen in Figs. 1 and 2. In contrast, the hypervariable
regions from a second crystallized Fab', New IgG (λ) (Poljak et al., 1974), are in
general shorter and form a shallow groove in contrast to the M603 cavity. Chemical studies in other systems, such as $\beta(1,6)$-D-galactan-binding myeloma proteins
(Jolley et al., 1974; Roy et al., 1981), indicate that these sites are also of a
"shallow" nature and the amino acid sequences from these proteins (Rao et al.,
1979; Rudikoff et al., 1980) reveal hypervariable region sequences shorter in
length than those found in M603. Two types of sites, both cavity and grooved,
have been suggested for $\alpha(1,6)$-binding myeloma proteins (Cisar et al., 1974,
1975; A. M. Wu et al., 1978; Bennett and Glaudemans, 1979), although no amino
acid sequence data are available to correlate type of site with hypervariable
region lengths.

  A second effect of hypervariable region lengths is to create potential interactions between segments of the immunoglobulin domains. In the M603 structure, the extended L1 loop is in intimate contact with residues in the H3 region,
as well as others in heavy chain framework segments. These interactions will
obviously effect functional characteristics displayed by the antibody and will
vary in individual antibodies with both the length of the hypervariable regions
and the nature of the amino acids contained therein. These two profound
effects of hypervariable region length are a means of influencing antibody
function and are in addition to the effect of amino acid substitution.

  In order to address the role of amino acid substitutions in antigen or hapten
binding, it is necessary first to define the interactions between antibody and
antigen as precisely as possible. From a detailed view of the M603 binding site

---

[*]L1, L2, L3, H1, H2, and H3 refer to the three light and heavy chain hypervariable or
complementarity-determining regions, respectively.

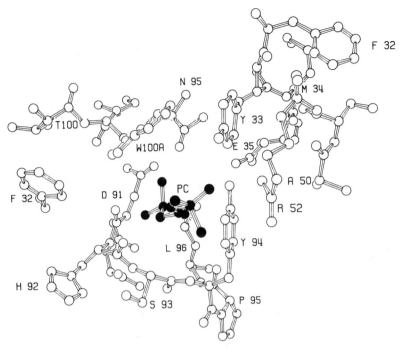

Figure 2. M603 binding site. Heavy chain complementarity-determining regions are located in the upper portion. Light chain contributions are mainly from L3 (lower portion). PC hapten is indicated by solid circles. This figure was kindly provided by Dr. Enid Silverton from the data of D. R. Davies, Y. Satow, E. A. Padlan, and G. H. Cohen (in preparation).

(Fig. 2) it can be seen that the PC hapten is bound asymmetrically with most of the contacts involving amino acids in the heavy chain (Segal *et al.*, 1974). The choline portion of the hapten is bound deep in the cavity with the phosphate group toward the exterior. The positively charged trimethylammonium (choline) interacts primarily with the main chain atoms of residues 91–94 and the side chain of Leu-96 in L3, as well as possibly the negatively charged carboxyl side chains of Glu-35 (H1) and Glu-58 (H2). The phosphate group interacts exclusively with heavy chain amino acids. One oxygen of the phosphate moiety is hydrogen-bonded to the phenolic hydroxyl of Tyr-33 (H1) and a second to the guanidinium of Arg-52 (H2). The negatively charged phosphate is also proximal to the positively charged side chains of Arg-52 and Lys-52b (H2). Extensive van der Waals contacts exist between the hapten and the side chains of Tyr-33 (H1) and Trp-100a (H3). In contrast, the binding of hydroxyvitamin K_1 by New Fab′ involves principally L1, L2, and H3 (Poljak *et al.*, 1974) and lacks the electrostatic interactions observed in M603. These two structures thus point out the extreme functional diversity inherent in antibody-combining sites in terms of both the particular hypervariable regions involved and the nature of the interactions between hapten and protein.

Using the structure of the M603 binding site it has now been possible to assess the likely effects associated with amino acid substitutions observed in other PC-binding myeloma proteins and hybridomas for which complete sequences are available. As mentioned previously, the murine immune response to PC is characterized by three different light chain species, represented by the myeloma proteins T15 (V_{K22}),* M603 (V_{K8}), and M167 (V_{K24}) (Barstad et al., 1974). Complete sequence analyses of these light chains (Rudikoff and Potter, 1978; Rudikoff et al., 1981; Kwan et al., 1981) have demonstrated that they differ extensively in both framework and hypervariable regions (Fig. 3), as predicted from their NH_2-terminal sequences. Proteins expressing these three light chains have different, characteristic specificity profiles for a series of choline analogs (Leon and Young, 1971; Claflin et al., 1981) even though their heavy chains are quite similar. This result suggests that the light chains may play a role in fine specificity determination, although most hapten (PC) antibody interactions are associated with the heavy chains. Furthermore, the observation that immunization with a variety of PC-containing antigens induces antibodies employing the same three light chains (Claflin, 1976; Claflin and Rudikoff, 1976) again substantiates the secondary nature of the role played by the light chain in response to PC. From a functional point of view it is important to note that these three light chains pair with the product of a single V_H gene (Crews et al., 1981), indicating that "combinatorial association" of three different light chains with a single heavy chain occurs routinely in the production of anti-PC antibodies. Exceptions to this pairing have been noted, albeit infrequently. In one case, a single CBA/N monoclonal antibody was found to express a V_{K3} light chain in combination with a T15 V_H region (S. H. Clarke, J. Kenney, and S. Rudikoff, in preparation). In another study BALB/c mice suppressed at birth with antisera to the T15 idiotype (Kocher et al., 1980) produced monoclonal anti-PC antibodies using the three common V_{K24}, V_{K8}, and V_{K22} sequences and, in addition, a fourth light chain homologous to V_{K15}. Furthermore an unusual V_H sequence was found in two of these hybridomas. Although the hybridomas expressing unusual light or heavy chains were specifically eluted from PC-immunoadsorbent columns, it is not known whether their fine specificity profiles are similar to those of conventional anti-PC antibodies. Whether or not pairing of V_L and V_H regions is completely random is unknown, but this question is potentially of major importance in the generation of functional diversity among antibodies.

Several important points concerning structure–function can be derived from an examination of the PC light chain sequences (Fig. 3). First, although these three light chains differ greatly in their V_L regions, they all employ the same J_L sequence (J5). In addition, an M167 identical light chain from a second genotype,

*V_{K22}, V_{K8}, and V_{K24} represent different κ-chain subgroups as defined by Potter (1977).

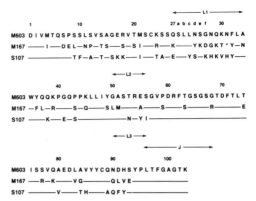

Figure 3. Amino acid sequence of κ light chains from the three major subgroups used in the anti-PC immune response. Solid lines indicate identity with topmost sequence and numbering in all figures is according to Kabat et al. (1979).

C57BL, also employs the J5 sequence (Clarke et al., 1983). There thus exists a direct correlation between PC binding and the use of J5 in these three light chain types. An examination of the M603 binding site (Fig. 2) reveals that Leu-96, the first amino acid of the J segment, is a light chain amino acid whose side chain is involved in hapten contact. J5 is the single J segment coding for Leu at this position. This datum provides the first example of a J_L segment involved in an apparently specificity-determining role, although this function cannot be generalized, as indicated by results in other systems. Second, all three light chains have the amino acid sequence Tyr-Pro-Leu at positions 94, 95, and 96. This sequence is not found at these positions in any light chains from non-PC-binding antibodies analyzed to date (Kabat et al., 1979). The function of Leu-96 has already been discussed. Tyr-94 appears to be a structurally important residue, as it is hydrogen-bonded to Glu-35 of the heavy chain and also is a hapten-contacting residue forming one side of the binding pocket. The hydrogen bond to Glu-35 is likely to play a significant role in stabilizing the surrounding areas of the binding pocket in which the choline portion of the hapten rests. The analysis of these light chain sequences has provided a correlation between the use of a specific J segment (which supplies a hapten-contacting amino acid) as well as amino acids in the third hypervariable region and PC binding. Furthermore, it is evident that three very different V_L regions could generate these required structures. It is interesting that all three of these light chains have unusually long L1 regions, although the existence of a possible structural requirement for this long L1 in PC-binding antibodies is unproven.

The heavy chains from the myeloma proteins T15, M603, and M167 are similar (Rudikoff and Potter, 1974, 1976), yet significant differences exist among these polypeptides (Fig. 4). These three heavy chains have been inferred to derive from the same V_H gene, which directly encodes the T15 V_H sequence (Crews et al., 1981). The V_H substitutions in M603 and M167 result from somatic mutations. Additional differences in the H3 region likely result from alterations

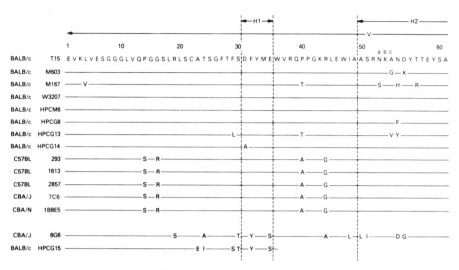

Figure 4. Heavy chain variable region sequences and association

in recombination sites between V_H-D_H and D_H-J_H segments (Early et al., 1980). Padlan et al. (1976a) in an analysis of these sequences have concluded that the PC-binding site is largely unaltered in spite of the observed amino acid variation. The critical hapten-contacting residues Tyr-33, Arg-52, Lys-52b, and Glu-58 are found in all three heavy chains. Alanine present at position 50 is also conserved. The presence of the small side chain associated with Ala-50 appears necessary to allow penetration of the hapten into the pocket. Trp-100a is the only contacting amino acid (missing in M167) not uniformly present. Affinity labeling studies of T15 using p-diazoniumphenylphosphocholine (Chesebro and Metzger, 1972) resulted in labeling of Tyr-32 and -92 of the light chain. While position 32L is probably not proximal to the PC-binding site, 92L is close to the hapten-contacting residue Leu-96L in the M603 structure. In other experiments, blocking of arginyl groups by glyoxylation or partial esterification of carboxyl groups either inactivated or largely reduced PC binding (Grossberg et al., 1974). These results are consistent with the X-ray analysis and further suggest the proposed conservation in the nature of the PC-binding sites. It is interesting that the sequence Phe-Tyr-Met-Glu in H1 has only been observed in PC-binding antibodies (Kabat et al., 1976). A human PC-binding myeloma protein was found to have the sequence Phe-Tyr-Met-Asp in this region (Riesen et al., 1976), demonstrating a remarkable conservation and pointing out the importance of this sequence to PC specificity.

Although the PC-binding site is similar in these three proteins, differences in fine specificity are likely associated with some of the observed amino acid substitutions (Padlan et al., 1976a). For example M167 has an Asp at position 97 that is not found in T15 (Fig. 4). This substitution may explain the lower affinity of

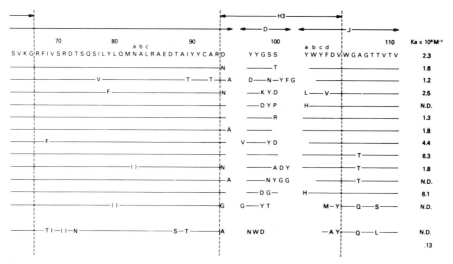

constants from anti-PC myeloma and hybridoma proteins.

M167 for PC (Metzger *et al.*, 1971), as this residue would result in an unfavorable electrostatic interaction with the phosphate group of the hapten. Conversely, these proteins would be expected to have a higher affinity for free choline, as has been observed, owing to the additional negative charge. This analysis suggests that, although the PC-binding site is remarkably conserved, somatic mutations such as those observed in M167 may alter fine specificities of given antibodies. These mutations either can originate as classical point mutations or be generated by alterations in recombination between V_H-D_H-J_H segments. It should be remembered that the relations between changes in fine specificity and the immune response to an antigen are at present unknown. For example, if antibodies such as T15, M603, and M167, which are routinely produced in the immune response to PC (Claflin, 1976), are also produced in the response to choline, the fine specificity differences of these antibodies become relatively unimportant in terms of the ability to induce a given functional antibody population.

Using the model of the M603 combining site in the context of the structural conservation described above, it is now possible to begin to assess the role of various processes involved in the generation of antibody diversity in terms of PC binding. A number of V_H sequences have been determined for PC-binding BALB/c myeloma proteins (Rudikoff and Potter, 1974, 1976; Hood *et al.*, 1976), BALB/c hybridomas (Gearhart *et al.*, 1981), C57BL hybridomas (Clarke *et al.*, 1983) and CBA/J hybridomas (Clarke *et al.*, 1982). Representative sequences are presented in Fig. 4. Eight additional V_H sequences have been found to be identical to T15 (Gearhart *et al.*, 1981). A comparison of the gene sequences encoding the BALB/c PC-V_H regions (Crews *et al.*, 1981) have suggested that essentially all of the BALB/c myeloma and hybridoma sequences are derived from the gene directly encoding the T15 V_H sequence. The V_H substitutions observed in IgG and IgA proteins were attributed to somatic mutations that appeared to correlate with the class-switching process. An examination of the amino acid sequences from positions 1 to 95 (the segment encoded by the V_H gene) reveals an array of substitutions occurring in both framework and hypervariable regions. Among the BALB/c proteins the M167 myeloma is the most divergent in the V_H region, with eight substitutions. The only replacement found in more than one protein is Thr at position 40 in M167 and HPCG13. All of the C57BL and CBA V_H regions share amino acid substitutions at positions 14, 16, 40, and 44. These substitutions, together with serological analyses demonstrating simple Mendelian segregation of antigenic markers associated with these V regions (Lieberman *et al.*, 1981), define the C57BL and CBA V regions as products of a gene allelic to T15 of BALB/c mice (Claflin and Rudikoff, 1979; Rudikoff and Potter, 1980; Clarke *et al.*, 1982, 1983). With the exception of the CBA/J 6G6 and BALB/c HPCG15, all of the remaining V_H regions contain the residues identified as critical to the PC-binding site: Tyr-33, Glu-35, and Arg-52. Since the binding affinities (Fig. 4) of all proteins for the PC hapten are quite similar, the data indicate that the substitutions in the BALB/c proteins generated by somatic mutations, and those in the C57BL and CBA proteins generated by mutations in the germline, have little, if any, effect on the binding of PC. As the binding assays were performed only with free PC, it is possible that some of these substitutions affect the interaction between antibody and other portions of macromolecular antigens of which PC is a haptenic determinant.

The CBA 6G6 sequence is interesting in that it differs from T15 V_H at 17 positions (Fig. 4). This sequence has been shown to be more homologous to a second gene of the PC V_H family (Clarke *et al.*, 1982), indicating that at least two V_H genes can be used in the immune response to PC. The BALB/c protein HPCG15 also expresses the linked amino acids Thr-30, Tyr-32, Ser-35, suggesting similarly, that it is the product of a PC-V_H gene other than T15. These proteins lack Glu-35, which is associated with PC binding. HPCG15 has the lowest affinity $(0.13 \times 10^5 \ M^{-1})$ of any PC-binding antibody and the possible significance of the Glu-Ser interchange at position 35 will be discussed later.

From Fig. 4 it can be seen that most of the sequence diversity occurs in the D region. The discovery that this region of the immunoglobulin heavy chain, which includes a portion of the third hypervariable region, was encoded by a separate genetic element (Early *et al.*, 1980) led to the speculation that D segments would play a significant role in the generation of the vast repertoire of antibody specificities. While it is clear that D segments can introduce extensive *structural* diversity in heavy chains, the relationship between this *structural* diversity and *functional* diversity in terms of the generation of new antigen-binding specificities is unclear. An evaluation of D segments from PC-binding immunoglobulins (Table I) indicates that multiple, different D segments can be employed. Proteins from different strains (T15 BALB/c and 293 C57BL) may use the same D segment, while, conversely, proteins from the same strain (T15, M167, HPCM6-BALB/c, and 293-, 1613-, and 2857-C57BL) may express very different D segments. Of 25 available D-segment sequences, 14 are different. Of the 14 different sequences as many as 9 may be encoded by different D genes. It is thus surprising (Table I) that proteins with such structurally different D segments have remarkably similar association constants for PC hapten. These data suggest that, as in the case of the V_H mutations, alterations in the D segment have at most minor effects on hapten binding. Furthermore, it can be seen that antibodies from animals immunized with PC on very different carriers—e.g., HPCM2 (PC-HCN), 293 (PC-KLH), 23169 (*Proteus morganii*)—have identical D regions. Similarly 6F9 (*Streptococcus pneumoniae*) and 7C6 (PC-KLH + PC-BGG) express identical D regions, which differ from those of HPCM2 and the T15 group. Conversely, immunization with a given antigen can produce antibodies with very different D segments. Also, it has been demonstrated that the myeloma proteins H8, which differs from T15 by one amino acid, and M603 bind PC on two completely different bacterial polysaccharide backbones in an identical manner (Glaudemans *et al.*, 1977). It thus appears that in the PC system the D segment plays no significant role in hapten binding, antibody–carrier interaction, or determining the repertoire of antibodies produced in response to

Table I. Diversity (D) Segment Sequences Found in Anti-PC Heavy Chains

Protein	Class	Strain	Immunogen	V_H	D	J_H	K_a ($\times 10^5$ M^{-1})
T15	IgA	BALB/c	–	RD	YYGS S	YWY	2.3
M167	IgA	BALB/c	–	—A	D—N–YFG	–	1.2
M603	IgA	BALB/c	–	–N	———T	——	1.6
HPCM1	IgM	BALB/c	PC-HCN	—	———	——	N.D.[a]
HPCM2	IgM	BALB/c	PC-HCN	—	———	——	3.5
HPCM6	IgM	BALB/c	PC-HCN	—	—DY P	H—	N.D.
HPCG8	IgG3	BALB/c	PC-HCN	—	———R	——	1.3
HPCG13	IgG1	BALB/c	PC-HCN	—A	———	——	1.8
HPCG14	IgG1	BALB/c	PC-HCN	—	V——YD	—	4.4
293	IgM	C57BL	PC-KLH	—	———	——	6.3
1613	IgM	C57BL	*Streptococcus pneumoniae*	–N	———ADY	——	1.8
23169	IgM	C57BL	*Proteus morganii*	–N	———	——	0.61
2857	IgM	C57BL	PC-KLH	—A	——NYGG	–	N.D.
6F9	IgM	CBA/J	*Streptococcus pneumoniae*	–N	—DG—	——	6.1
7C6	IgM	CBA/J	PC-KLH; PC-BGG	—	—DG—	H—	12.0

[a]N.D., not determined.

PC-containing antigens. Furthermore, there is no correlation between D-segment sequence and light chain type. Proteins T15, HPCG13, and 23169 (Table I) have identical D sequences and express respectively the T15-, M167-, and M603-type light chains. Similarly, proteins HPCM1, HPCM6, HPCG14, and 7C6 all employ T15 light chain but have different D sequences. The only correlation observed is that proteins expressing the T15 light chain all have D segments of the same length. D-segment length in other systems appears more critical than primary sequence and may reflect the primary contribution of this region of the heavy chain.

All anti-PC V_H regions derived from the T15 V_H (or its allelic form, C3) employ the J_H1 joining segment, with the exception of the CBA/N protein 1B8E5 (Fig. 4). The reason for the preferential use of J_H1 is unclear. The only interaction between residues in the J_H region and hapten are relatively weak van der Waals forces associated with Trp 100a. Trp is encoded at this position in both J_H1 and J_H3. The fact that this residue is deleted by the D_H-J_H recombination in proteins M167 and 2857 further suggests that this amino acid is not essential for PC binding. 1B8E5 employs the J_H4 joining segment (S. H. Clarke, J. Kenney, and S. Rudikoff, in preparation), indicating that at least two J_H regions can pair with the T15 V_H gene product in PC-binding antibodies. This protein is unusual in that it employs a light chain other than those normally found in other PC antibodies. As in the case of the D segments, no correlation is seen between immunogen (Table I, Fig. 4) and the use of J_H1, suggesting that the J_H region is not involved in carrier specificity. The CBA/J protein 6G6, which is the product of a PC-V_H gene other than that encoding the T15 sequence, pairs with a J_H3 segment.

While the above analysis of hybridoma and myeloma proteins indicates that extensive *structural* diversity need not generate corresponding *functional* diversity, these systems have a major drawback as the basis for attempts to correlate amino acid substitutions with specificity changes in that they are positively selected by antigen. Thus, only proteins that do, in fact, bind a given antigen with an appropriate affinity are selected. This process likely selects proteins displaying varying numbers of amino acid replacements as long as the substitutions do not significantly alter binding specificity or affinity. The hybridoma and myeloma proteins described above are examples of this selection. All antibody systems positively selected by antigen will in general not detect variants exhibiting altered specificity regardless of the number of amino acid substitutions present in the variant molecules.

In order to detect potential antigen-binding variants two systems involving negative selection have recently been described. In the first, variants are selected on the basis of altered antigenic (idiotypic or allotypic) determinants as detected by analysis using the fluorescence-activated cell sorter (Radbruch *et al.*, 1980). This technique has been used to identify constant region variants and is currently

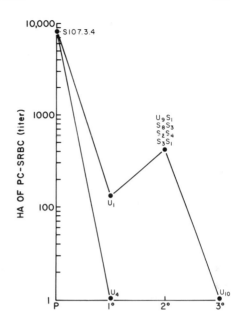

Figure 5. Derivation of somatic variants from the PC-binding S107 myeloma cell line. Variants are characterized by ability to agglutinate PC-coupled sheep red blood cells.

being employed to detect V-region mutants by analysis with antiidiotypic monoclonal antibodies. The second system for which significant structural data are currently available involves "negative" antigen selection, again using PC-binding myeloma proteins.

Variants of the PC-binding IgA myeloma protein S107[*] have been identified in an *in vitro* culture system. The S107 myeloma was cloned in soft agar and mutants were selected following overlay with PC-KLH antigen. Cells that are not surrounded by antigen–antibody precipitates are presumed to be antigen-binding variants and may be selected for further characterization. Detectable variants arise at the surprisingly high frequency of 0.1–1% and approximately 70% of these appear to secrete normal amounts of IgA molecules (Cook and Scharff, 1977). A set of such mutants has been described as depicted in Fig. 5. U_1 and U_4 are first-generation variants with altered ability to agglutinate PC-coupled sheep red blood cells (SRBC). A series of revertants derived from U_1 that agglutinate better than the U_1 parent but less well than the "wild-type" S107 have also been isolated. Binding characteristics have been determined for the U_1 and U_4 variants and are presented in Table II. U_1 was found to react less well than parent with PC coupled to a variety of carriers (Cook *et al.*, 1982), although affinity for free hapten was indistinguishable. These results suggest that the hapten-binding site is identical in the two proteins but that U_1 has a

---

[*]S107 is a myeloma protein that appears to be identical to T15.

Table II. Binding Characteristics of S107 Variants[a]

Cell line	HA titer[b]	RIA PC-KLH (percent relative binding[c])	K_a ($\times 10^5$ M^{-1})	Tryptic peptide differences H	L
S107.3.4	8192	100%	2.3		
U$_4$	0	0.01	0	+	–
U$_1$	128	9.0	2.5	+	–
S$_3$S$_1$	512	26	2.1	+	–

[a] Adapted from Cook *et al.* (1981).
[b] 250 μg of purified protein examined in twofold dilutions.
[c] Percent relative binding = $\dfrac{\text{ng parent required for 50\% inhibition}}{\text{ng variant required for 50\% inhibition}} \times 100.$

defect in the region involved in interaction with the carrier portion of the antigenic molecule. This defect is not carrier-specific in that a variety of PC-carrier conjugates show the same effect. Detailed biochemical characterization revealed that the light chains of U$_1$ and parent were identical by tryptic peptide mapping and NH$_2$-terminal sequence analysis of the first 50 residues. The heavy chain amino acid sequence of U$_1$ (Fig. 6) differs from the parent at a single position, the fifth residue of the J segment, at which an Ala-Asp substitution occurs. While the data do not rule out the possibility that additional substitutions have also occurred in the carboxy-terminal portion of the light chains, the evidence suggests that the phenotypic alterations seen in U$_1$ are associated with the single substitution observed in J$_H$. Analysis of the three-dimensional structure of the

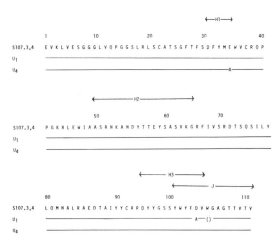

Figure 6. Heavy chain variable region sequences from S107 parent and variants U$_1$ and U$_4$.

binding site of the related M603 protein (Fig. 1) indicates that the fifth residue of J is not within the hapten-binding site. This finding is consistent with the observation that the affinity of U_1 for free hapten and its reactivity with PC analogs are similar to those of the parent. It appears as thouth the U_1 variant may be an example of a substitution in a region of the immunoglobulin heavy chain normally thought of as "framework" but which, in fact, interacts with a segment of the antigen adjacent to the PC moiety (i.e., a carrier determinant). Thus, substitutions in framework segments may in some instances produce alterations in specificity.

An additional first-generation variant, U_4, was characterized (Table I) (Rudikoff et al., 1982) and shown to have lost the ability to agglutinate PC-SRBC; furthermore, it did not bind free PC hapten in equilibrium dialysis. Serological analysis using conventional antisera to the PC-binding site as well as monoclonal anti-PC variable region antibodies revealed that some reagents could discriminate between U_4 and parent (Maximum difference approximately tenfold) while others failed to distinguish between the two. These data indicate that changes have occurred in the antigen-binding site that significantly alter specificity but only minimally effect antigenic determinants (idiotypes). The defect in antigen binding was further localized to the heavy chain by analysis of heterologous recombinant molecules between U_4 and parent. Recombinants employing the U_4 heavy chain failed to react with PC or PC-containing antigens. Sequence analysis of the U_4 heavy chain identified a single amino acid substitution of Ala for Glu at position 35 in the first hypervariable or complementarity-determining region (Fig. 6). As may be recalled, Glu-35 has been designated a critical residue in the PC-binding site. In the M603 structure (Fig. 2) the role of Glu-35 in direct hapten contact is somewhat uncertain as it appears to be at the distance limits acceptable for interaction with the phosphate moiety (D. R. Davies, personal communication). However, the side chain of Glu-35 is hydrogen-bonded to the phenolic hydroxyl of Tyr-94 in the light chain. This bond is important in stabilizing the region of the binding pocket containing hapten-contacting residues Tyr-33 and Arg-52 from the heavy chain and Leu-96 from the light chain. Not only does the substitution of Ala for Glu remove the hydrogen bond, but the decrease in side chain volume would further distort this region of the binding pocket. As previously noted, PC-binding antibodies may employ three structurally different light chains, yet all three have Tyr at position 94 and can thus form this hydrogen bond. Two of the hybridoma heavy chains described earlier (6G6 and HPCG15) were noted to be encoded by a PC V_H gene other than T15. Both of these proteins have Ser at position 35. HPCG15 has the lowest association constant for PC (Gearhart et al., 1981) of all hybridomas and myelomas tested to date, suggesting that the size of the Ser side chain may partially compensate for the Glu, whereas the small Ala side chain in the U_4 variant cannot perform this function. The preferential use of the T15 V_H gene may stem from the fact that this is the only functional gene in this family encoding Glu at position 35.

The results obtained from the S107 antigen-binding variants demonstrate that small numbers of amino acid substitutions, such as those presumed to arise by somatic mutations, can potentially produce alterations in antigen binding specificities. The U_1 variant may be an example of a substitution in a portion of the V region not normally thought of as involved in antigen binding that may, in some instances, alter specificity by affecting interactions with regions of the carrier portion of macromolecular antigens. The substitution in U_4 provides a striking structural correlation for the complete loss in antigen binding resulting from a single amino acid replacement. It should be clearly emphasized that the results of the hybridoma and myeloma sequence analyses indicate that many, and possibly most, amino acid substitutions do not significantly effect specificity or affinity.

B. $\beta(1,6)$-D-Galactan

A second set of homogeneous immunoglobulins for which structure–function studies are being undertaken consists of myeloma and hybridoma proteins that bind $\beta(1,6)$-D-galactan-containing antigens. Six myeloma and ten hybridoma proteins exhibiting this specificity have been characterized to varying degrees. Both the light and heavy chains from all of the $\beta(1,6)$-D-galactan-binding antibodies fall into single subgroups (Rudikoff *et al.*, 1973; Pawlita *et al.*, 1982). Complete light chain sequences from sixteen of these molecules (Rudikoff *et al.*, 1980; Pawlita *et al.*, 1982) have revealed that in the variable region 12 are identical, one differs by a single framework substitution, two differ by the identical two framework substitutions, and the fourth variant differs at three positions in hypervariable and two positions in framework regions (Fig. 7). Complete heavy chain sequences from four of the myeloma proteins (Rao *et al.*, 1979) have demonstrated that two (X44 and T601) are identical in the variable region (positions 1–95) and the remaining two differ at three and four positions, respectively. These substitutions occur in both framework and hypervariable regions (Fig. 8).

Several interesting comparisons can be made to the PC system described in the previous section:

1. Whereas three different light chain subgroups are commonly employed in the response to PC, only a single subgroup is found in the antigalactan response, suggesting a strict functional correlation with this particular variable region.
2. All three light chains employed in the PC response use the J5 joining segment and residue 96 encoded by the first trinucleotide of the J5 gene is a hapten-contacting amino acid. Among the antigalactan light chains (Fig. 7) all four J segments are potentially used. Fifteen of these light chains have an Ile at position 96 and a Trp is found in the sixteenth (X-24). The association constant of X-24 for galactotriose hapten (Rudikoff *et al.*,

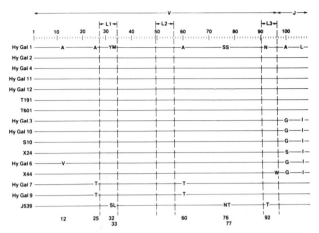

Figure 7. Light chain variable region sequences from $\beta(1,6)$-D-galactan-binding myeloma and hybridoma proteins.

1980) is similar to that of proteins with Ile at position 96, indicating that position 96 and the light chain J segment play no significant role in hapten binding.

3. As in the anti-PC heavy chains, scattered substitutions are found throughout the antigalactan V_H regions. Considerable sequence variation is generated at the points of V_H-D and D-J_H joining, but, in contrast to the anti-PC heavy chains, the length of the D segment and the third hypervariable region is constant. This result suggests that the length of the third hypervariable or complementarity-determining region may be of more importance in the antigalactan proteins than the actual primary sequence. It cannot be determined at this point whether the observed length correlation is directly related to antigen binding or possibly to the proper association of heavy and light chains.

4. Antigalactan heavy chains employ at least three different J segments, in contrast to anti-PC heavy chains encoded by the T15 V_H gene, which show a restricted association with J_H1. At present, it is unknown whether the antigalactan heavy chains are encoded by more than one V_H gene.

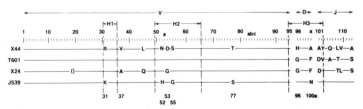

Figure 8. Heavy chain variable region sequences from $\beta(1,6)$-D-galactan-binding myeloma proteins.

This may prove to be an important point, as the use of particular J_H regions may be related to the gene structure of the V_H and D regions with which they pair, as well as their potential functional role in either antigen binding or light-chain/heavy-chain association.

Although one of the galactan-binding myeloma proteins (J539) has been crystallized and a low-resolution map determined (Navia et al., 1979), a detailed, three-dimensional analysis, as in the PC system, must await high-resolution X-ray analysis. A number of biochemical studies have, however, defined many of the parameters of $\beta(1,6)$-D-galactan–antibody interaction. Two of the myeloma proteins, J539 and X24, have been studied in considerable detail. These two proteins reveal identical specificity profiles for 30 carbohydrate haptens (Jolley et al., 1974) despite nine amino acid substitutions in complementarity-determining regions (Figs. 7 and 8). Many of the interchanges in these proteins result in the occurrence of amino acids with structurally very different side chains as represented by the following examples: Tyr-Ser in L1; Asn-Thr in L3; Asn-His in H2; Gly-Asp in H2; Ser-Gly in H2; Gly-His in H3; Phe-Asn in H3. Thus, as many as nine substitutions, some of which introduce structurally and functionally unrelated amino acids, can be accommodated without gross alterations in the specificity profiles of these antibodies. It should be noted that these two proteins can be differentiated at the fine specificity level (Jolley et al., 1974) in that J539 binds mono- and disaccharide haptens with slightly higher affinities than X-24. In the case of both proteins the termainal nonreducing galactosyl residue contributes most of the binding energy for oligosaccharide interaction and little additional increase occurs between the tri- and tetrasaccharides, indicating that three to four sugar residues is the maximum size of the combining surface interacting with $\beta(1,6)$-linked galactose moieties. The functional similiarities of these molecules are further evidenced by the ability of heterologous recombinants (Manjula et al., 1976) to display binding properties similar to those of the parent molecules.

Using a series of galactopyranosyl derivatives, deductions have been made as to the nature and importance of various portions of galactopyranosyl haptens in binding to antibody. It appears that interactions occur along the polysaccharide chain and involve predominantly the first three galactosyl subunits. For proteins X-24 and J539 the contributions of binding energy for the tetrasaccharide are: terminal nonreducing sugar > residue 2 > residue 3 >> residue 4. The conformation of the binding site based on this data was suggested to be an extended "groove," with binding occurring predominantly along one side of the galactosyl tetrasaccharide (Jolley et al., 1974; Roy et al., 1981). Specific amino acids involved in hapten or antigen binding have not as yet been elucidated.

The antigalactan system potentially addresses a number of questions that will, in the future, be key to an analysis of structure-function relations. Since suitable crystals have been obtained from J539, the high-resolution structure of this Fab, when determined, will provide a test for conclusions drawn from biochemical experiments. Of equal importance is the potential of this structure to test the feasibility of model-building for use in assessment of structure–function problems. It seems clear from the fact that only two Fab structures from known antigen-binding proteins have been solved since 1974 that we cannot expect to see a significant number of new structures determined in the near future. Some investigators have therefore employed model-building as an alternative means of constructing immunoglobulin-binding sites. All of these experiments are based on the premise of using the structures determined from X-ray crystallography and modifying these structures in relation to the particular protein being studied. The observation that the frameworks of immunoglobulins are remarkably conserved, as was shown in comparisons of human and mouse κ chains (Davies *et al.*, 1975a), has provided impetus to this approach. It should be cautioned that, while the conservation of framework regions is readily apparent, modeling of hypervariable regions is an entirely different problem. In most model-building studies the structure of hypervariable or complementarity-determining regions has been based on the use of corresponding segments of equal length from proteins whose structure has been determined by X-ray diffraction. Although X-ray diffraction analysis is the basis for complementarity-determining loop structure in these models, it must be pointed out that X-ray analysis in many instances does not provide absolute and unambiguous structures. Therefore, a number of assumptions whose validity has yet to be tested are necessarily made in the construction of models.

Recently, a second approach has been used to obtain a model of the galactan-binding J539 myeloma protein (Feldmann *et al.*, 1981). This model was constructed on a computer display system using the M603 backbone structure, but not employing hypervariable region structures derived from other crystallized proteins. The hypervariable region sequences of J539 were instead "grafted" onto the backbone by visual analysis so as to cause the least possible perturbation of the polypeptide chain. It is important that in three hypervariable regions J539 is shorter than M603, thus requiring the introduction of deletions and subsequent rejoining of segments in the M603 structure to produce the J539 model. Using the model generated in this fashion, a hypothetical binding site, although not a unique solution, has been postulated. The importance of this model is that the predictions made are testable. The determination of a high-resolution X-ray map, which is in progress, will permit a more accurate assessment of the potential role of modeling studies in generating structures of sufficient accuracy to be valid experimental tools.

IV. STRUCTURAL CORRELATES OF IDIOTYPES

Variable region antigenic determinants (idiotypes), originally described in humans (Slater *et al.*, 1955) and rabbits (Oudin and Michel, 1963), have proven to be valuable markers in the study of immunoglobulin genetics, structure, and regulation. As the interest in idiotypy has grown a certain confusion associated with this term has also developed. Idiotypes were originally considered to be individual antigenic determinants located within the immunoglobulin variable regions. Subsequently two classes of "idiotypes" have been functionally identi- fied: (1) those that are unique to a homogeneous species (individual idiotypes) and (2) those that are shared among several molecular species (cross-reacting idio- types). Proteins that share cross-reacting idiotypes are usually functionally related in that they bind the same haptenic determinant. The variable region idiotypes are distinct from allotypes, which are usually found in the constant region al- though variable region allotypes have been described in the rabbit (reviewed by Mage *et al.*, 1973). A serological marker in the variable region of murine heavy chains has also been reported (Bosma *et al.*, 1977) which may be analogous to the rabbit variable region allotypes (see Mage *et al.*, 1973, for a review of allotypes). A number of allotypic determinants have been structurally characterized and in general are represented by single amino acid substitutions or small numbers of substitutions.

Structural characterization of idiotypes has proven to be a difficult task for a number of reasons. First, few systems have been characterized containing closely related members, some of which are positive while others are negative, for a given idiotype. Second, idiotypes may be located on the light chain or the heavy chain or be produced by a combination of the two chains. These determinants may therefore be predominantly determined either by primary structure or by con- formational interactions, which may be highly complex. Idiotypes may further be associated either with hypervariable regions, which may or may not be in the combining site, or with framework segments. The determination of the structural basis of idiotypes is still in a very early stage and only two systems have, to date, been developed to the point of making feasible deductions concerning the struc- tural basis of these markers. However, the potential role of these determinants in networks involved in the regulation of the immune response as proposed by Jerne (1974) makes an understanding of the structural basis of these antigens key to an assessment of the biology of the proposed regulation.

A. Antiinulin

One of the most extensive idiotype systems characterized to date consists of mouse myeloma proteins that bind bacterial levans. These proteins can be divided into two groups. The first and largest consists of 11 proteins that bind fructosans, such as inulin, which are linear polysaccharides with $\beta(2,1)$ linkages. The second includes two proteins that are thought to react with $\beta(2,6)$ linkages on bacterial levans (Cisar *et al.*, 1974). Mouse antiidiotypic antisera prepared to nine of the inulin-binding myeloma proteins were found to cross-react with several other members of this group, identifying a number of cross-reactive idiotypic (IdX) determinants (Lieberman *et al.*, 1975). Absorption of a given antiserum with one of the cross-reactive molecules rendered it specific for the immunizing protein and thus defined individual idiotypes (IdI) associated with each of the myeloma proteins. Thus, the IdX and IdI determinants on the same molecule were clearly distinguishable and no two proteins shared the same IdI determinant. Based on these observations 10 IdX systems were defined by coating SRBC with a myeloma protein with which the antiserum reacted but which was not the immunizing protein (a cross-reacting protein) and assaying the ability of 12 levan-binding myeloma proteins to inhibit the various systems. One half of the IdI systems involving inulin-binding myeloma proteins were inhibitable by $\beta(2,1)$-fructosan trisaccharide, as were all of the IdX systems, suggesting that the corresponding determinants were associated with the combining site. Subsequent studies using heterologous recombinant molecules prepared by "mixing" the heavy and light chains from two different proteins were able to localize several of the IdI and IdX determinants to either light or heavy chains (Lieberman *et al.*, 1977). Even though the determinants were associated with either the light or heavy chains, it was found that the second chain had to be from an inulin-binding myeloma, as recombinants using a heavy or light chain from a protein with a different binding specificity failed to bind inulin or express idiotypes. This result indicates that the expression of idiotypes by antiinulin light or heavy chains requires a specific partner chain structure, which likely provides a conformation necessary for idiotype expression. The localization of idiotypes to specific chains by use of recombinant molecules is key to an assessment of the structural basis of these markers.

Idiotypes from antiinulin myeloma proteins for which corresponding protein structure data are available are presented in Tables III and IV. Corresponding light (Vrana *et al.*, 1979; Johnson *et al.*, 1982) and heavy (Vrana *et al.*, 1978; Rudikoff and Potter, 1981; Johnson *et al.*, 1982) chain sequences are presented in Figs. 9 and 10. Furthermore, a model has been constructed of the E109 variable region (Potter, 1977), and it has been used in the deductions of idiotype localization. The E109 IdI is localized to the light chain (Table III) and is not hapten-inhibitable. An examination of the light chain sequences (Fig. 9) reveals that E109 differs from the others at positions 56, 65, and 106. All three of these

Table III. Distribution of Antiinulin IdI Determinants

Determinant	Hapten inhibition	Determinant chain location			
		E109L	E109H	U61L	U61H
E109IdI	−	+	−	−	−
U61IdI	−	−	−	+	−

Table IV. Distribution of Antiinulin IdX Determinants

Determinant	Hapten inhibition	Protein location							
		U61	A4	J606	A47N	W3082	E109	AM1	T957
IdXA	+	+	+ (H)	–	–	+	+	–	–
IdXB	+	+ (L)	–	–	–	+	–	–	–
IdXC	+	+	+	–	–	+	+	+	N.D.[a]
IdXD	+	+	–	+	–	+	+	+	N.D.

[a]N.D., not determined.

residues are external in the theoretical model and could form the basis of the antigenic determinant. In addition positions 56 and 65 are close enough that they could probably be bridged by an antibody, combining site and could both participate in determinant formation. A further possibility is that any of these substitutions in proximity to other nonvariant amino acids could produce the determinant. Thus, the amino acid substitutions in the E109 light chain are limited to three positions, any of which could form the basis of the E109 IdI.

The U61 IdI is similarly located on the light chain and is not hapten-inhibitable. An examination of the light chain sequences reveals no position at which U61 expresses unique amino acids. Therefore, this determinant either may be complex in nature or possibly may not be located in the variable region. Since U61 and J606 differ by only a single amino acid at position 53 and U61 and W3082 are identical in this region, there is no obvious pattern to be associated with a possible complex determinant.

The IdXA specificity is found on the heavy chain of A4 and is shared among proteins U61, A4, W3082, and E109. Since proteins J606, A47, and AM1, which lack the determinant, do not share substitutions (Fig. 10), the marker must be determined by several amino acids. It has been suggested (Johnson et al., 1982) that position 53 is involved in this determinant since A4, which expresses IdXA, and J606, which does not, differ by this single amino acid. However, AM1,

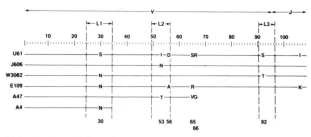

Figure 9. Light chain variable region sequences from inulin-binding myeloma proteins.

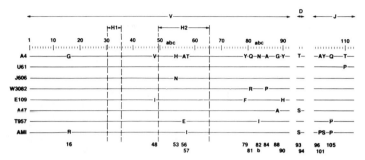

Figure 10. Heavy chain variable region sequences from inulin-binding myeloma proteins.

which is identical to A4 at this position, is also negative for IdXA, indicating that if this position is involved it is part of a complex involving several amino acids that may be located in both hypervariable and framework regions.

The IdXB determinant (Table IV) was found to be hapten-inhibitable and located on the U61 light chain. This marker was originally proposed to result from the proximity of Ser-30 and Ser-92 in the first and third hypervariable regions (Vrana *et al.*, 1979). The addition of the W3082 and J606 sequences revealed that the W3082 light chain had Asn and Thr at positions 30 and 92 and was positive for the idiotype while J606 was identical to U61 at these positions and negative for the marker (Johnson *et al.*, 1982). The idiotypic determinant thus is unlikely to be associated with these two positions. Since there are no positions at which U61 and W3082 are identical but differ from all other light chains, it appears as though the IdXB determinant must be complex in nature and involve more than one amino acid. It has been suggested (Johnson *et al.*, 1982) that positions 53 and 56 may both be involved in the determinant, although contributions from other positions in the chain cannot be ruled out.

The IdXC idiotype, while not localized to a given chain, appears to correlate most closely with the presence of Ile-53 in the light chains, although this analysis should be considered somewhat tenuous in view of the lack of chain recombination experiments and the different distribution of IdXD, which also appears to correlate with Ile-53. A number of additional idiotypes have been serologically characterized in this system. However, attempts to deduce structural correlates become increasingly difficult and speculative and must await more precise experimental data.

The antiinulin system is another example of the potential role of model-building in structure–function analysis. A hypothetical three-dimensional model has been constructed of the E109 protein using the backbone of M603 and "grafting" on hypervariable regions. This model has played a significant role in attempts to deduce the structure of idiotypes associated with inulin-binding antibodies (Vrana *et al.*, 1979). For example, from the heavy chain sequences (Fig. 10) it is tempting to associate the IdXA marker with position 93, which contains substitutions in two of the proteins (A47 and AM1) that are negative for the determinant. However, the three-dimensional model suggests an internal position for this amino acid, so that conservative substitutions, such as the observed Thr-Ser interchange, would not be expected to alter idiotypic determinants. This particular point draws attention to one of the significant limitations of modeling. The antiinulin proteins are extremely "short" in the third heavy chain hypervariable region when compared to other heavy chains. No other structures are available with an equivalent length in H3, so that the construction of this region requires a number of assumptions. Since residue 93 is located in this segment an erroneous placement of this amino acid would greatly affect the interpretation of its potential role in the determination of idiotypes. It must therefore be emphasized that *hypothetical* models are no more than the name implies and must be used in such a context.

While the antiinulin idiotype systems discussed above do not unambiguously provide structural correlates, they do provide the basis for two general conclusions concerning idiotypes:

1. Idiotypes such as the E109 IdI are probably determined by no more than two amino acids and are thus relatively simple in nature. This is analogous to many of the constant region allotypes described in other species (Mage *et al.*, 1973).
2. In contrast the IdX markers all appear to be complex in nature and in most cases involve residues both inside and outside of the hypervariable regions. The complexity of the IdX markers is not necessarily surprising since these markers were identified in systems designed to detect the broadest possible reactivity among this group of proteins by coating test cells with a cross-reactive protein rather than the immunogen and analyzing inhibition by other members. Thus, the antisera are possibly recognizing a collection of determinants that may be associated with the same amino acids, i.e., antibodies in the same antisera may recognize alternative or overlapping sites of the same determinant or physically distinct antigenic entities. The observation that pairs of proteins such as U61-J606 differ by more idiotypes than amino acid substitutions supports the concept that a single amino acid can be involved in multiple antigenic determinants.

Considering the present complexity of the IdX systems it would be of extreme interest to analyze these determinants with monoclonal antibodies. Such reagents may considerably simplify the observed IdX patterns and facilitate correlation with amino acid sequence.

B. $\alpha(1,3)$ Dextran

Three myeloma proteins, M104E (Leon *et al.*, 1970), J558 (Blomberg *et al.*, 1972, 1973), and UPC102 (Cisar *et al.*, 1974) have been described that bind $\alpha(1,3)$ dextrans. The size of the M104E combining site was found to be optimally complementary to three sequential $\alpha(1,3)$-D-glucopyranosyl residues (Leon *et al.*, 1970). Although the protein is easily inhibited by nigerosyl$(1,3)$nigerose (Young *et al.*, 1971), suggesting specificity for the 1,3 linkage, M104E has also been found to precipitate with dextrans containing varying proportions of other glucose linkages [i.e., $\alpha(1,6)$, $\alpha(1,4)$, and $\alpha(1,2)$] as well as dextrans supposedly lacking $\alpha(1,3)$ linkages (Leon *et al.*, 1970). The basis for this reactivity is unknown. J558 appears to be more complementary to a pentasaccharide and, while demonstrating a preference for $\alpha(1,3)$ linkages, also precipitates with dextrans apparently lacking $\alpha(1,3)$ linkages (Lundblad *et al.*, 1972). This protein furthermore binds to $\alpha(1,4)$-linked dextrans. The binding site of UPC102 appears to be similar to that of M104E (Cisar *et al.*, 1974).

In addition to these myeloma proteins a series of $\alpha(1,3)$ dextran-binding hybridomas have been generated following immunization with the branched dextran B1355. The $\alpha(1,3)$ dextran system is especially interesting in that, as in the case of the $\beta(1,6)$ galactan antibodies, it potentially addresses both the question of the structural basis of antibody–antigen interactions and the structural basis of idiotypes.

Fourteen $\alpha(1,3)$ dextran-binding hybridomas as well as the myeloma proteins M104E and J558 have been characterized in detail (Schilling *et al.*, 1980; Clevinger *et al.*, 1980, 1981). All fourteen of the hybridoma antibodies express λ light chains and the M104E and J558 myeloma light chains have been shown to be identical by amino acid sequence analysis (Weigert *et al.*, 1970). The hybridoma light chains have identical isoelectric focusing patterns to the sequenced myeloma proteins, but have as yet not been shown to be invariant by sequence analysis. Complete heavy chain variable region amino acid sequences have been determined for the $\alpha(1,3)$ dextran-binding proteins and are summarized in Fig. 11.

From the amino acid sequence data it can be seen that M104E and J558 differ only at positions 96 and 97 (which comprise the heavy chain D segment) in their entire variable regions. Thus, the apparent difference in the size and specificity of these two combining sites must be related to the amino acid substitutions at these positions. These positions may either directly effect antigen binding or change conformation by, for example, producing an altered interaction with light chain. Further examination of the heavy chain variable region sequences reveals that, with the exception of the hybridoma proteins Hdex 8, 9, 10, 13, and 14, all V-region diversity occurs in the D segment (residues 96 and 97). Several inferences can be drawn from these sequences and the observed D-segment diversity:

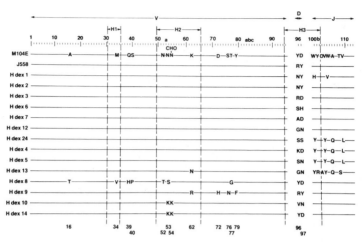

Figure 11. Heavy chain variable region sequences from $\alpha(1,3)$ dextran-binding myeloma and hybridoma proteins.

1. Since all of the hybridomas were generated by dextran immunization the variation in amino acids found in the D segment suggests that primary sequence in this region is not critical to the response to dextran B1355. These residues may, however, produce fine specificity differences that discriminate among related oligosaccharides.

2. All proteins have D segments that are two amino acids long. The conserved size of the D segment [which is similarly observed in the $\beta(1,6)$-galactan system but not found in the PC system] suggests that length in this region may be more important than primary amino acid sequence in generating this combining site.

3. The occurence of three different J segments in the antidex hybridomas indicates that particular J-segment sequences, as in the $\beta(1,6)$galactan antibodies, are not required in these molecules.

4. The Hdex 10 and 14 substitutions in the second hypervariable region indicate that the carbohydrate moiety probably is not involved in antigen binding.

The relative simplicity in the pattern of variation among the anti-dextran antibodies has provided a unique opportunity to assess precisely the structural basis of idiotypes in this system. Idiotypic antisera have been prepared that recognize IdI determinants on either M104E or J558 or that recognize an IdX determinant shared by M104E, J558, and most of the antidex hybridomas (Blomberg et al., 1972, 1973; Carson and Weigert, 1973; Clevinger et al., 1980). Using mouse antiidiotypic antisera to J558 to assay recombinant molecules prepared by pairing various λ chains of known sequence with the J558 heavy chain, it was found (Carson and Weigert, 1973) that recombinant molecules with the S178 λ chain were only 15% as effective in binding to antiidiotype as homologous recombinants or recombinants with other λ chains. The S178 λ chain differs from the parental J558 λ chain at three positions: an Asn-for-Ser substitution at residue 25 in L1, an Asn-for-Gly substitution at position 52 in L2, and an Arg-for-His substitution at position 97 in L3. The S176 λ chain has the identical Asn substitution at position 25 and recombinants using this λ chain inhibit as well as J558, suggesting that this position is not involved in the alteration of the idiotypic determinant. The J558 determinant therefore appears to involve either or both residues 52 and 97. The location of these residues in hypervariable regions is consistent with the observation that binding of J558 to anti-J558 was inhibited by antigen. Furthermore, since the J558 and M104E λ chains are identical and M104E protein only weakly inhibits the J558:anti-J558 idiotype assay, the determinant must be generated by the amino acid sequence difference in the heavy chain D segment (Fig. 11). The J558 idiotype is not inhibited by isolated chains and, based on the above data, must involve amino acids on both the λ and heavy chain even though the heavy chain substitutions provide the molecular basis of this marker.

A detailed analysis of antidextran idiotypes has been performed for M104E and J558 IdI determinants recognized by rabbit antisera, an IdX determinant (shared by M104E and J558) recognized by goat antisera, and a J558 IdI determinant recognized by mouse monoclonal antibodies (Schilling et al., 1980; Clevinger et al., 1980, 1981). The reactivity of the various antiidiotypic reagents is summarized in Table V. An examination of the IdX expression in terms of the heavy chain protein sequences (Fig. 11) reveals a correlation with the Asn residues at positions 53 and 54 and the carbohydrate attached to Asn-54. Hdex 8 with a Ser substitution at position 53 weakly expresses the IdX. Hdex 10 and 14, which have Lys substitutions at both 53 and 54 and which lack the carbohydrate moiety do not express IdX. The IdX determinant in the dextran system thus appears much less complex than the IdX markers described for antiinulin proteins.

Since 104E and J558 differ only in their heavy chain D segments, these substitutions would be expected to form the basis of the respective IdIs. The M104E IdI correlates with the D-segment sequence Tyr-Asp (Table V). Hdex 8 and 14, which have an identical D sequence (although substitutions are found in the V segment), fully express the determinant. Interestingly, Hdex 7, which has an Ala substituted for the Tyr at position 96, also expresses the marker, indicating that the negatively charged Asp is the dominant contributor to the determinant and that the replacement of the bulky aromatic Tyr side chain by the small methyl group of Ala does not alter expression. In contrast proteins Hdex 3 and 4, which both have Asp at 97, are both idiotype-negative. As can be seen, at position 96 in both proteins the Tyr is replaced by a positively charged Arg (Hdex 3) or Lys (Hdex 4), suggesting that these side chains interact with either

Table V. Expression of Anti-α(1,3)Dextran Idiotypes

Protein	D-region sequence 96–97	IdX	J558 IdI		M104E IdI
			Heterologous	Monoclonal	
J558	RY	++	++	++	–
Hdex 9	RY	++	++	++	–
Hdex 1	NY	++	+	++	
Hdex 2	NY	++	+	++	–
Hdex 6	SH	++	–	++	–
Hdex 12	GN	++	–	++	–
Hdex 13	GN	++	–	++	–
Hdex 24	SS	++	–	++	–
M104E	YD	++	–	–	++
Hdex 8	YD	+	–	–	++
Hdex 14	YD	–	–	–	++
Hdex 3	RD	++	–	–	–
Hdex 4	KD	++	–	–	–
Hdex 5	SN	++	–	–	–
Hdex 7	AD	++	–	–	++
Hdex 10	VN	–	–	–	–

Asp-97 or other portions of the molecule to alter the idiotype expression normally found associated with this residue.

Similarly, the J558 IdI detected by heterologous antisera is expressed on Hdex 9, which has an identical D-segment sequence (Arg-96, Tyr-97). Hdex 1 and 2 partially express the determinant and have the identical Asn-Tyr D-region sequence, indicating that, as in the case of the M104E IdI, position 97 is the major contributor to the determinant, although Arg-95 is clearly important. The presence of Arg-96 in association with other amino acids at 97 (Hdex 3) is apparently not sufficient for even partial expression.

A surprisingly different pattern of idiotypic reactivity was found using a monoclonal antibody recognizing a J558 IdI. The monoclonal antibody reacted with the same set of molecules as the heterologous antisera, but the reaction with Hdex 1 and 2 was approximately equivalent to that with J558 and Hdex 9. Furthermore, this reagent reacted strongly with proteins Hdex 6, 12, 13, and 24. As can be seen from Table V these molecules have D-segment sequences that are extremely different from the Arg-Tyr found in J558. Structurally, the D-segment amino acids found in this group are extremely diverse and no correlation can be seen between D segment and reactivity. Thus, the monoclonal antibody shows a broader range of specificity than a heterologous antiserum. The structural basis for this observation is unclear although it is interesting to speculate as to the nature of the reactivity. One possibility is that the D segment produces multiple idiotypic determinants and that the idiotypes recognized by the heterologous antisera and the monoclonal antibody are different. An important correlate to this interpretation is that very different amino acid sequences, as represented by the different D segments, can produce the same determinant. It will be extremely informative to determine whether or not these various reagents in fact react with the same determinant.

In the antidextran system both IdX and IdI determinants appear to correlate with at most two amino acid substitutions. It must be remembered that, even though the number of amino acid substitutions is small, the actual antigenic determinant being recognized may be quite complex. For example, the J558 IdI recognized by mouse antisera is generated by the heavy chain D segment yet clearly involves residues in the light chain. It is also not known whether, as for example in the case of J558, IdI determinants recognized by homologous, heter-ologous, or monoclonal antibodies are the same. Thus, while we have now begun to identify the molecular basis of idiotypes, we are still far from understand-ing the complexity of these determinants and their possible roles in biological systems. The potential existence of multiple idiotypes (both IdX and IdI) on the same molecule further complicates proposed regulatory systems that involve the recognition of these determinants.

C. Other Systems

1. Nitrophenylacetyl

Recent studies of monoclonal antibodies against nitrophenylacetyl (NP) have begun to develop this system in terms of both structure–function and idiotype analysis. Nucleotide sequences for the heavy chains of two λ-expressing anti-NP hybridomas of C57BL origin have been determined (Bothwell *et al.*, 1981). The heavy chain from one of these antibodies, B1-8 (IgM), is directly encoded in the NP V_H gene family. The second, S43 (IgG2a), differs from B1-8 at six positions in the heavy chain variable region and has a markedly different D segment, but appears to derive from the B1-8 V_H gene by somatic mutation. The translated heavy chain amino acid sequences from the two anti-NP antibodies were found to be similar to the antidextran M104E heavy chain (Fig. 12), which, as may be recalled, also has a λ light chain. B1-8 differs from M104E at 18 positions in the V_H segment (amino acids 1-95), nine of which occur in H1 and H2. Binding studies with the related hapten nitroiodophenylacetate (NIP) have shown that B1-8 and S43 have identical fine-specificity profiles (Reth *et al.*, 1978) although their affinities for NIP differ more than ten fold. Furthermore, neither of the two bind dextran, nor does M104E bind NIP.

Based on these observations it has been suggested (Reth *et al.*, 1981) that hypervariable region substitutions shared by B1-8 and S43 that differentiate this

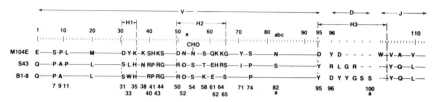

Figure 12. Heavy chain variable region sequences of anti-PC hybridomas compared to the dextran-binding M104E sequence. The anti-PC sequences are translated from corresponding gene segments.

pair from M104E are likely to be important in NIP binding. B1-8 and S43 are identical at two such positions in H1 (31 and 35), five in H2 (50, 52, 54, 61, and 65) and one at the V_H-D_H boundary (95). Based on the model of the DNP binding site from M315 and the assumption that the NIP binding site would be similar, it was further suggested that the substitutions at positions 54, 61, and 65 were probably not in the binding site and consequently not involved in specificity determination. This interpretation should be considered speculative as the validity of the proposed model has clearly not been demonstrated and is subject to many problems associated with modeling. Since the D regions of B1-8 and S43 are quite different this area is presumably not critical to NIP binding or specificity for related haptens. Thus, the substitutions at some of these H1 and H2 positions are probably involved in the change in specificity from dextran to NIP binding. This analysis is in the preliminary stages and several assumptions inherent in the conclusions should be kept in mind. First, although all three proteins express λ chains, the possibility that critical differences will exist in the dextran λ chains as compared to the NIP λ chains has not been ruled out. Second, the proposed association between hypervariable region substitutions and changes in specificity assumes that the nine framework region substitutions are netural. Since it has been shown in the PC-binding variant U_1 (Cook et al., 1982) that substitutions in regions normally considered framework may affect antigen binding, this question remains open. Third, the M104E heavy chain has a carbohydrate moiety attached to Asn-54 in H2. The role of the carbohydrate as well as its influence on the structure of the binding site is unknown.

A series of monoclonal antiidiotype reagents directed against the B1-8 protein has been generated (Reth et al., 1979). These antibodies fall into two general classes—one that is inhibited by free hapten and a second that is not inhibited by free hapten but is inhibited by hapten–carrier conjugates. Both classes of idiotypes are expressed on B1-8 but are absent from S43 and M104E. A comparison of the amino acid sequences reveals amino acids unique to B1-8 at positions 33 and throughout the D region. In addition the combinations of Glu-Lys at residues 61, 62 and Lys-Ser at 64, 65 are found only in B1-8. Reth et al. (1981) have speculated that, based on the M315 model and the assumption of similarity to anti-NIP antibodies, the class I idiotypes are possibly associated with D-segment differences and the class II idiotypes with H2 differences. This conclusion is based largely on the presumed proximity of the respective regions to the NIP binding site, which has not been experimentally established. In fact, since based on previous arguments the D region appears not to be involved in NIP binding, it might be considered surprising that if the class I idiotypes were located in this region they would be hapten-inhibitable. Clearly, additional experiments will be necessary to define precisely the heavy chain segments involved, as well as the potential contribution of the light chain to these determinants.

2. Arsonate

Antibodies induced to the arsonate (Ars) hapten in A/J mice have been found to express serological determinants comprising a cross-reactive idiotype (CRI) on 20-70% of the antibody population (Kuettner et al., 1972). Since this observation a number of studies have been undertaken to examine the molecular basis of anti-Ars idiotypes. Surprisingly, sequence analyses available to date indicate a marked degree of heterogeneity among CRI$^+$ monoclonal antibodies in both heavy and light chains (Estess et al., 1980; Marshal-Rothstein et al., 1980; Alkan et al., 1980; Margolies et al., 1981). These results suggest that CRI determinants will be present on a family of Ars-binding antibodies that display significant heterogeneity. While complete light chain sequences have been determined for five anti-Ars hybridomas (Siegelman and Capra, 1981) it is clear that an understanding of the anti-Ars idiotypes at the molecular level will require additional complete light and heavy chain sequences.

V. CONCLUDING REMARKS

In the present review I have attempted to present structural correlates of antigen binding and idiotypy. In an analysis such as this, it quickly becomes obvious that many of the conclusions are based on extrapolations from a small number of determined structures. It is unfortunate that X-ray analyses are, as yet, not available for additional immunoglobulins with known antigen-binding activity. Further structures are clearly needed to aid in interpretations such as these and to test the feasibility of model-building as a partial substitute for detailed X-ray analysis. Nonetheless, a number of interesting observations can be derived from the available information. It is surprising that in all systems examined a relatively large number of substitutions can occur in hypervariable regions without apparent alteration in binding specificity. In the case of PC binding it appears as though the conservation of a small number of hapten-contacting amino acids is sufficient to maintain specificity. It is unknown whether the hypervariable region substitutions in these molecules create additional specificity, as this is difficult to test. Furthermore, in most of the systems being studied the haptenic groups are relatively small. The interaction of these antibodies with macromolecular antigens may therefore be altered by substitutions that do not affect hapten binding. In contrast, from the studies of the S107 variants it is clear that in some instances single amino acid substitutions, such as those originating by somatic mutation, may alter antigen or hapten binding. The observation that one of the variants, with a substitution in the heavy chain J segment, appeared to have an alteration in the portion of the variable region associated with carrier specificity suggests that substitutions in regions of the molecule normally thought of as "framework" in nature may produce changes affecting antigen binding. This potential effect of framework substitutions adds an entirely new dimension to our concepts of the generation of functional diversity. In general, it appears that the *structural* diversity in antibody sequences is far greater than the *functional* diversity in terms of detectable specificity differences.

In virtually all of the systems analyzed the greatest degree of structural diversity appears to be associated with the heavy chain D segment. Surprisingly, however, no functional differences, in terms of specificity changes or V_L-V_H association, correlated with this D-segment diversity. In $\beta(1,6)$-D-galactan- and $\alpha(1,3)$dextran-binding antibodies the lengths of the D segment and third hypervariable region were invariant, suggesting that in some antibodies D-segment length may be more important structurally than primary amino acid sequence. These results point out the danger in trying to generalize as to the functional role of given antibody segments. For example, in some specificities the D segment may play a critical role in antigen binding while in others it may be of little importance.

The study of the structural basis of idiotypy is still in a very early stage with the best-defined markers being found in the $\alpha(1,3)$dextran system. Even in this case, where the markers are generated by a very few amino acid changes, the antigenic determinant appears to be complex in nature and to involve other portions of the variable region. The entire subject of how antibodies interact with protein antigens, such as idiotypes, has yet to be examined at the structural level and provides one of the most interesting areas of structure–function relations to be explored.

VI. REFERENCES

Alkan, S. S., Knecht, R., and Braun, D. G., 1980, *Hoppe-Seylers Z. Physiol. Chem.* **361:** 191–195.

Barstad, P., Rudikoff, S., Potter, M., Cohn, M., Konigsberg, W., and Hood, L., 1974, *Science* **183:**962–964.

Bennett, L. G., and Glaudemans, C. P. J., 1979, *Carbohydr. Res.* **72**:315–319.
Bernard, O., and Gough, N. M., 1980, *Proc. Natl. Acad. Sci. U.S.A.* **77**:3630–3634.
Bernard, O., Hozumi, N., and Tonegawa, S., 1978, *Cell* **15**:1133–1144.
Blomberg, B., Geckler, W. R., and Weigert, M., 1972, *Science* **177**:178–180.
Blomberg, B., Carson, D., and Weigert, M., 1973, in *Specific Receptors of Antibodies, Antigens, and Cells, Third International Convocation on Immunology* (D. Pressman, T. B. Tomasi, Jr., A. L. Grossberg, and N. R., Rose, eds.), pp. 285–293, S. Karger, New York.
Bosma, M. J., DeWitt, C., Hausman, S. J., and Potter, M., 1977, *J. Exp. Med.* **146**:1041–1053.
Bothwell, A., Paskind, M., Reth, M., Imanishi-Kari, T., Rajewsky, K., and Baltimore, D., 1981, *Cell* **24**:625–637.
Brack, C., Hirowa, A., Lenhard-Schueller, R., and Tonegawa, S., 1978, *Cell* **15**:1–14.
Braun, D. G., and Jaton, J. C., 1974, *Curr. Top. Microbiol. Immunol.* **66**:29–76.
Briles, D. E., Nahm, M., Schroer, K., Davie, J., Baker, P., Kearney, J., and Barletta, R., 1981a, *J. Exp. Med.* **153**:694–705.
Briles, D. E., Claflin, J. L., Schroer, K., and Forman, C., 1981b, *Nature (London)* **294**:88–90.
Carson, D., and Weigert, M., 1973, *Proc. Nat. Acad. Sci. U.S.A.* **70**:235–239.
Cesari, I. M., and Weigert, M., 1973, *Proc. Natl. Acad. Sci. U.S.A.* **70**:2112–2116.
Chesebro, B., and Metzger, H., 1972, *Biochemistry* **11**:766–771.
Cisar, J., Kabat, E. A., Liao, J., and Potter, M., 1974, *J. Exp. Med.* **139**:159–179.
Cisar, J., Kabat, E. A., Dorner, M. M., and Liao, J., 1975, *J. Exp. Med.* **142**:435–459.
Claflin, J. L., 1976, *Eur. J. Immunol.* **6**:669–674.
Claflin, J. L., and Rudikoff, S., 1976, *Cold Spring Harbor Symp. Quant. Biol.* **41**:725–734.
Claflin, J. L., and Rudikoff, S., 1979, *J. Immunol.* **122**:1402–1406.
Claflin, J. L., Hudak, S., and Maddelena, A., 1981, *J. Exp. Med.* **153**:353–364.
Clarke, S. H., Claflin, J. L., and Rudikoff, S., 1982, *Proc. Natl. Acad. Sci. U.S.A.* **79**:3280–3284.
Clarke, S., Claflin, J. L., Potter, M., and Rudikoff, S., 1983, *J. Exp. Med.* **157**:98–113.
Clevinger, B., Schilling, J., Hood, L., and Davie, J. M., 1980, *J. Exp. Med.* **151**:1059–1070.
Clevinger, B., Thomas, J., Davie, J., Schilling, J., Bond, M., Hood, L., and Kearney, J., 1981, in: *Immunoglobulin Idiotypes and Their Expression*, ICN-UCLA Symposium on Molecular and Cellular Biology, Volume 20 (C. Janeway, E. E. Sercarz, H. Wigzell, and C. F. Fox, eds.), pp. 159–168, Academic Press, New York.
Cohn, M., 1967, *Cold Spring Harbor Symp. Quant. Biol.* **32**:211–221.
Cook, W. D., and Scharff, M. D., 1977, *Proc. Natl. Acad. Sci. U.S.A.* **74**:5687–5691.
Cook, W., Desaymand, C., Giusti, A., Kwan, S. P., Thammana, P., Yelton, D., Zack, D., Rudikoff, S., and Scharff, M. D., 1981, in: *Immunoglobulin Idiotypes and Their Expression*, ICN-UCLA Symposium on Molecular and Cellular Biology, Volume 20 (C. Janeway, E. E. Sercarz, H. Wigzell, and C. F. Fox, eds.), pp. 281–292, Academic Press, New York.
Cook, W. D., Rudikoff, S., Giusti, A., and Scharff, M. D., 1982, *Proc. Natl. Acad. Sci. U.S.A.* **79**:1240–1244.
Cory, S., and Adams, J. M., 1980, *Cell* **19**:37–51.
Cory, S., Tyler, B. M., and Adams, J. M., 1981, *Mol. Appl. Genet.* **1**:103–116.
Crews, S., Griffin, J., Huang, H., Calame, K., and Hood, L., 1981, *Cell* **25**:59–66.
Davies, D. R., Padlan, E. A., and Segal, D. M., 1975a, *Annu. Rev. Biochem.* **44**:639–667.
Davies, D. R., Padlan, E. A., and Segal, D. M., 1975b, in: *Contemporary Topics in Molecular Immunology*, Volume 4 (F. P. Inman and W. J. Mandy, eds.), pp. 127–155, Plenum Press, New York.
Davis, M. M., Calame, K., Early, P. W., Livant, D. L., Joho, R., Weisman, I. L., and Hood, L., 1980, *Nature (London)* **283**:733–739.

Dower, S. K., Wain-Hobson, S., Gettins, P., Givol, D., Jackson, R., Perkins, S. J., Sunderland, C. A., Sutton, B., Wright, C., and Dwek, R. A., 1977, *Biochem. J.* **165**:207–223.

Dwek, R. A., Knott, J. C. A., Marsh, D., McLaughlin, A. C., Press, E. M., Price, N. C., and White, A. I., 1975, *Eur. J. Biochem.* **53**:25–39.

Dwek, R. A., Wain-Hobson, S., Dower, S., Gettins, P., Sutton, B., Perkins, S. J., and Givol, D., 1977, *Nature (London)* **266**:31–37.

Early, P., Huang, H., Davis, M., Calame, K., and Hood, L., 1980, *Cell* **19**:981–992.

Eichmann, K., 1972, *Eur. J. Immunol.* **2**:301–307.

Eisen, H. N., 1971, in: *Progress in Immunology, First International Congress of Immunology* (B. Ames, ed.), pp. 243–251, Academic Press, New York.

Eisen, H. N., Simms, E. S., and Potter, M., 1968, *Biochemistry* **7**:4126–4134.

Estess, P., Lamoyi, E., Nisonoff, A., and Capra, J. D., 1980, *J. Exp. Med.* **151**:863–875.

Feldmann, R. J., Potter, M., and Glaudemans, C. P. J., 1981, *Mol. Immunol.* **18**:683–698.

Gearhart, P., Johnson, N. D., Douglas, R., and Hood, L., 1981, *Nature (London)* **291**:29–34.

Givol, D., Strausbauch, P. H., Hurwitz, E., Wilchek, M., Haimovich, J., and Eisen, H. N., 1971, *Biochemistry* **10**:3461–3466.

Glaudemans, C. P. J., Manjula, B. N., Bennett, L. G., and Bishop, C. T., 1977, *Immunochemistry* **14**:675–679.

Goetzl, E. J., and Metzger, H., 1970, *Biochemistry* **9**:3862–3871.

Good, A. H., Traylor, P. S., and Singer, S. J., 1967, *Biochemistry* **6**:873–881.

Gough, N. M., and Bernard, O., 1981, *Proc. Natl. Acad. Sci. U.S.A.* **78**:509–513.

Grossberg, A. L., Krasz, L. M., Rendina, L., and Pressman, D., 1974, *J. Immunol.* **113**:1807–1814.

Harber, E., 1971, *Ann. N.Y. Acad. Sci.* **190**:283–305.

Haimovich, J., Eisen, H. N., and Givol, D., 1970, *Proc. Natl. Acad. Sci. U.S.A.* **67**:1656–1661.

Haimovich, J., Eisen, H. N., Hurwitz, E., and Givol, D., 1972, *Biochemistry* **11**:2389–2398.

Haselkorn, D., Friedman, S., Givol, D., and Pecht, I., 1974, *Biochemistry* **13**:2210–2222.

Honjo, T., and Kataoka, T., 1978, *Proc. Natl. Acad. Sci. U.S.A.* **75**:2140–2144.

Hood, L., Loh, E., Hubert, J., Barstad, P., Eaton, B., Early, P., Fuhrman, J., Johnson, N., Kronenberg, M., and Schilling, J., 1976, *Cold Spring Harbor Symp. Quant. Biol.* **41**:817–836.

Jaffe, B. M., Simms, E. S., and Eisen, H. N., 1971, *Biochemistry* **10**:1693–1699.

Jerne, N., 1974, *Ann. Inst. Pasteur* **125C**:373–389.

Johnson, N., Slankard, J., Paul, L., and Hood, L., 1982, *J. Immunol.* **128**:302–307.

Jolley, M. E., Glaudemans, C. P. J., Rudikoff, S., and Potter, M., 1974, *Biochemistry* **13**:3179–3184.

Kabat, E. A., 1956, *J. Immunol.* **77**:377–385.

Kabat, E. A., 1957, *J. Cell. Comp. Physiol.* **50**(Suppl. 1):79–102.

Kabat, E. A., 1960, *J. Immunol.* **84**:82–85.

Kabat, E. A., and Wu, T. T., 1971, *Ann. N.Y. Acad. Sci.* **190**:382–393.

Kabat, E. A., Wu, T. T., and Bilofsky, H., 1976, *Proc. Natl. Acad. Sci. U.S.A.* **73**:617–619.

Kabat, E. A., Wu, T. T., and Bilofsky, H., 1979, Sequences of Immunoglobulin in Chains, U.S. Department of Health, Education and Welfare, NIH Publication No. 80-2008.

Kocher, H. P., Berek, C., Schreier, M. H., Cosenza, H., and Jaton, J. C., 1980, *Eur. J. Immunol.* **10**:264–267.

Kohler, G., and Milstein, C., 1975, *Nature (London)* **256**:495–497.

Kohler, G., and Milstein, C., 1976, *Eur. J. Immunol.* **6**:511–519.

Krause, R. M., 1970, *Fed. Proc.* **29**:59–65.

Krause, R. M., 1971, *Adv. Immunol.* **12**:1–56.

Kuettner, M. G., Wang, A. L., and Nisonoff, A., 1972, *J. Exp. Med.* **135**:579–597.

Kurosawa, Y., and Tonegawa, S., 1982, *J. Exp. Med.* **155**:201–218.

Kwan, S. P., Rudikoff, S., Seidman, J. G., Leder, P., and Scharff, M. D., 1981, *J. Exp. Med.* **153**:1366–1370.

Lenhard-Schuller, R., Hohn, B., Brack, C., Hirama, M., and Tonegawa, S., 1978, *Proc. Natl. Acad. Sci. U.S.A.* **75**:4709–4713.

Leon, M. A., and Young, N. M., 1971, *Biochemistry* **10**:1424–1428.

Leon, M. A., Young, N. M., and McIntire, K. R., 1970, *Biochemistry* **9**:1023–1030.

Lieberman, R., Potter, M., Humphrey, W., Mushinski, E. B., and Vrana, M., 1975, *J. Exp. Med.* **142**:106–119.

Lieberman, R., Vrana, M., Humphrey, W., Chien, C. C., and Potter, M., 1977, *J. Exp. Med.* **146**:1294–1304.

Lieberman, R., Rudikoff, S., Humphrey, W., and Potter, M., 1981, *J. Immunol.* **126**:172–176.

Lundblad, A., Steller, R., Kabat, E. A., Hirst, J. W., Weigert, M. G., and Cohn, M., 1972, *Immunochemistry* **9**:535–544.

Mage, R., Lieberman, R., Potter, M., and Terry, W. D., 1973, in: *The Antigens*, Volume 1 (M. Sela, ed.), pp. 300–376, Academic Press, New York.

Manjula, B. N., Glaudemans, C. P. J., Mushinski, E. B., and Potter, M., 1976, *Proc. Natl. Acad. Sci. U.S.A.* **73**:932–936.

Margolies, M. N., Marshak-Rothstein, A., and Gefter, M. L., 1981, *Mol. Immunol.* **18**: 1065–1077.

Marquardt, M., Deisenhofer, J., Huber, R., and Palm, W., 1980, *J. Mol. Biol.* **141**:369–391.

Marshak-Rothstein, A., Siekevitz, M., Margolies, M. N., Mudgett-Hunter, M., and Gefter, M. L., 1980, *Proc. Natl. Acad. Sci. U.S.A.* **77**:1120–1124.

Max, E., Seidman, J. G., and Leder, P., 1979, *Proc. Natl. Acad. Sci. U.S.A.* **76**:3450–3454.

Metzger, H., and Potter, M., 1968, *Science* **162**:1398–1400.

Metzger, H., Wofsy, L., and Singer, S. J., 1963, *Biochemistry* **2**:979–991.

Metzger, H., Wofsy, L., and Singer, S. J., 1964, *Proc. Natl. Acad. Sci. U.S.A.* **51**:612–618.

Metzger, H., Chesebro, B., Hadler, N. M., Lee, J., and Otchin, N., 1971, in: *Progress in Immunology, First International Congress of Immunology* (B. Ames, ed.), pp. 243–251, Academic Press, New York.

Michaelides, M. C., and Eisen, H. N., 1974, *J. Exp. Med.* **140**:687–702.

Navia, M. A., Segal, D. M., Padlan, E. A., Davies, D. R., Rao, D. N., Rudikoff, S., and Potter, M., 1979, *Proc. Natl. Acad. Sci. U.S.A.* **76**:4071–4074.

Oudin, J., and Michel, M., 1963, *C. R. Acad. Sci.* **257**:805–808.

Padlan, E. A., Davies, D. R., Rudikoff, S., and Potter, M., 1976a, *Immunochemistry* **13**: 945–949.

Padlan, E. A., Davies, D. R., Pecht, I., Givol, D., and Wright, C., 1976b, *Cold Spring Harbor Symp. Quant. Biol.* **41**:627–637.

Pawlita, M., Potter, M., and Rudikoff, S., 1982, *J. Immunol.* **129**:615–618.

Pecht, I., Givol, D., and Sela, M., 1972, *J. Mol. Biol.* **68**:241–247.

Poljak, R. J., Amzel, L. M., Chen, B. L, Phizackerley, L. P., and Saul, F., 1974, *Proc. Natl. Acad. Sci. U.S.A.* **71**:3440–3444.

Potter, M., 1970, *Fed. Proc.* **29**:85–91.

Potter, M., 1973, in: *Multiple Myeloma and Related Disorders*, Volume 1 (H. A. Azar and M. Potter, eds.), pp. 194–246, Harper and Row, Hagerstown, Maryland.

Potter, M., 1975, in: *Cancer: A Comprehensive Treatise*, Volume 1 (F. F. Becker, ed.), pp. 161–179, Plenum Press, New York.

Potter, M., 1977, *Adv. Immunol.* **25**:141–211.

Potter, M., and Leon, M. A., 1968, *Science* **162**:369–371.

Potter, M., and Lieberman, R. I., 1970, *J. Exp. Med.* **132**:737–751.

Potter, M., Pumphrey, J. G., and Bailey, D. W., 1975, *J. Natl. Cancer Inst.* **54**:1413–1417.

Rabbitts, T. H., Forster, A., Dunnick, W., and Bentley, D. L., 1980, *Nature (London)* **283**: 351–356.

Radbruch, A., Liesegang, B., and Rajewsky, K., 1980, *Proc. Natl. Acad. Sci. U.S.A.* **77**: 2909-2913.

Rao, D. N., Rudikoff, S., Krutzsch, H., and Potter, M., 1979, *Proc. Natl. Acad. Sci. U.S.A.* **76**:2890-2894.

Reth, M., Hammerling, G. J., and Rajewsky, K., 1978, *Eur. J. Immunol.* **8**:393-400.

Reth, M., Imanishi-Kari, T., and Rajewsky, K., 1979, *Eur. J. Immunol.* **9**:1004-1013.

Reth, M., Bothwell, A. L. M., and Rajewsky, K., 1981, in: *Immunoglobulin Idiotypes and Their Expression*, ICN-UCLA Symposium on Molecular and Cellular Biology, Volume 20 (C. Janeway, E. E. Sercarz, H. Wigzell, and C. F. Fox, eds.), pp. 169-178, Academic Press, New York.

Riesen, W. F., Braun, D. G., and Jaton, J. C., 1976, *Proc. Natl. Acad. Sci. U.S.A.* **73**:2096-2100.

Roy, A., Manjula, B. N., and Glaudemans, C. P. J., 1981, *Mol. Immunol.* **18**:79-84.

Rudikoff, S., and Potter, M., 1974, *Biochemistry* **13**:4033-4037.

Rudikoff, S., and Potter, M., 1976, *Proc. Natl. Acad. Sci. U.S.A.* **73**:2109-2112.

Rudikoff, S., and Potter, M., 1978, *Biochemistry* **17**:2703-2707.

Rudikoff, S., and Potter, M., 1980, *J. Immunol.* **124**:2089-2092.

Rudikoff, S., and Potter, M., 1981, *J. Immunol.* **127**:191-194.

Rudikoff, S., Mushinski, E. B., Potter, M., Glaudemans, C. P. J., and Jolley, M. E., 1973, *J. Exp. Med.* **138**:1095-1106.

Rudikoff, S., Rao, D. N., Glaudemans, C. P. J., and Potter, M., 1980, *Proc. Natl. Acad. Sci. U.S.A.* **77**:4270-4274.

Rudikoff, S., Satow, Y., Padlan, E., Davies, D., and Potter, M., 1981, *Mol. Immunol.* **18**: 705-711.

Rudikoff, S., Giusti, A. M., Cook, W. D., and Scharff, M. D., 1982, *Proc. Natl. Acad. Sci. U.S.A.* **79**:1979-1983.

Sakano, H., Huppi, K., Heinrich, G., and Tonegawa, S., 1979, *Nature (London)* **280**:288-294.

Sakano, H., Maki, R., Kurosawa, Y., Roeder, W., and Tonegawa, S., 1980, *Nature (London)* **286**:676-683.

Sakano, H., Kurosawa, Y., Weigert, M., and Tonegawa, S., 1981, *Nature (London)* **290**: 562-565.

Schilling, J., Clevinger, B., Davie, J. M., and Hood, L., 1980, *Nature (London)* **283**:35-40.

Segal, D. M., Padlan, E. A., Cohen, G. H., Rudikoff, S., Potter, M., and Davies, D. R., 1974, *Proc. Natl. Acad. Sci. U.S.A.* **71**:4298-4302.

Seidman, J. G., Leder, A., Nau, M., Norman, B., and Leder, P., 1978, *Science* **202**:11-17.

Seligmann, M., and Brouet, J. C., 1973, *Semin. Hematol.* **10**:163-177.

Selsing, E., and Storb, U., 1981, *Cell* **25**:47-58.

Sher, A., and Tarikas, H., 1971, *J. Immunol.* **106**:1227-1233.

Shimazu, A., Takahashi, N., Yamawaki-Kataoka, Y., Nishida, Y., Kataoka, T., and Honjo, T., 1981, *Nature (London)* **289**:149-153.

Siegelman, M., and Capra, J. D., 1981, *Proc. Natl. Acad. Sci. U.S.A.* **78**:7679-7683.

Singer, S. J., and Thorpe, N. O., 1968, *Proc. Nat. Acad. Sci. U.S.A.* **60**:1371-1378.

Slater, R. J., Ward, S. M., and Kunkel, H. G., 1955, *J. Exp. Med.* **101**:85-107.

Sutton, B., Gettins, P., Givol, D., Marsh, D., Wain-Hobson, S., William, K. J., and Dwek, R. A., 1977, *Biochem. J.* **165**:177-197.

Vicari, G., Sher, A., Cohn, M., and Kabat, E. A., 1970, *Immunochemistry* **7**:829-838.

Vrana, M., Rudikoff, S., and Potter, M., 1978, *Proc. Natl. Acad. Sci. U.S.A.* **75**:1957-1961.

Vrana, M., Rudikoff, S., and Potter, M., 1979, *J. Immunol.* **122**:1905-1910.

Wain-Hobson, S., Dower, S. K., Gettins, P., Givol, D., McLaughlin, A. C., Pecht, I., Sunderland, C. A., and Dwek, R. A., 1977, *Biochem. J.* **165**:227-235.

Weigert, M., Cesari, M., Yonkovich, S. J., and Cohen, M., 1970, *Nature (London)* **228:** 1045–1047.

Weigert, M., Gatmaitan, L., Loh, E., Schilling, J., and Hood, L., 1978, *Nature (London)* **276:** 785–790.

Weigert, M., Perry, R., Kelley, D., Hunkapiller, T., Schilling, J., and Hood, L., 1980, *Nature (London)* **283:** 497–499.

Wofsy, L., and Parker, D. C., 1967, *Cold Spring Harbor Symp. Quant. Biol.* **32:** 111–116.

Wu, A. M., Kabat, E. A., and Weigert, M. G., 1978, *Carbohydr. Res.* **66:** 113–124.

Wu, T. T., and Kabat, E. A., 1970, *J. Exp. Med.* **132:** 211–250.

Yaoita, Y., and Honjo, T., 1980, *Nature (London)* **286:** 850–853.

Young, N. M., Jocius, J. B., and Leon, M. A., 1971, *Biochemistry* **10:** 3457–3460.

Homologs of CRP: A Diverse Family of Proteins with Similar Structure

John E. Coe

Laboratory of Persistent Viral Diseases
Rocky Mountain Laboratories
National Institute of Allergy and Infectious Diseases
National Institutes of Health
Public Health Service
U.S. Department of Health and Human Services
Hamilton, Montana 59840

I. INTRODUCTION

Human C-reactive protein (CRP) was first noted over 50 years ago (Tillet and Francis, 1930) as a serum protein that rapidly increased in concentration in diseased patients. Inflammation or injury will nonspecifically cause a variety of serum constituents to fluctuate from normal levels; these proteins are designated acute phase reactants (Owen, 1967). However, human CRP is regarded as the archetype acute phase protein because of its relatively long history and impressive serum changes as an acute reactant. Since the discovery of CRP, numerous investigators have puzzled over its function in inflammation. Another protein, a constituent of human amyloid called amyloid P (AP) component, has been shown to be homologous to CRP (Osmand *et al.*, 1977a; Levo *et al.*, 1977). Because these proteins have been the subject of several excellent current reviews (Koj, 1974; Kushner, 1981; Gewurz *et al.*, 1982; Pepys, 1981; Kushner *et al.*, 1982), this chapter will deal primarily with the expression of proteins homologous with human CRP and AP that have been identified in other animals. In general, these two proteins are represented in a wide variety of species, from fishes to mammals, and a conservative evolution has resulted in functional characteristics similar to those of their human counterparts. These proteins also have a similar unique structure.

211

This chapter will focus on a recently defined pentraxin present in serum of the Syrian hamster. This novel protein is called female protein (FP) (Coe, 1977) and displays functional attributes characteristic of both CRP and AP. Furthermore, FP has a variety of unique characteristics when compared to other members of the CRP-AP family. Indeed, the unusually high normal serum levels and peculiar sex hormone control of FP would indicate that this protein has little in common with CRP and AP. Yet the similarities in structure (Coe et al., 1981) provide fascinating evidence of the diversity that can evolve within descendants of a common ancestral gene. Whether these homologous proteins have functional roles analogous to that of their common ancestor and common to each other is unknown but will be of great interest when their raison d'être is finally established.

II. ISOLATION AND BINDING SPECIFICITY OF CRP HOMOLOGS

Human CRP was originally detected because of its capacity to bind to pneumococcal C substance, C polysaccharide (CPS) (Abernethy and Avery, 1941; MacLeod and Avery, 1941) in the presence of Ca^{2+}. The specificity of this reaction was found to be directed to the phosphorylcholine residue (PC) (Volanakis and Kaplan, 1971). This known specificity of human CRP has been utilized to define CRP homologs in a variety of species, which exhibit a similar Ca^{2+}-dependent binding to immobilized CPS, PC, or PC derivatives. Some of the isolated CRPs, e.g., CRP from rabbit and plaice (a teleost fish) (Baldo and Fletcher, 1973) have been partially sequenced and show significant homologies with human CRP (Osmand et al., 1977a; Levo et al., 1977; Oliveira et al., 1979; Pepys et al., 1980). However, many of the CRP homologs found in other species, e.g., monkey, dog, pig, mouse, rat, chicken, and fish (Pepys et al., 1978a; Oliveira et al., 1980; DeBeer et al., 1982) have been isolated and essentially defined because of their binding specificity to CPS or PC in the presence of Ca^{2+}. As noted later in this chapter, data from hamster FP suggests that this PC specificity cannot be used as an absolute criterion for a CRP homolog. CRP homologs usually are present as minor constituents in normal serum—less than 1-2 µg/ml in human, rabbit, and mouse, although higher levels (50 µg/ml) were reported in a marine teleost, the plaice (White et al., 1981) and the highest levels (0.5 mg/ml) were detected in rat (DeBeer et al., 1982). Isolation of CRP can be facilitated by use of acute phase serum; for example, in humans, CRP levels may increase to 0.3-0.5 mg/ml during active inflammation (Claus et al., 1976). However, CRP in some species, such as the mouse, does not act as an acute phase protein (Pepys et al., 1979a).

III. ISOLATION AND BINDING SPECIFICITY OF SAP HOMOLOGS

Human AP originally was isolated from amyloid, in which it was found as a constant minor component, even though the major component, fibrillar protein, may be of diverse origin (immunoglobulin L chains, AA protein, etc.) (Skinner *et al.*, 1974; Bladen *et al.*, 1966; Cathcart *et al.*, 1965; Glenner, 1980). AP is also present in normal serum (where it is called SAP); this protein is very similar or identical to AP in amyloid (Skinner *et al.*, 1980). The recent description of Ca^{2+}-dependent binding of human SAP to agarose (Pepys *et al.*, 1977) has facilitated isolation of this serum component; in the presence of Ca^{2+}, SAP is selectively bound on agarose and after washing, can be eluted with ethylenediaminetetra-acetic acid. This binding specificity has also been utilized to define and isolate SAP homologs from serum in a variety of other species, including mammals, amphibians, and fishes (Pepys *et al.*, 1978b). In the human, mouse, and rat, SAP is a minor constituent of normal serum (30–40 $\mu g/ml$) (Pepys *et al.*, 1978b; DeBeer *et al.*, 1982).

A useful distinguishing feature between human CRP and AP is that AP does not have the PC-binding specificity (Pepys *et al.*, 1977) and CRP does not bind strongly to agarose (Volanakis and Narkates, 1981) (Table I). Similarily, SAP homologs (mouse, rat, plaice, etc.) do not bind PC, and this ability to bind PC with Ca^{2+} has frequently been used as a criterion to distinguish CRP (+) from AP (−) homologs. From an operational standpoint, this is a useful nomenclature. However, one must be mindful of this rather arbitrary categorization based on limited knowledge of their binding specificities and real functions. Even now, the heterogeneity expressed by these homologs in various species is impressive, and eventual sequence comparisons will probably produce some surprising associations and also a more valid classification. For example, three laboratories have isolated what appears to be the same protein from rat serum. Pontet (1981) iso-

Table I. Comparison of CRP, FP, and AP:
Major Features

	CRP	FP	AP
Pentraxin structure	+	+	+
Acute phase reactant	+	+	+
PC binding	+	+	0
Agarose binding	±	+	+
Amyloid component	0	+	+
Sex hormone control	−	+	−
Polymorphic forms	−	+	−

lated a PC–Sepharose-binding protein that was thought to be structurally more similar to human AP than CRP and was therefore called rat SAP. Nagpurkar and Mookerjea (1981) also defined a PC–Sepharose-binding protein that was structurally similar to the CPS-binding protein found by DeBeer *et al.* (1982). A more typical SAP homolog (agarose-binding) was also isolated from rat serum by De-Beer *et al.* (1982), so they called the CPS-binding protein rat CRP, even though aberrant features were noted. That is, rat CRP was glycosylated, did not precipitate CPS or fix complement, and displayed a covalent binding of some monomer subunits. So far, experimental results in various species are consistent with this dualism of pentraxin expression, but this ideology should not preclude other patterns of representation within a particular animal, such as one or two AP homologs and no CRP homolog, nor deny the existence of other pentraxin subfamilies distinct from human CRP and AP, such as rat CRP or hamster FP.

IV. ISOLATION AND BINDING SPECIFICITY OF HAMSTER FP

Hamster FP originally was noted because it was a prominent protein only in female sera; a fast α-precipitin arc was detected in female but not male sera when whole hamster sera were examined by immunoelectrophoresis (Fig. 1). Anti-FP was a significant constituent in rabbit or sheep antisera to whole hamster serum, so that antisera specific for FP initially were made by simply adding whole male sera to sheep anti-whole-hamster. Subsequently, FP was purified by preparative Pevikon block electrophoresis–Sephadex filtration and also by affinity chromatography. Thus, hamster FP is unusual because of high normal levels and sex distribution. Normal adult females have a mean value of 1.25 mg/ml (range 0.7–3.0) and normal males 50- to 100-fold less (0.010–0.020 mg/ml).

After structural studies suggested that this sex-limited protein was a CRP–AP

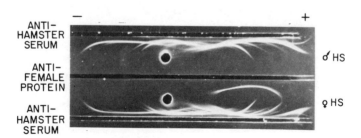

Figure 1. A comparison of serum FP in normal adult male and female hamsters. Immunoelectrophoresis of normal male (top well) and female (bottom well) Syrian hamster sera developed with specific rabbit anti-FP (center trough) and rabbit anti-whole-hamster serum (outside troughs). Female protein is a prominent fast α protein only in the female sera.

homolog, the ability of FP to bind to PC was tested. PC covalently bound to Sepharose was used and the results showed that hamster FP does bind to PC and requires Ca^{2+} for this interaction (Coe *et al.*, 1981). Figure 2 shows by immunoelectrophoresis (IEP) the results of passing normal female hamster serum (HS) (center well) through a PC-Sepharose column in 0.5 mM Ca^{2+}. The passthrough material (PT, top well) essentially was devoid of FP, which was found in the subsequent EDTA eluate (EDTA-E, bottom well). This EDTA eluate also contained trace amounts of two or three other serum proteins (B_1C, albumin) not seen on IEP but detectable with appropriate reagents on simple gel diffusion and on polyacrylamide gel electrophoresis. However, elution of the column with free PC (10^{-3} M) in the same Ca^{2+} buffer used for washing the column (0.1 M Tris HCl, 0.5 mM $CaCl_2$) resulted in complete elution of FP alone. The subsequent EDTA eluate contained only the other trace proteins (Table II). In regard to the question of whether FP is the sole CRP-AP homolog expressed in Syrian hamsters, we have examined both the PC and EDTA eluates of normal and acute phase hamster serum for other CRP-AP homologs; so far, none has been detected.

Like human CRP, hamster FP binds to PC in a Ca^{2+}-dependent fashion. However, unlike human CRP, FP does not bind to CPS. A similar phenomenon has been reported with rat CRP (DeBeer *et al.*, 1982). However, only a limited spectrum of CPS derivatives has been tried with FP, so that this interaction cannot be ruled out. For example, comparison of human and rabbit CRP has shown differences in their specificity for various CPS (H. C. Anderson and McCarty, 1951) and PC derivatives (Oliveira *et al.*, 1980).

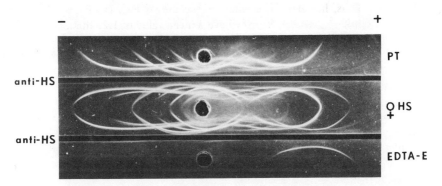

Figure 2. Isolation of FP by selective binding on PC–Sepharose. Normal female hamster serum (center well) was filtered (0.5 mH $CaCl_2$) through a PC–Sepharose column. The serum that passed through (PT, top well) was devoid of FP. The bound FP in the column was detected in the subsequent EDTA eluate (EDTA-E, bottom well). Immunoelectrophoresis developed with a sheep anti-whole-hamster serum that has little antibody to albumin, so that FP appears as the most anodal major protein. Reproduced from Coe *et al.* (1981) by permission of The Rockefeller University Press.

**Table II. Differential Elution of FP and Other Proteins
from PC–Sepharose and Plain Sepharose Columns**

Elution scheme	PC–Sepharose		Plain Sepharose	
	FP	Other proteins	FP	Other proteins
EDTA	+[a]	+	+	+
PC 10^{-3} M	+	0	+	0
EDTA after PC	0	+	0	+
PC after EDTA	0	0	0	0

[a]+, Present; 0, absent.

Not only does FP bind to PC like CRP, but it also binds to plain Sepharose (agarose) like SAP, and this interaction requires the presence of Ca^{2+} (Table II). However, comparison of PC-Sepharose and plain Sepharose revealed about 15-fold greater binding of FP and PC-Sepharose. Apparently the PC binding site of FP is involved in this reaction with agarose, since FP again was completely eluted by free PC in the presence of Ca^{2+}. In addition to the relatively low binding capacity of plain Sepharose for FP, a less avid binding was suggested by successful elution with 10^{-4} PC versus the 10^{-3} M usually required for PC-Sepharose (Coe, 1982). Thus, although FP and SAP both bind to agarose, the binding differs since SAP (human and murine) cannot be eluted from agarose with free PC (unpublished results in collaboration with H. Gewurtz). As previously mentioned, CRP binds weakly to agarose, and this weak interaction, which is inhibited by free PC, may be detected only by relative retardation of CRP passage through an agarose column (Volanakis and Narkates, 1981). Absolute comparison of agarose binding studies done in different laboratories is difficult because various preparations of agarose may contain several agar impurities and variable amounts of accessible galactose, hydrogalactose, or sulfates, which have been found to influence SAP binding capacity (DeBeer et al., 1982; R. Painter, personal communication) and also CRP binding (C. O. Kindmark, personal communication).

Extensive binding studies have not yet been done with FP. However, FP has been noted to bind to zymosan. This was detected earlier during production of anti-hamster B_1C by the zymosan absorption procedure (Mardiney et al., 1965). In this regard, FP is similar to AP, which also binds to zymosan, whereas CRP does not (Kindmark, 1972; Pepys et al., 1979a).

V. MOLECULAR STRUCTURE

The molecular size of FP in whole female serum was calculated from the diffusion coefficient (4.4×10^7) obtained by filtration through G200 Sephadex

(FP eluted just after 7 S OD peak) and from the sedimentation value (7.3 S) in sucrose density gradient ultracentrifugation (FP eluted coincident with rabbit gamma globulin marker). The value obtained, a molecular weight of 150,000 for FP in whole serum, was very similar to results obtained with purified FP that was analyzed by high-speed equilibrium centrifugation (151,000). In addition, this latter technique showed the isolated FP to be a homogeneous monodisperse preparation (Coe et al., 1981).

However, when FP was analyzed on sodium dodecyl sulfate-polyacrylamide gel electrophoresis, it migrated as a single band of 30,000-molecular-weight size with or without 2-mercaptoethanol reduction. A similar result was obtained by high-speed equilibrium sedimentation of FP in 5 M guanidine-HCl. This result indicated that FP is a pentamer of five 30,000-molecular-weight subunits that are noncovalently assembled. This rather unusual structure was the first hint that this sex-limited protein of Syrian hamster was related to CRP and AP, which are also noncovalently assembled pentamers with a subunit molecular size (23,000-27,000) (Gotschlich and Edelman, 1965; Pinteric et al., 1976; Levo et al., 1977) somewhat smaller than that of FP monomer. The intact human CRP molecule accordingly is smaller (120,000-140,000) than FP, whereas human AP is larger (9.5 S), as it characteristically forms face-to-face doublets of pentamers (Pinteric et al., 1976; Painter, 1977).

When examined by electron microscopy, FP appeared as a pentagonal structure with a configuration very similar to that of CRP and SAP (Fig. 3). The term *pentraxin* (Osmand et al., 1977a) has been proposed to describe proteins with this unique polygonal ultrastructure as seen by electron microscopy. This characteristic pentraxin appearance of the single pentameric molecule has been detected in CRP-AP homologs from a variety of species and appears to be a diagnostic feature of this family of proteins. SAP and some CRP (e.g., plaice) preparations, however, will stack up by face-to-face interactions (Painter et al., 1976; Osmand et al., 1977a; Pepys et al., 1978a).

Comparison of amino acid sequences has been especially informative in showing relationships within the pentraxin family. The 50–60% homology of human CRP and human SAP indicate their common gene ancestry (Osmand et al., 1977a; Levo et al., 1977). This gene duplication apparently occurred at or below the evolutionary level of teleost fish since both CRP and AP homologs are described in plaice (*Pleuronectes platessa*) (Pepys et al., 1978a). The conservative evolution of these pentraxins is evidenced by the human CRP-AP relationship and also by comparison within the respective homologs; for example, plaice SAP is reported to be about 50% homologous with human SAP, whereas the homology of plaice CRP to human CRP is less (Pepys et al., 1980). The serum (and eggs) of another teleost, the lumpsucker (*Cyclopterus lumpus*) contains a protein antigenically similar to plaice CRP. Like plaice CRP, lumpsucker CRP does exhibit Ca^{2+}-dependent precipitation with pneumococcal CPS (Fletcher and Baldo, 1976) and is structurally similar to human CRP (Fletcher

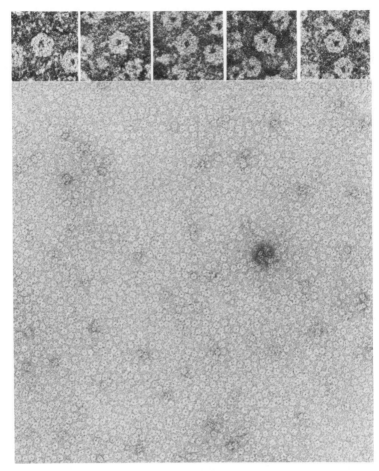

Figure 3. Electron micrographs of Syrian hamster FP negatively contrasted with uranyl acetate. FP appeared as individual pentagonal objects with a diameter around 10 nm. Field magnified 134,784× and insets 494,208×. Reproduced from Coe *et al.* (1981) by permission of The Rockfeller University Press.

et al., 1981); however, an amino acid sequence has not been published. A particularly fascinating sequence for comparison will be that of limulin, a PC (Ca^{2+}-dependent)-binding protein of an invertebrate, the horseshoe crab (*Limulus polyphemus*) (Robey and Liu, 1981), which is reported to have significant homologies with human CRP and SAP from positions 50 to 80 (Liu *et al.*, 1982, T. Liu, personal communication).

The amino acid composition of FP is very similar to that of CRP, but the NH_2-terminal 26-amino-acid sequence of FP is clearly closer to that of AP, with an identical sequence from positions 2 to 14 (Table III) (Coe *et al.*, 1981). Thus, of 25 identified residues, 20 sequences were identical to AP (80% homology). Further sequence data on FP (collected in collaboration with J. A. Sogn) substantiate the homology with AP, although it is less striking than that at the very beginning of the amino terminus. However residues 39–47 of FP (Ala, Tyr, Ser, Asp, Leu, Ser, DG, DG, Arg) are identical to those reported in human AP, (J. K. Anderson and Mole, 1982) when deletion gaps (DG) are added at positions 45 and 46. This is the sequence area of CRP (Phe_{39}-Tyr_{40}-Thr_{41}-Glu_{42}) postulated to contain the greatest homology (Young and Williams, 1978) to the Phe-Tyr-Met-Glu sequence common to PC-binding myeloma proteins in the first hypervariable region (Kabat *et al.*, 1976). The substitution of Asp in SAP for Glu in CRP has been postulated to explain the lack of PC binding by SAP (J. K. Anderson and Mole, 1982). However, the presence of the same sequence in SAP (non-PC-binding) and FP (PC-binding) indicates that the PC binding site of FP is not in this area of the molecule. This would also suggest another sequence for PC binding in CRP. Completion of the FP sequence, with its many similarities to SAP, will provide another non-Ig protein with PC binding capacity that can be used for localization of a PC binding site presumably common to FP and CRP and also perhaps common to PC-binding myeloma proteins.

A common antigenic specificity shared by CRP and PC-binding monoclonal immunoglobulins has been detected by the use of antiidiotype reagents specific for TEPC 15 PC-binding idiotypes (Volanakis and Kearney, 1981). Of particular

Table III. NH_2-Terminal Amino Acid Sequence of FP Compared with Those of Amyloid P Component, Human CRP, and Rabbit CRP[a]

	Reference[b]	Sequence					
		1	5	10	15	20	25 26
FP	–	P C A T D L S G K V F V F P R Q S E T D Y V K L I X X L					
C1t[c]	1	H————————————————E—V——H—N——T P—					
AP component	2	[ ] X———————————————E—V—$\frac{Y}{H}$—N——T P—					
Human CRP	3	————M—R—A————K E—D—S——S—K A P—					
Rabbit CRP	1	[ ] A $\frac{G}{V}$ M H K—A————K E—D B S——S—B—G—					

[a] X, no identification; [ ], deletion (no residue present); line indicates homology to top sequence; two letters (e.g., $\frac{Y}{H}$) indicate that a mixed sequence is found at that step. A, Ala; B, Asx; D, Asp; E, Glu; F, Phe; G, Gly; H, His; I, Ile; K, Lys; L, Leu; M, Met; N, Asn; P, Pro; Q, Gln; R, Arg; S, Ser; T, Thr; V, Val; Y, Tyr.
[b] References for sequences: (1) Osmand *et al.* (1977a); (2) Levo *et al.* (1977); (3) Oliveira *et al.* (1979).
[c] C1t is now known to be AP (Painter, 1977).

interest was the finding that CRP required Ca^{2+} for this antiidiotype reaction, suggesting a Ca^{2+}-dependent antigenic site on CRP. CRP has been shown to bind Ca^{2+} (Gotschlich and Edelman, 1967) and Ca^{2+}-dependent conformational changes have been detected by circular dichroism studies (Young and Williams, 1978). The presence on FP of the same or another specificity common to the PC-binding Ig idiotype will be of great interest.

Monomer FP appears somewhat larger (30,000) than AP or CRP monomer (23,000–27,000). Preliminary results of the FP sequence determination do indicate that the C terminus is different from that of SAP (J. A. Sogn, personal communication). Thus, the apparent larger size of monomer FP may be a longer chain, although it is apparent that one or more carbohydrate groups may also be present. However, other subunit structures in FP have not been detected; for instance, electrophoresis of $[^{125}I]$-FP on disc SDS–PAGE revealed only a single peak of radioactivity at 30,000 molecular weight.

The monomer subunit of FP has some special properties. This isolated subunit is difficult to work with because it is very hydrophobic. This property may explain the capacity of the monomer subunits to reassociate and form appropriate-sized (7 S) and -appearing (pentraxin) parent molecules when the dissociating agent (5 M guanidine) is removed by dialysis. This reassociation is concentration-dependent but quite significant at higher concentration (1 mg/ml). In contrast, preliminary attempts to reassemble monomer CRP have not been successful (E. Gotschlich, personal communication), and our attempts with isolated murine SAP have also been unsuccessful. Perhaps SAP or CRP can be incorporated into an FP molecule during reassembly. The production of an SAP-FP or CRP-FP hybrid pentamer would be of great interest for binding and functional studies. Also, if such a hybrid molecule could be constructed *in vitro*, a similar phenomenon would be conceivable *in vivo* if two similar pentraxins are synthesized in the same cell. An *in vivo* hybrid pentamer of FP has been obtained with a polymorphic form of FP found in wild Syrian hamsters (detailed in Section XII).

VI. BIOLOGICAL ACTIVITIES

CRP is frequently compared to antibody, and PC-binding Ig have been detected in normal serum (Lieberman *et al.*, 1974) and in myeloma proteins (Cohn, 1967). As previously mentioned, some evidence of a common structure in the PC binding site of CRP and Ig has been published. The PC ligand is found in many microbial products (Baldo *et al.*, 1979) and is ubiquitous in cell wall constituents (lecithin, sphingomyelin). This prominent PC specificity and also polycation specificity (DiCamelli *et al.*, 1980) have prompted the suggestion that the role of CRP is to participate in the inflammatory reaction and to facilitate clearance of products from damaged tissues (Volanakis and Kaplan, 1971; Volanakis and Wirtz, 1979; Pepys, 1981).

The analogy of CRP with Ig is especially poignant when complement interaction is considered. CRP, like antibody, is an effective activator of the classical complement cascade after reacting (precipitation or agglutination) with an appropriate ligand (Kaplan and Volanakis, 1974; Siegel et al., 1974). Even plaice CRP is reported to activate complement (cited in DeBeer et al., 1982). This amplification, starting with C1q, permits a wide variety of potential biological effects to be generated (phagocytosis enhancement, cytolytic phenomena, and inflammatory reactions) (reviewed by Gerwurz et al., 1982). This antibodylike activity prompted the suggestion that CRP and IgG (C_H3 domain) were evolutionarily related, and N-terminal sequence comparisons supported the idea (Osmand et al., 1977b); however, this theory was disputed when the complete CRP sequence was compared (Oliveira et al., 1979).

Although activation of complement has not been described for any SAP representatives, human SAP will bind to complement (C3bi) fixed on erythrocytes (Hutchcraft et al., 1981) and C4bp fixes to aggregated human SAP (DeBeer et al., 1981). In collaboration with H. Gewurz and C. Mold, we are currently testing FP for fixation of complement and binding to C3 breakdown products.

AP (or a very similar protein) has been found in human vascular basement membranes and elastic fibers (Dyck et al., 1980; Breathnach et al., 1981). The results of these studies indicated that AP is covalently linked to collagen or other matrix proteins and suggested that AP is a normal constituent of basement membrane. In addition, aggregated AP will bind fibronectin in a Ca^{2+}-dependent fashion (DeBeer et al., 1981). This relationship may have great significance because plasma fibronectin is an important opsonin (called α_2 surface-binding glycoprotein) (for review, see Saba and Jaffe, 1980). Also, cell-surface fibronectin has important functions in cell-to-cell interactions and in cell-to-substratum adhesions (for review, see Pearlstein et al., 1981).

Binding of CRP to cells (T cells, macrophages, platelets) and alteration (enhancement, depression) of their functions (Gerwurz et al., 1982) has stimulated attempts to find corresponding functions in SAP. A recent report does indicate that SAP binds to human lymphocytes; its presence was correlated with suppression of various antigen-specific and nonspecific cellular functions (Li et al., 1982). In collaboration with J. J. Li and P. W. J. McAdam, FP has been tested in this system and preliminary results indicate that, similarly to SAP, FP also can inhibit the phytohemagglutinin proliferative response.

As previously mentioned, Nagpurkar and Mookerjea (1981) isolated and defined a PC-binding protein in rat serum (a putative CRP homolog). This protein was notable because it prevented the usual complexing of lipoproteins by heparin and Ca^{2+}. Presumably this protein interacted with the free PC molecules on the surface of lipoprotein, as its inhibitory effect was counteracted by addition of free PC. In collaboration with A. Nagpurkar and S. Mookerjea, FP has been tested in this sytem and initial results indicate that FP can also inhibit the lipoprotein-heparin interaction. The Syrian hamster, with its hormonally controllable FP, may be useful as a model to define the role of these lipoprotein complexes in the pathogenesis of atherosclerosis.

VII. SPECIFIC PROTECTIVE EFFECTS

The role of pentraxins as a nonspecific defense mechanism is still unclear, although deposits of CRP have been found in areas of injury (Kushner et al., 1963) and inflammation (DuClos et al., 1981; Parish, 1977). However, one example of specific protection can be cited; CRP has recently been shown to protect mice from lethal *Streptococcus pneumoniae* infection (Mold et al., 1981). This is a logical result, considering the ability of CRP to bind to pneumococci (PC determinant), initiate complement (C1) cascade, and enhance phagocytosis (Kindmark, 1971). Because FP also has the PC binding site, we are looking, in collaboration with D. Briles, for a possible protective effect of FP in mice and hamsters. Binding of [^{125}I]-FP to *S. pneumoniae* has been demonstrated, although complement consumption and enhanced phagocytosis have not been tested. If hamster FP did have a comparable protective effect, one would expect female hamsters to be especially resistant to pneumococci, considering their high FP levels. However, preliminary results do not support this idea; the LD$_{50}$ after i.v. injection of female hamsters with *S. pneumoniae* was not extraordinary and so far not significantly different from the LD$_{50}$ in male hamsters (5 × 10^3 type 5; 10^7 strain A66 type 3). However, a typical acute phase response of FP was detected (FP decrease in females and increase in males) after pneumococcal injection, which partially nullified the large sex difference of FP levels in normal animals. Comparison of FP with CRP (and IgG with anti-PC specificity) in regard to specificity of binding and ultimate deposition of pneumococci would be of considerable interest.

VIII. HORMONAL CONTROL

At the present time, FP is the sole CRP-SAP homolog that is clearly under sex hormone control, although human SAP levels have been noted to be somewhat higher in males (43 μg/ml) versus females (33 μg/ml) (Pepys et al., 1978b). Serum proteins controlled by sex hormones are not that rare; some of the more obvious examples (e.g., those in cockroaches and chickens) are proteins important in egg production (Engelman, 1969; Laskowski, 1935; Schjeide and Urist, 1956). Sex hormone control of sex-limited protein expression in the mouse has been particularly well characterized (Passmore and Shreffler, 1971). Also, other mammalian serum proteins have been shown to be influenced by sex (IgM, complement components) (Rhodes *et al.*, 1969; Urbach and Cinader, 1966; Churchill *et al.*, 1967); however, no particular sex-related need or function has been correlated with these differences.

During the first few weeks of life, male and female hamsters have similar concentrations of FP in serum (Fig. 4). It is first easily detected in both male and female hamsters 5–10 days of age and rapidly increases in serum concentration in the next week or so. Male FP levels peak between 15 and 25 days after birth and then decline to normal adult levels (10–20 μg/ml) by 45 days of age. The decline in serum level during this phase correlates inversely with the rise in serum testosterone and its effects on seminal vesicles (F. Turek, personal communication). However, the increasing levels in males until weaning at 21 days suggested possible transfer of FP or a specific stimulus via maternal milk. The evidence indicates that this is not the case (Coe, 1977), since FP was not detectable in maternal milk. However, more definitive proof was obtained by foster-rearing a litter of Syrian hamsters on a Chinese hamster mother; Chinese hamsters were used because FP has not been detected in their sera. The FP levels in the foster litter were compared with those of control littermates that remained with the original Syrian mother. The Chinese- and Syrian-reared babies had comparable FP at weaning. Furthermore, Chinese hamster babies foster-reared by Syrian mothers did not contain FP in their sera at weaning. Thus, serum levels reflect a similar FP synthesis occurring in both male and female hamsters during the first few weeks. Although the decrease in FP coincides with increased endogenous serum testosterone, repeated administration of exogenous testosterone to young male hamsters (starting 2 days after birth) has not inhibited synthesis during the first few weeks of life. This result is in marked contrast to the capacity of testosterone administration to depress FP levels in adult castrated males. Therefore, it appears that maturation of a "testosterone receptor" (or some other mediator mechanism), in addition to endogenous testosterone production, is required to effect suppression of FP synthesis in the developing male hamster. Exogenous testosterone will also depress FP levels in normal adult females; however, prolonged treatment is required, in contrast to the finding in castrated males. This result suggests the absence or relatively inefficiency of the so-called "testosterone receptor" mechanism, also in female hamsters.

The role of testosterone suppression of FP in normal adult males has been shown by castration (Fig. 5); after orchiectomy, FP levels increased from 10–20 μg/ml to approximately 0.5 mg/ml within 8–10 days and were maintained at that concentration. Subsequent injection of exogenous testosterone depressed FP to normal male levels and cessation of testosterone injection resulted in a return to typical castrated high levels (Fig. 5). Diethylstilbesterol (DES) (15-mg pellet) administration subcutaneously will produce similar results, even in non-castrated hamsters. Presumably this is a result of the testosterone antagonism

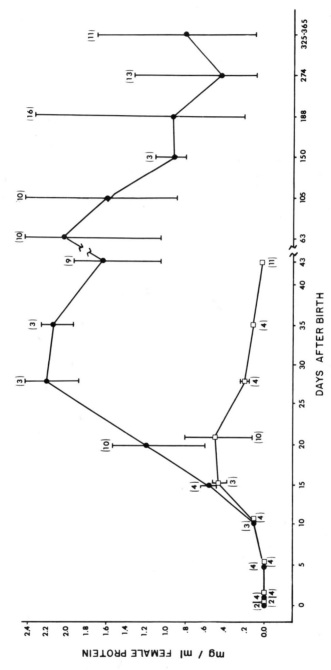

Figure 4. Ontogeny of hamster FP in serum of normal females (●) and males (□). Serum levels were measured by ring diffusion assay and mean levels were plotted at various days after birth. Brackets denote range of values obtained and associated figure indicates number of individual sera assayed.

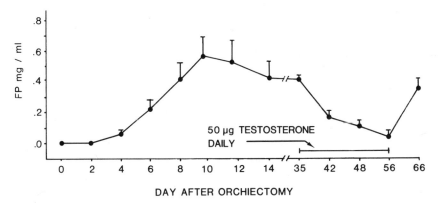

Figure 5. Effect of castration and testosterone on FP levels of male hamsters. Five adult male Syrian hamsters were castrated on day 0 and the mean FP concentration in serum was determined at various intervals during the experiment. The mean value was plotted and brackets denote +1 SEM value. Increased FP levels after castration were depressed during administration of exogenous testosterone (50 μg daily).

effect of DES (Kirkman, 1957), as no synergistic effect was detected when combinations of DES plus castration were tested. That is, comparable levels of FP were attained in males with either castration or DES or both treatments (Coe, 1982). The level of FP attained in these "desuppressed" males was usually about 50% that of females, suggesting that other hormonal elements are involved or that a separate sex-limited homeostatic control mechanism exists. We have observed that castration of weanling male hamsters will result in higher FP levels (but still less than those in females) than will castration of old male hamsters, so that this "homeostatic control suppression" does increase as intact males mature. Only in the first few weeks of life does synthesis of FP in males appear to be without suppression (i.e., similar to that in females).

In contrast to the findings in males, female castration had no effect on mean FP level. However, administration of testosterone did suppress FP concentration in females (a result similar to its effect on castrated males) although more time was required in females. Depotestosterone (2.5 mg) administered weekly resulted in mean FP levels of 0.250 mg after 10 weeks and 0.020 mg/ml after 21 weeks of injections (Coe and Ross, 1983).

Females are apparently synthesizing FP at essentially maximal rates under normal circumstances. That is, administration of DES did not cause an increase in FP levels, even at a dose of 36 mg (12-mg pellets $\times$ 3). Other hormonal manipulations have not had impressive effects on FP levels. Progesterone (5 mg/week $\times$ 4) did result in increased FP in males (0.09 mg/ml) and cause a slight increase in females. Cortisone acetate (1.5 mg/day) results in lower FP levels in females and a moderate increase in males after 10–15 days. A similar effect was seen after hypophysectomy (FP decrease in females, increase in males), although adrenalectomy was without effect.

IX. BIOSYNTHESIS AND CATABOLISM

In general, only small amounts of CRP and AP are present in normal serum of mammals (that is, CRP less than 1-2 μg/ml and SAP ~30-50 μg/ml). However, high levels of rat CRP (0.5 mg/ml) (DeBeer *et al.*, 1982) and especially of FP in female hamsters (1-2 mg/ml) suggest that a wide variation of serum expression will be found as more homologs are defined in other species. Whether higher serum levels are indicative of a larger role in analogous functions or reflect the evolution of a new functional role will be of considerable interest.

FP in normal Syrian hamster females has a peculiar variability in serum concentration. Whereas hamster serum Ig classes (IgG1, IgG2, IgA, IgM), B_1C, and albumin are maintained at relatively constant levels, as in other mammals (Coe, 1978), FP can vary within an individual by ±50% within a 48-hr period. This was noted when sequential 6-hr plasma bleeds of 10 female hamsters were quantified for FP; over a 6-day period, FP levels in individual females randomly increased, decreased, or remained relatively stable. However, variability or stability was not constant within individuals, as a repeat assessment of the same group during 3 weeks of observation showed a statistically random individual variation; that is, variability was found in all females without any obvious periodicity. This variability was not related to time of day or estrous cycle. Nor was it related to caging (individual versus group) and cagemates did not display any synchronism. Because of the short half-life of FP ($T_{1/2}$ = 10-14 hr), these changes of serum concentration could be explained by fluctuations in synthesis and the relatively consistent $T_{1/2}$ of [^{125}I]-FP found after testing numerous females is compatible with this idea. On the other hand, castrated (or DES-treated) male hamsters with elevated FP levels do not have such variability. As female hamsters get older, FP levels generally decline, with a corresponding decrease in variability. Also, mean FP levels in females will vary somewhat according to season of the year, although an established pattern has not evolved. The Syrian hamster's endocrine system is affected by photoperiod (Reiter, 1974), and a short light–long dark cycle in winter may have an effect on FP levels via hormone control. For example, short-light cycles are known to result in testicular atrophy and accessory sex organ involution in male hamsters owing to decreased serum testosterone (Turek *et al.*, 1975). This photosensitivity is apparently mediated by the pineal gland, since pinealectomy will abolish this response. Preliminary results indicate that photoperiod can affect FP levels in male hamsters, presumably through regulation of testosterone production, although other hormones may be involved. The variability of FP levels in serum may be a reflection of an unusually complex control system for FP synthesis.

CRP has been shown to be synthesized in the liver of rabbits and humans (Hurlimann et al., 1966; Kushner et al., 1980) and AP has been seen by the fluorescent antibody technique in the cytoplasm of hepatocytes (Baltz et al., 1980b). The origin of FP at present is unknown, although the relatively large amount of FP produced in normal female hamsters suggests the liver as a probable source. Our difficulty in finding the site of FP synthesis may be explained by (1) the relatively weak interaction of anti-FP with the monomer subunit of FP, which is known, and (2) a hypothetical penultimate assembly of FP just prior to secretion. These factors may account for the absence of convincing cytoplasmic fluorescence in liver and other tissues after reaction with fluorescein-labeled antibody to FP.

Recent investigations of CRP metabolism have determined a very short half-life ($T_{1/2}$ = 4.5 hr) for radiolabeled rabbit CRP in normal rabbits, and similar $T_{1/2}$ was found during the acute phase elevation of CRP in rabbits (Chelladurai et al., 1982). Therefore the constant fractional catabolic rate (FCR) (0.14) did not indicate accelerated consumption of CRP during the acute phase. Similarly, the half-life of murine [^{125}I]-SAP in normal mice ($T_{1/2}$ = 7.5-9.5 hr) was not affected during the acute phase increase in serum levels (Baltz et al., 1980c). Normal plasma catabolism of human and mouse AP in rabbits and mice respectively indicated a $T_{1/2}$ of 8.5-8.75 hr with a similar $T_{1/2}$ in amyloidotic mice (Skinner et al., 1982).

We have recently evaluated the catabolism of FP in hamsters, primarily to determine if accelerated catabolism in males could be responsible for the observed low serum levels (Coe and Ross, 1983). The results indicated that sex differences in FP levels were indeed a reflection of the rate of synthesis, as similar $T_{1/2}$ (12-14 hr) were calculated from the terminal slope of the plasma disappearance curve. However, the initial extravascular distribution of [^{125}I]-FP during the first 18-22 hr was consistently different in males and females; that is, more [^{125}I]-FP was lost from the intravascular compartment of males (70-85%) than females (~40%). This accelerated egress of intravascular [^{125}I]-FP in males is probably related to their low FP levels and may indicate the existence of (1) a saturable transport system for FP or (2) saturable extravascular FP receptors (T. Waldman, personal communication). It would be of great interest to know the amount and location of FP bound in tissues, considering the known presence of SAP in vascular basement membrane and the capacity of SAP to bind fibronectin. The sex difference in FP distribution may also be explained by the existence of another sex-limited protein that complexes with circulating FP, or may even represent a recognition by males of a female-derived FP. These studies have all been done with FP derived from female serum, which may differ in some way from normal male FP. However, differences between FP from males (normal or castrated) and FP from females have not been detected for a variety of parameters (antigenicity, electrophoresis mobility, PC-binding characteristics).

Evaluation of the overall plasma disappearance of [^{125}I]-FP did result in slightly greater FCR/hr in males (0.13) versus females (0.07), but this would not account for the 50- to 100-fold difference in serum concentration. However, these studies did indicate a substantial synthesis (assuming synthesis = catabolism) of FP in females; calculations from FCR and plasma FP content indicated 80.4 mg/kg synthesized per day, which is more than the synthetic rate for the major IgG class of hamsters, IgG2, of 55 mg/kg per day (J. Converse and J. E. Coe, unpublished observations).

X. ACUTE PHASE RESPONSE

As previously noted, the first member of this family of proteins, CRP, was detected because of its impressive increase in the serum of diseased patients. Even 50 years later, human CRP remains the acute phase protein par excellence, as its potential 500- to 1000-fold increase after injury or infection has not been surpassed by other acute phase reactants. CRP and AP proteins described in other animals also share this property of acute phase increase in concentration after inflammation, although not of the magnitude of human CRP. However, in various species either the CRP or the SAP homolog (but usually not both) appears to increase in serum concentration after injury. Thus, the acute phase response of human, rat, and plaice involves CRP (not SAP) (Pepys et al., 1978b; DeBeer et al., 1982; White et al., 1981), whereas mouse SAP (and not mouse CRP) is the acute phase protein (Pepys et al., 1979a).

FP has been found (Coe and Ross, 1983) to react as a typical acute phase protein in male hamsters with a prompt serum increase ($\sim$500%) after injection of turpentine or croton oil (Fig. 6). However, an opposite response was found in females; noxious stimuli were typically followed by a transient decrease ($\sim$50%) in serum concentration (Fig. 7). Additional daily injection of turpentine (days 1, 2, 3) did not further depress FP levels of females, but did prolong the phase of depression. An acute phase decrease in serum concentration is typical for certain proteins (e.g., transferrin and albumin) (Owen, 1967) but heretofore has not been described in the CRP-AP homologs. Also, to my knowledge, such a sex-limited divergent response has not been reported in any of the acute phase proteins. FP in the Syrian hamster provides an example of the potential diversity that pentraxins may display in an acute phase response.

Acute phase stimulus of CRP synthesis is apparently hormonally mediated by endogenous pyrogen and prostaglandins (Merriman et al., 1975; Bornstein and Walsh, 1978; Whicher et al., 1980). Could the divergent response of FP indicate a sex-limited opposite stimulus resulting from injury in males and females? To resolve this question partially, FP levels were hormonally elevated in males (DES treatment or castration) and depressed in females (testosterone injection). The response to injury (0.5 ml turpentine i.m.) in these hamsters was found to be a function of starting serum levels of FP rather than sex; thus, a

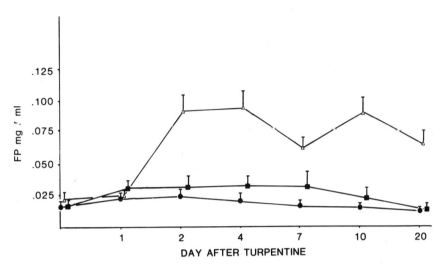

Figure 6. Acute phase increase of serum FP in male hamsters after turpentine injection. In groups of 10 each, male hamsters were injected on day 0 with 0.5 ml turpentine (△), 0.5 ml saline (■), or nothing (●), and FP levels in serum were determined at various intervals thereafter. The mean levels of FP were plotted and the bracket represents +1 SEM.

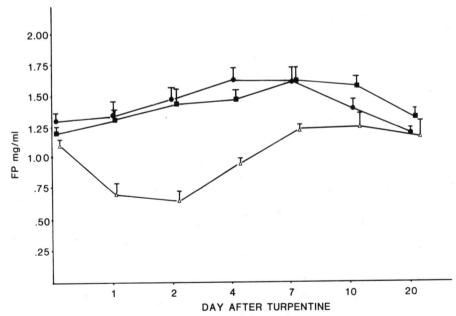

Figure 7. Acute phase decrease of serum FP in female hamsters after turpentine injection. In groups of 10 each, female hamsters were injected on day 0 with 0.5 ml turpentine (△), 0.5 ml saline (■), or nothing (●), and FP levels in serum were determined at various intervals thereafter. The mean levels of FP were plotted and the bracket represents +1 SEM.

typical decrease was found in the high-FP males and a substantial increase was detected in low-FP females. Presumably, the mediator released from the injury site or its effect on FP synthesis also was influenced by hormonal treatment or by the resulting circulating FP levels. Obviously this hormonal manipulation did more than reverse the normal FP concentration, but at least it provides an

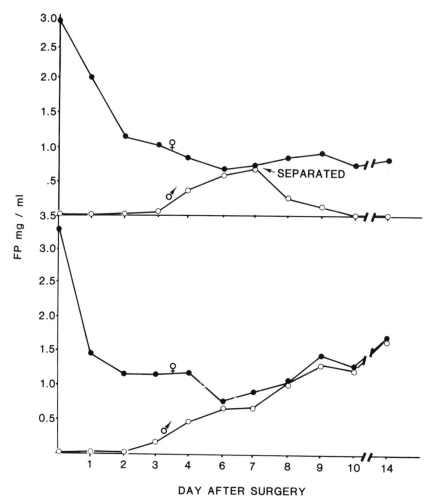

Figure 8. FP levels in individual female (♀) and male (♂) hamsters after male–female parabiosis on day 0. FP concentration in males was similar to that of their respective female partner's after 5 days of parabiosis and was maintained with continuing union (pair in bottom graph). However, male FP decreased promptly after surgical separation from the female (pair in top graph).

example of the extra parameter of hormonal control that is available in studies on the functional role of this AP homolog in Syrian hamsters.

The transient decrease of FP in acute phase females suggested a consumption of FP after injury. However, we have no evidence for this attractive explanation, and recent studies on catabolism of $[^{125}I]$-FP during this interval have not shown a significant shortening of half-life. Therefore, it appears that decreased synthesis is responsible for the acute phase decrease of FP.

The acute phase decrease of FP in females may be related to a "stress" hormonal influence. However, we have evaluated the effect of injecting cortisone acetate on FP and cannot reproduce the transient acute decrease found after injury.

Acute phase increase of serum CRP is a characteristic response in humans after surgery. In a consistent (albeit contrary) fashion, FP levels decrease in female hamsters as a response to surgery. This was observed in early studies on FP, when male and female hamsters were surgically parabiosed to determine if males could inhibit FP expression in parabiosed females. Actually, after establishment of vascular communication (4-5 days), male FP levels increased to the female partner's level and were maintained only with continuing parabiosis (Fig. 8). However, within 24 hr after surgery FP concentration in females typically decreased 50-60%, and this puzzling change was even observed with female-female parabiosis. A similar reduction after sham surgery (Fig. 9) confirmed that the nonspecific stimulus was from the surgery itself, as anesthesia was without effect.

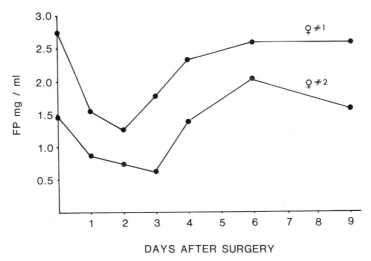

DAYS AFTER SURGERY

Figure 9. FP levels in two individual females after sham parabiosis surgery.

XI. AMYLOID

AP was originally isolated from amyloid and is a constant minor constituent of all forms of amyloid. Indeed, the consistent presence of AP with various major fibrillar components (L chains, AA, etc.) has led to the suggestion that AP may have a framework role in amyloid deposition, as amyloid has a similar ordered structure regardless of the origin of fibrillar protein. The framework role of AP is supported by studies in which AP has been shown to form various ordered structures by itself when in the presence of Ca^{2+} (Pinteric and Painter, 1979). Elevation of SAP levels correlated more closely with amyloid deposition in mice than levels of serum AA, the presumed serum precursor of AA fibrillar component of amyloid (Baltz et al., 1980a). However, SAP has also been shown to bind in a Ca^{2+}-dependent fashion to amyloid fibrils and therefore could be deposited secondarily (Pepys et al., 1979b). In the hamster, FP has been detected in amyloid both by quantitative extraction and also by direct fluorescent antibody measurements using a specific rabbit anti-FP. It would appear that FP resembles AP as a constituent of hamster amyloid, and, from preliminary observations, FP appears to be the only AP homolog present in hamster amyloid. Our studies so far confirm reports about other hamster colonies that indicate that the incidence of amyloid is much higher in normal females than in normal males (Parviz Pour et al., 1976). This relationship suggests a positive influence of higher FP levels in amyloid deposition. We currently are studying the influence of FP levels on hamster amyloid deposition utilizing the unique advantage of this AP homolog, i.e., that its synthesis (serum levels) can be manipulated by sex hormones.

XII. FP PHYLOGENY

Whereas the typical CRP and AP homologs are ubiquitous and have been detected in a variety of animals (mammals, birds, and fish) by functional and morphological criteria, FP as such has only been detected in other hamster species (Coe, 1981). An antigenically similar protein has not been found in a variety of other rodents (mouse, rat, *Peromyscus*, gerbil, *Microtus*, guinea pig). Furthermore, these rodents show no evidence of a comparable major sex-limited protein, as detectable with rabbit antisera to one sex or the other and cross-absorbed. A close relative of the Syrian hamster, the Turkish hamster (*Mesocricetus brandti*), does have a serum FP that appears to be very similar to that of the Syrian. Turkish hamster FP is antigenically identical to that of the Syrian when analyzed with rabbit anti-Syrian FP, and it has similar molecular size (7 S) and PC-binding characteristics (Ca^{2+}-dependent). Furthermore, Turkish hamster FP is testosterone-suppressed in males. Some electrophoretic variation of FP in individual Turkish females has been detected, which may be similar to the electrophoretic polymorphism of FP detected in wild Syrian hamsters.

Of the other hamster species examined, Armenian (*Cricetulus migratorius*), Chinese (*Cricetulus griseus*), European (*Cricetus cricetus*), and Djzungarian (*Phodopus songorus*) do not have serologically detectable FP, even when assayed by hemagglutination inhibition with rabbit anti-FP; this assay will detect Syrian hamster FP at 0.002 mg/ml. This result was somewhat surprising, as extensive Ig cross-reactivity can be detected in these hamsters with antisera specifically directed to the IgG1, IgG2, IgA, and IgM classes of Syrian hamster (Coe, 1981), and CRP-AP appears to have evolved in a more conservative fashion than did immunoglobulins. However, one must bear in mind that conservatively evolved proteins may prejudice the specificity of the antisera because of shared self determinants in the antibody source. Thus, a paradoxial situation may arise in which antisera to the more conservative protein (e.g., FP) can detect fewer homologs than antisera to the less-conserved proteins (e.g., Ig). Therefore, homologs of FP certainly may exist in these other hamsters but not be detected with rabbit antisera, which are directed to a limited number of FP determinants. In an attempt to provide greater immunological perspective by using phylogenetic distance, bullfrogs are currently being immunized with FP and other CRP-AP preparations. Previous studies with bullfrog anti-rabbit IgG showed marked cross-reactivity among all mammalian Ig (Coe, 1970), whereas comparable mouse or guinea pig anti-rabbit IgG were relatively specific for lagomorph Ig.

In general, serological techniques have been of limited help in showing relatedness within the family of pentraxins; this may be due to the conservative evolution of pentraxins. Thus, human CRP and AP do not show any cross-reactions when tested with heterologous antisera (Levo *et al.*, 1977). However, some other mammalian CRPs (monkey, rabbit, dog) have been found to share detectable common antigens with human CRP (Gotschlich and Stetson, 1960; Gotschlich, 1962; Oliveira *et al.*, 1980). Serological cross-reactions within the AP homologs have not been reported, and hamster FP does not share detectable antigens with human AP (or CRP) when tested with heterologous antisera (Coe, 1981). However, in collaboration with B. Hansen and H. Gerwurz, we have recently found some cross-reactivity between FP and murine SAP preparations.

Chinese hamster sera are currently being assayed for potential PC- and agarose-binding proteins detectable in either normal or acute phase sera. A more typical CRP and SAP homolog (i.e., like mouse) in this and other non-FP hamsters would be extremely interesting, especially if its structure were very similar to that of FP.

The conservative evolution of CRP homologs has apparently resulted in little polymorphism, as no examples have been reported, although both Gly and Val were detected at position 3 in rabbit CRP (Osmand *et al.*, 1977a). However, we have recently found an electrophoretic variant of FP in a new capture of wild hamsters made in Syria by M. Murphy in 1970 (Murphy, 1971). The purpose of this expedition was to obtain hamsters with greater genetic heterogeneity, as all of the commercially available Syrian hamster strains (outbred and inbred) are derived from a 1930 capture of two females and one male, which were litter-mates (Adler, 1948). The limited gene pool represented in these descendants has been thought to account for some of the surprising histocompatibility among outbred hamsters (Robinson, 1968). All of the commercially available inbred and outbred Syrian hamsters we have examined do have an antigenically and electrophoretically identical FP. From the new catch of wild hamsters, seven strains of hamsters were bred at MIT, and of these, three were found to have an electrophoretically slower 7 S FP, although it was antigenically identical with standard "fast" FP. Electrophoretic mobility of FP in whole sera was assayed by immunofixation using an overlay of specific anti-FP after electrophoresis on agarose. This electrophoretic mobility difference was not due to variations in sialic acid content, as a corresponding slight decrease in electrophoretic mobility was seen with both fast and slow FP after neuraminidase treatment. Hybrid offspring from fast $\times$ slow FP mating consistently showed a single FP with an electrophoretic migration intermediate between the two parental mobil-ities (mixtures of fast and slow parent sera resolved into the usual fast and slow peak without detectable intermediates). Therefore, it appears that both fast and slow allelic forms of FP are co-produced with random assemblage within the cell. The parents of these three "slow FP" strains were predominantly from one of the two capture areas (M. Murphy, personal communication), suggesting that other FP polymorphisms may be present on a regional basis.

XIII. CONCLUSIONS

The CRP-AP genes have been stably conserved through vertebrate evolution. Even in invertebrates, such as the horseshoe crab, a homologous protein has been defined. Obviously, the conservative maintenance of these genes implies a signif-icant functional role for their proteins. However, it is also apparent that within this family of pentraxins a significant diversity has evolved. Hamster FP is per-haps the best example of nonconformity, and suggests that other examples of CRP-AP homologs, which superficially bear little resemblance to classical proto-types, will also be shown to be pentraxins. Indeed, studies with the aberrant forms may indicate the true functional role of pentraxins in general, especially if the anomalous protein fulfills a more vital biological need. One might specu-late that the prominence of FP in serum of female Syrian hamsters augurs for its special importance in that sex. Actually, if FP were a *beneficial* acute phase protein, one should expect numerous examples of female superiority to occur in the literature, considering the hamsters' widespread use in various experimental disease models. We cannot find evidence to support this. On the other hand, high levels of FP may be a necessity in females, satisfying a deficiency not present in the "complete" male. If so, the role of this pentraxin in these "deficient" females would be of considerable interest. Such reasoning is probably specious, although a valid model of that sort would be warmly welcomed by pentraxinologists and may be found in some species as an "experiment of nature."

Definition of a protein as a member of the pentraxin family is relatively straightforward, since the characteristic structure and electron microscopic morphology so far have been diagnostic. However, true determination of a CRP or AP homolog (or a new subfamily) may ultimately require an amino acid sequence analysis rather than categorization based on functional criteria. For example, a pentraxin with Ca^{2+}-dependent PC binding specificity heretofore has been classified as homologous with CRP. It is apparent from Table I that FP functionally would be classified as a CRP homolog with its capacity to bind to PC. Yet structural analysis indicates a closer AP relationship, and this is supported by the presence of FP in hamster amyloid. Such a combination of CRP-AP functions in one protein is unique at present and may indicate the existence of another pentraxin subfamily (i.e., FP in addition to CRP and AP). It is unlikely that FP represents an unmatched combinatorial event not evident in other species, considering the overall conservative evolution of pentraxins; however, FP expression, even in other hamsters, appears limited. Of course, the peculiar sex hormone control of this pentraxin is also without precedent, although, since the definition of FP, other sex-limited proteins may be shown to have a pentraxin structure. It is to be hoped that expansion of the CRP-AP family with increasing information on functional capacity will provide insight into the ultimate biological role of these ancient proteins.

XIV. REFERENCES

Abernethy, T. J., and Avery, O. T., 1941, *J. Exp. Med.* **73**:173.
Adler, S., 1948, *Nature (London)* **162**:256.
Anderson, H. C., and McCarthy, M., 1951, *J. Exp. Med.* **93**:25.
Anderson, J. K., and Mole, J. E., 1982, *Ann. N.Y. Acad. Sci.* **389**:216.
Baldo, B. A., and Fletcher, T. C., 1973, *Nature (London)* **246**:145.
Baldo, B. A., Krilis, S., and Fletcher, T. C., 1979, *Naturwissenschaften* **66**:623.
Baltz, M. L., Gomer, K., Davies, A. J. S., Evans, D. J., Klaus, G. G. B., and Pepys, M. B., 1980a, *Clin. Exp. Immunol.* **39**:355.
Baltz, M. L., Dyck, R. F., and Pepys, M. B., 1980b, *Immunology* **41**:59.
Baltz, M. L., Rogers, S. L., Gomer, K., Davies, A. J. S., Doenhoff, M. J., Klaus, G. G. B., and Pepys, M. B., 1980c, in: *Amyloid and Amyloidosis* (G. G. Glenner, P. Pinho e Costa, and A. F. de Freitas, eds.), p. 534, Excerpta Medica, Amsterdam.

Bladen, H. A., Nylen, M. V., and Glennev, G. G., 1966, *J. Ultrastruct. Res.* **14**:449.

Bornstein, D. L., and Walsh, E. C., 1978, *J. Lab. Clin. Med.* **91**:236.

Breathnach, S. M., Bhogal, B., Dyck, R. F., DeBeer, F. C., Black, M. M., and Pepys, M. B., 1981, *Br. J. Dermatol.* **105**:115.

Cathcart, E. S., Comerford, I. R., and Cohen, A. S., 1965, *N. Engl. J. Med.* **273**:143.

Chelladurai, M., MacIntyre, S. S., and Kushner, I., 1982, *Fed. Proc.* **41**:868 (abstr.).

Churchill, W. H., Jr., Weintraub, R. M., Borsos, T., and Rapp, H. J., 1967, *J. Exp. Med.* **125**:657.

Claus, D. R., Osmand, A. P., and Gewurz, H., 1976, *J. Lab. Clin. Med.* **87**:120.

Coe, J. E., 1970, *J. Immunol.* **104**:1166.

Coe, J. E., 1977, *Proc. Natl. Acad. Sci. U.S.A.* **74**:730.

Coe, J. E., 1978, *Fed. Proc.* **37**:2030.

Coe, J. E., 1981, in: *Hamster Immune Responses in Infectious and Oncological Diseases* (J. W. Streilein, D. A. Hart, J. Steinz Streilein, W. R. Duncan, and R. E. Billingham, eds.), p. 95, Plenum Press, New York.

Coe, J. E., 1982, *Ann. N.Y. Acad. Sci.* **389**:299.

Coe, J. E., and Ross, M. J., 1983, *J. Exp. Med.* (in press).

Coe, J. E., Margossian, S. S., Slayter, H. S., and Sogn, J. A., 1981, *J. Exp. Med.* **153**:977.

Cohn, M., 1967, *Cold Spring Harbor Symp. Quant. Biol.* **32**:211.

DeBeer, F. C., Baltz, M. L., Holford, S., Feinstein, A., and Pepys, M. B., 1981, *J. Exp. Med.* **154**:1134.

DeBeer, F. C., Baltz, M. L., Munn, E. A., Feinstein, A., Taylor, J., Bruton, C., Clamp, J. R., and Pepys, M. B., 1982, *Immunology* **45**:55.

DiCamelli, R., Potempa, L. A., Siegel, J., Suyehira, L., Petras, K., and Gewurz, H., 1980, *J. Immunol.* **125**:1933.

DuClos, T. W., Mold, C., Paterson, P. K., Alroy, J., and Gewurz, H., 1981, *Clin. Exp. Immunol.* **43**:565.

Dyck, R. F., Lockwood, C. M., Kershaw, M., McHugh, N., Duance, V., Baltz, M. L., and Pepys, M. B., 1980, *J. Exp. Med.* **152**:1162.

Engelman, F., 1969, *Science* **165**:407.

Fletcher, T. C., and Baldo, B. A., 1976, *Experientia* **32**:1199.

Fletcher, T. C., White, A., Youngston, A., Pusztai, A., and Baldo, B. A., 1981, *Biochim. Biophys. Acta* **671**:44.

Gewurz, H., Mold, C., Siegel, J., and Fiedel, B., 1982, *Adv. Intern. Med.* **27**:345.

Glenner, G. G., 1980, *N. Engl. J. Med.* **302**:1283.

Gotschlich, E. C., 1962, *Fed. Proc.* **21**:14.

Gotschlich, E. C., and Edelman, G. M., 1965, *Proc. Natl. Acad. Sci. U.S.A.* **54**:558.

Gotschlich, E. C., and Edelman, G. M., 1967, *Proc. Natl. Acad. Sci. U.S.A.* **57**:706.

Gotschlich, E. C., and Stetson, C. A., 1960, *J. Exp. Med.* **111**:441.

Hurlimann, J., Thorbecke, G. J., and Hochwald, G. M., 1966, *J. Exp. Med.* **123**:367.

Hutchcraft, C., Gewurz, H., Hansen, B., Dyck, R. F., and Pepys, M. B., 1981, *J. Immunol.* **126**:1217.

Kabat, E. A., Wu, T. T., and Bilofsky, H., 1976, *Proc. Natl. Acad. Sci. U.S.A.* **73**:617.

Kaplan, M. H., and Volanakis, J. E., 1974, *J. Immunol.* **112**:2135.

Kindmark, C.-O., 1971, *Clin. Exp. Immunol.* **8**:941.

Kindmark, C.-O., 1972, *Clin. Exp. Immunol.* **11**:283.

Kirkman, H., 1957, *Cancer* **10**:757.

Koj, A., 1974, in: *Structure and Function of Plasma Proteins*, Volume 1 (A. C. Allison, ed.), p. 73, Plenum Press, New York.

Kushner, I., 1981, in: *Textbook of Rheumatology* (W. N. Kelley, E. D. Harris, Jr., S. Ruddy, and C. B. Sledge, eds.), p. 669, W. B. Saunders, Philadelphia.

Kushner, I., Rakita, L., and Kaplan, M. H., 1963, *J. Clin. Invest.* **42**:286.

Kushner, I., Ribich, W. N., and Blair, J. B., 1980, *J. Lab. Clin. Med.* **96**:1037.

Kushner, I., Volanakis, J. E., and Gewurz, H. (eds.), 1982, C-Reactive Protein and the Plasma Protein Response to Tissue Injury, *Ann. N.Y. Acad. Sci.* **389**.

Laskowski, M., 1935, *Biochem. Z.* **278**:345.

Levo, Y., Frangione, B., and Franklin, E. C., 1977, *Nature (London)* **268**:56.

Li, J. J., McAdam, P. W. J., Miercio, E. A., and Pereira, J., 1982, *Fed. Proc.* **41**:813 (abstr.).

Lieberman, R., Potter, M., Mushinski, E. B., Humprey, W., Jr., and Rudikoff, S., 1974, *J. Exp. Med.* **139**:983.

Liu, T., Robey, F. A., and Wang, C. H., *Ann. N.Y. Acad. Sci.* **389**:151.

MacLeod, C. M., and Avery, O. T., 1941, *J. Exp. Med.* **73**:183.

Mardiney, M. R., Muller-Eberhard, J. R., and Muller-Eberhard, H. J., 1965, *J. Immunol.* **94**:877.

Merriman, C. R., Pulliam, L. A., and Kampschmidt, R. F., 1975, *Proc. Soc. Exp. Biol. Med.* **149**:782.

Mold, C., Nakayama, S., Holzer, T. J., Gewurz, H., and DuClos, T. W., 1981, *J. Exp. Med.* **154**:1703.

Murphy, M. R., 1971, *Am. Zool.* **11**:632.

Nagpurkar, A., and Mookerjea, S., 1981, *J. Biol. Chem.* **256**:7440.

Oliveira, E. B., Gotschlich, E. C., and Liu, T.-Y., 1979, *J. Biol. Chem.* **254**:489.

Oliveira, E. B., Gotschlich, E. C., and Liu, T.-Y., 1980, *J. Immunol.* **124**:1396.

Osmand, A. P., Friedenson, B., Gewurz, H., Painter, R. H., Hoffman, T., and Shelton, E., 1977a, *Proc. Natl. Acad. Sci. U.S.A.* **74**:739.

Osmand, A. P., Gewurz, H., and Friedenson, B., 1977b, *Proc. Natl. Acad. Sci. U.S.A.* **74**:1214.

Owen, J. A., 1967, in: *Advances in Clinical Chemistry*, Volume 9 (H. Sobotka and C. P. Stewart, eds.), p. 1, Academic Press, New York/London.

Painter, R. H., 1977, *J. Immunol.* **119**:2203.

Painter, R. H., Pinteric, L., Hotman, T., Kells, D. I. C., and Katz, A., 1976, *J. Immunol.* **116**:1745.

Parish, W. E., 1977, in: *Bayer Symposium IV: Experimental Models of Chronic Inflammatory Diseases* (L. E. Glynn and H. D. Schlumberger, eds.), p. 117, Springer-Verlag, Berlin.

Parviz Pour, N., Moch, K., Greiser, E., Mohr, U., Althoff, J., and Cardesa, A., 1976, *J. Natl. Cancer Inst.* **56**:931.

Passmore, H. C., and Shreffler, D. C., 1971, *Biochem. Genet.* **5**:201.

Pearlstein, E., Gold, L. I., and Garcia-Pardo, A., 1981, *Mol. Cell. Biochem.* **29**:103.

Pepys, M. B., 1981, *Lancet* **1**:653.

Pepys, M. B., Dash, A. C., Mumm, E. A., Feinstein, A., Skinner, M., Cohen, A. S., Gewurz, H., Osmand, A. P., and Painter, R. H., 1977, *Lancet* **1**:1029.

Pepys, M. B., Dash, A. C., Fletcher, T. C., Richardson, N., Mumm, E.A., and Feinstein, A., 1978a, *Nature (London)* **273**:168.

Pepys, M. B., Dash, A. C., Markham, R. E., Thomas, H. C., Williams, B. D., and Petrie, A., 1978b, *Clin. Exp. Immunol.* **32**:119.

Pepys, M. B., Baltz, M., Gomer, K., Davies, A. J. S., and Doenhoff, M., 1979a, *Nature (London)* **278**:259.

Pepys, M. B., Dyck, R. F., DeBeer, F. C., Skinner, M., and Cohen, A. S., 1979b, *Clin. Exp. Immunol.* **38**:284.

Pepys, M. B., Baltz, M. L., Dyck, R. F., DeBeer, F. C., Evans, D. J., Feinstein, A., Milstein, C. P., Mumm, E. A., Richardson, N., Murch, J. F., Fletcher, T. C., Davies, A. J. S., Gomer, K., Cohen, A. S., Skinner, M., and Klaus, G. G. B., 1980, in: *Amyloid and Amyloidosis* (G. G. Glenner, P. Pinho e Costa, and A. F. de Freitas, eds.), p. 373, Excerpta Medica, Amsterdam.

Pinteric, L., and Painter, R. H., 1979, *Can. J. Biochem.* **57**:727.

Pinteric, L., Assimeh, S. N., Kells, D. I. C., and Painter, R. H., 1976, *J. Immunol.* **117**:79.

Pontet, M., D'Asnieres, M., Gache, D., Escaig, J., and Engler, R., 1981, *Biochim. Biophys. Acta* **671**:202.

Reiter, R. J., 1974, *Chronobiologia* **1**:365.

Rhodes, K., Markham, R. L., Maxwell, P. M., and Monk-Jones, M. E., 1969, *Br. Med. J.* **3**:439.

Robey, F. A., and Liu, T.-Y., 1981, *J. Biol. Chem.* **256**:969.

Robinson, R., 1968, in: *The Golden Hamster: Its Biology and Use in Medical Research* (R. A. Hoffman, P. F. Robinson, and H. Magalhaes, eds.), p. 41, Iowa State University Press, Ames.

Saba, T. M., and Jaffe, F., 1980, *Am. J. Med.* **68**:577.

Schjeide, O. A., and Urist, M. R., 1956, *Science* **124**:1242.

Siegel, J., Rent, R., and Gewurz, H., 1974, *J. Exp. Med.* **140**:631.

Skinner, M., Cohen, A. S., Shirahama, T., and Cathcart, E. S., 1974, *J. Lab. Clin. Med.* **84**:604.

Skinner, M., Pepys, M. B., Cohen, A. S., Heller, L. M., and Lian, J. B., 1980, in: *Amyloid and Amyloidosis* (G. G. Glenner, P. Pinho e Costa, and A. F. de Freitas, eds.), p. 384, Excerpta Medica, Amsterdam.

Skinner, M., Sipe, J., Cohen, A. S., and Yood, R., 1982, *Ann. N.Y. Acad. Sci.* **389**:190.

Tillett, W. S., and Francis, T., Jr., 1930, *J. Exp. Med.* **52**:561.

Turek, F. W., Elliott, J. A., Alvis, J. D., and Menaker, M., 1975, *Biol. Reprod.* **13**:475.

Urbach, G., and Cinader, B., 1966, *Proc. Soc. Exp. Biol. Med.* **122**:779.

Volanakis, J. E., and Kaplan, M. H., 1971, *Proc. Soc. Exp. Biol. Med.* **136**:612.

Volanakis, J. E., and Kearney, J. F., 1981, *J. Exp. Med.* **153**:1604.

Volanakis, J. E., and Narkates, A. J., 1981, *J. Immunol.* **126**:1820.

Volanakis, J. E., and Wirtz, K. W. A., 1979, *Nature (London)* **281**:155.

Whicher, J. T., Martin, J. F. R., and Dieppe, P. A., 1980, *Lancet* **2**:1187.

White, A., Fletcher, T. C., Pepys, M. B., and Baldo, B. A., 1981, *Comp. Biochem. Physiol.* **69**:325.

Young, N. M., and Williams, R. E., 1978, *J. Immunol.* **121**:1893.

Index

239